Low Molecular Weight Heparin Therapy

Low Molecular Weight Heparin Therapy

An Evaluation of Clinical Trials Evidence

edited by
Monique Sarret
André Kher
Francis Toulemonde

MARCEL DEKKER, INC.   NEW YORK · BASEL

ISBN: 0-8247-8213-5

This book is printed on acid-free paper.

Headquarters
Marcel Dekker, Inc.
270 Madison Avenue, New York, NY 10016
tel: 212-696-9000; fax: 212-685-4540

Eastern Hemisphere Distribution
Marcel Dekker AG
Hutgasse 4, Postfach 812, CH-4001 Basel, Switzerland
tel: 41-61-261-8482; fax: 41-61-261-8896

World Wide Web
http://www.dekker.com

The publisher offers discounts on this book when ordered in bulk quantities. For more information, write to Special Sales/Professional Marketing at the headquarters address above.

Current printing (last digit):
10 9 8 7 6 5 4 3 2 1

PRINTED IN THE UNITED STATES OF AMERICA

Foreword

In a recent review on low molecular weight heparins, Jeffrey Weitz (N. Engl. J. Med. 1997, 337: 668–698) stated:

> After almost two decades of intensive ressearch, low-molecular-weight heparins have established their niche as an important class of antithrombotic compounds.

How true this statement is! Heparin was discovered in the very early part of this century and although many antithrombotic compounds have been discovered since, it remains one of the most commonly used therapeutic agents. The development of its low molecular weight form undoubtedly led to the further utilization of heparin.

Heparin, fractionated or not, is not the only antithrombotic drug. In the last decade, as thrombotic pathways and determinants were discovered, we have seen an explosion of new antithrombotic drugs that will greatly ameliorate the prevention and treatment of thrombosis. Should low-molecular-weight heparins be abandoned? The expert community rightfuly and forcefully says no! There are many good reasons for this belief. Indeed, many conditions can successfully be treated with low-molecular-weight heparin regimens.

This book is a powerful vehicle to assist physicians to decide where, and how, to use this therapy. It brings together in one place a discussion and evaluation of the evidence that this therapy is safe and effective. The authors and editors are well-known experts from many countries. This is an added value to this volume as low-molecular-weight heparin utilization differs somewhat between Europe and America. We can be sure that ultimately the patients will be the beneficiaries of this book.

Claude Lenfant, M.D.
Bethesda, Maryland

Preface

Just as the Nile becomes the mighty river that it is only by the convergence of its two major tributaries, the modern era of heparin therapy only began in the early 1970s, with the simultaneous development of a reliable diagnostic method for venous thrombosis and a suitable pharmaceutical preparation.

Indeed, the development of the radiolabelled-fibrinogen test extensively used by V.V. Kakkar (1970) produced a radical change: this new practical method, as opposed to the invasive venography technique proposed by C. Dos Santos in 1939, revealed that deep venous thrombosis (DVT) is even more common than previously suspected, often asymptomatic, and in many cases resolves spontaneously: a truly revolutionary concept.

Concomitantly, the concentrated calcium heparin salt available for subcutaneous administration demonstrated encouraging biological (J. Hirsh 1970) and antithrombotic properties (V.V. Kakkar 1971). Then began a period of ongoing debate which pitted advocates and opponents of laboratory monitoring during prophylaxis. Subsequent to the clinical outcome observed, it now was evident that the incidence of DVT could be significantly lowered by a simple regimen without the need for laboratory monitoring.

During this period, biochemists were successful in identifying the molecular structure of heparin chains and in understanding their specific mechanism of action on the serine proteases of the blood coagulation. The idea of fractionating heparin to produce low molecular weight moieties endowed with biological properties different from those of standard or "unfractionated" heparin (UFH) began to emerge.

Based on a simplified hypothesis, but which in hindsight approximates reality, it seemed possible to differentiate heparin's main properties, i.e. its antithrombotic activity from its anticoagulant one, maintaining its inhibitory effect on factor Xa while having less effect on factor IIa.

The era of low molecular weight heparins (LMWHs) had begun, and the first clinical paper on this topic was published by V.V. Kakkar in 1982 (Br Med J 284: 375-379); the first LMWHs were launched in the mid-1980s for two different indications: the first for hemodialysis, the second for prophylaxis of DVT in general surgery. During this period the clinical development of these compounds was essentially performed in Europe and thereafter extended to North America and other countries.

Subsequently, there followed a large number of publications which currently are now decreasing as if the majority of useful knowledge on LMWHs has been acquired, at least in the field of venous thrombosis. However, promising results with LMWHs in acute coronary syndromes are currently emerging.

More than fifteen years later, it is a good time to compile in a single volume clinical studies conducted with all available LMWHs to provide medical practitioners with a comprehensive review.

To achieve this goal, the reviewers have chosen the most relevant published studies or those of specific interest. It was decided to omit most abstracts and studies which involved combinations of products (i.e. LMWH plus dihydroergotamine) or heparinoid compounds (i.e. danaparoid).

Even though the interest of LMWHs in hemodialysis is well established, this topic has not been discussed because it was considered a particular clinical situation.

Each study is presented on two pages: the first page contains the overall description, including key elements such as study design, number of patients, type of surgery and anesthesia and assessment criteria. The second page lists the results taken from tables or text of the publication cited.

It should be mentioned that no specific data were reported regarding patient characteristics or risk factors because surprisingly, in almost every instance, no correlation was established by the authors between these factors and the reported results. Only concise comments regarding the studies are provided by the reviewers.

Obviously there is another method to evaluate the overall results: meta-analysis. However, meta-analyses do not provide a clear picture of each study. Recently, J. Bailar stated (N. Engl. J. Med. 1997: 337-559): "on my own review of selected meta-analysis, problems were so frequent and so serious that...I still prefer conventional narrative review, a type of summary familiar to the readers...". This is the objective of this study.

The editors and contributors have had the opportunity of being actively involved in the development of these compounds, witnessing doubts and satisfaction. It has been a source of much satisfaction to reexamine each trial and to commemorate a number of these authors who have contributed to such therapeutic progress represented by more simplified, safer and effective antithrombotic treatments with LMWHs.

Monique Sarret, Andre Kher, Francis Toulemonde.

The editors are indebted to Myriam de Barros and Daniel Fouché for their excellent technical assistance and diligence.

Introduction

Heparin is fairly unique in medicine since it was discovered by chance, by a medical student in 1916. More than 80 years later, it remains the most widely used agent for the immediate management of most thromboembolic disorders. Continued progress in its purification, understanding of chemistry and mode of action have resulted in ever-increasing therapeutic indications.

Exciting events in the mid 1970's laid the foundation for significant advances that allowed the development of low molecular weight heparins (LMWHs). Numerous clinical trials had established that a fixed regimen of low dose heparin provides effective prophylaxis, not only against deep vein thrombosis, but also against death from postoperative pulmonary embolism - a fact which was clearly demonstrated in the International Multicentre Trial involving over four thousand patients, and published in July, 1975. Three different groups of investigators (Lam, Silbert and Rosenberg; Höök, Björk, Hopwood et al; Andersson, Barrowcliffe, Holmer et al) independently, but almost simultaneously, announced their discovery in 1976 that heparin was not the homogeneous solution of identical molecules as thought previously, but instead a hetero-geneous mixture of linear polysaccharide chains that varied in molecular weight and in biological activity. Furthermore, only about one-third of the molecules in preparations of heparin had the ability to bind to antithrombin and the anticoagulant activity of the starting material resided mainly in the antithrombin-binding fraction.

In subsequent years, further elucidation of the structure-activity relationship culminated in the discovery by Lindahl et al (1980) that the biological activity is encoded in a pentasaccharide segment of unique structure in which a 3-0-sulphated glucosamine residue is an essential component. Either chemical or enzymatic hydrolysis was used to convert large heparin species into small molecules, the LMWHs. The pharmacological studies that followed clearly established their unique properties; i.e., they are readily absorbed following their subcutaneous administration and have a longer plasma half-life than conventional heparin and therefore need to be administered once daily. LMWH preparations currently in use are produced by different techniques and have variable molecular weight distribution, and therefore are likely to have different pharmacokinetic properties, which may have important clinical implications, particularly with respect to the associated risk of bleeding.

Impressed by these unique pharmacological properties of LMWHs, clinical investigators undertook studies to evaluate their efficacy and safety in preventing and treating venous thromboembolic disease. The first prospective study of the effiicacy of LMWHs in patients was published in 1982. This pivotal study paved the way for the many studies that have followed, confirming the original observation that a single daily dose of a low molecular weight heparin prevented most postoperative venous thrombolic episodes. Before any prophylactic therapy can be widely adopted, it is essential that it be easily administered, of low cost and, above all, of negligible risk. There is good reason to believe, based on current evidence, that the benefits of LMWH prophylaxis far outweigh the risk of hemorrhage. Its use has now become mandatory in all "high risk" patients.

LMWHs are also revolutionizing the treatment of extensive deep vein thrombosis. For the first time, it is possible to treat such patients at home, with major financial benefits for health care providers. A significant reduction in overall mortality for patients with deep vein thrombosis secondary to underlying cancer is once again testing scientific minds for possible explanation. The benefit of this therapy may also considerably improve management of arterial thromboembolic disease, in particular unstable coronary artery syndromes and acute stroke.

We are just beginning to realize the benefits of this unique therapy. This book contains not only detailed information but also critical reappraisal of the most relevant published clinical trials of LMWHs. The editors should be congratulated for adopting such a unique approach. The information will prove invaluable not only to all investigators, but also to clinicians dealing with thromboembolic disease in their daily practice.

Vijay V. Kakkar

Contents

Contributors

ACSADY György, M.D., Ph.D., D. Sc.
Associate Professor, Department of Cardiovascular Surgery, Semmelweis Medical University, Budapest, Hungary

BÉGUIN Suzette, Ph.D.
Department of Biochemistry, Cardiovascular Research Institute and University of Limburg,Maastricht, The Netherlands

BERGQVIST David, M.D., Ph.D.
Professor of Vascular Surgery, Department of Surgery, University Hospital, Uppsala, Sweden

BLASKO György, M.D., D. Sc.
Senior Consultant, Saint Emerich Teaching Hospital, Budapest, Hungary

BODA Zoltán, M.D., Ph.D., D.Sc.
Senior Lecturer,Department of Internal Medicine, University Medical School, Debrecen, Hungary

BONEU Bernard, M.D.
Professor of Medicine, Laboratoire d'Hématologie-Hémostase, Hôpital de Rangueil, Toulouse, France

BOUNAMEAUX Henri, M.D.,
Associate Professor of Medicine, Chief Division of Angiology and Hemostasis, Department of Internal Medicine, University Hospitals of Geneva, Switzerland

BOREL-DERLON Annie, M.D., Ph.D.
Laboratoire d'Hématologie-Hémostase, Centre Hospitalier Universitaire Côte de Nacre, Caen, France

BOUSSER Marie-Germaine, M.D.,
Professor, Department of Neurology, Hôpital Lariboisière, Paris, France

BREDDIN Hans Klaus, M.D.
Professor of Medicine, International Institute of Thrombosis and Vascular Disease, Frankfurt am Main, Germany

FAREED Jawed, Ph.D.
Professor of Pathology and Pharmacology, Director Hemostasis and Thrombosis Research Laboratories, Loyola University Medical Center, Maywood, Illinois, USA

FIESSINGER Jean-Noël, M.D.
Professor, Department of Vascular Medicine, Hôpital Broussais, Paris, France

GEERTS William H., M.D.
Clinical Epidemiology Unit, Sunnybrook Health Science Centre, University of Toronto, Canada

HAAS Sylvia, M.D.
Professor of Medicine, Institute for Experimental Surgery, University of Munich, Germany

HARENBERG Job, M.D.
Professor of Medicine, Faculty of Clinical Medicine Mannheim, University of Heidelberg, Mannheim, Germany

HEMKER Coenraad H., M.D., Ph.D.
Professor, Department of Biochemistry, Cardiovascular Research Institute and University of Limburg, Maastricht, The Netherlands

HIRSH Jack, M.D. F.R.A.C.P., F.R.C.P., F.A.C.P.
Professor of Medicine, McMaster University, Chedoke McMaster Hospitals, Hamilton, Ontario, Canada

HULL Russell, M.D., Mbbs, M.Sc.
Thrombosis Research Unit, Faculty of Medicine,
University of Calgary, Foothills Hospital, Calgary, Canada

KAKKAR Ajay K., BSc MbbS , PhD, F.R.C.S.
Professor, Department of Surgery, Imperial College
School of Medicine, Hammersmith Hospital, London, UK

KAKKAR Vijay V., F.R.C.S., F.R.C.S.E.,
Professor, Director Thrombosis Research Institute,
London, UK

KHER André, M.D.
Consultant in Clinical Development of Antithrombotics
and Thrombolytics Euthemis, Paris, France

KISS Robert Gabor, M.D., Ph.D.
Senior Lecturer in anesthesiology and intensive
medicine, Haynal Imre University of Health Sciences,
Budapest, Hungary

LECLERC Jacques R., M.D, F.R.C.P.C.
Senior Clinical Research Physician, Lily Research
Laboratories, Indianapolis, USA

MISMETTI Patrick, M.D., Ph.D.
Unité de Pharmacologie Clinique, Centre Hospitalier
Universitaire, Saint-Etienne, France

MONREAL Manuel, M.D.
Professor, Facultat de Medicina, Hospital Universitari,
« Germans Trias i Pujol », Barcelona, Spain

NENCI Giuseppe, M.D.
Professor of Internal Medicine, International Inter
University Centre for Thrombosis and Haemostasis,
Perugia, Italy

NICOLAIDES Andrew N., M.Sc., F.R.C.S., F.R.C.S.E.
Professor of Vascular Surgery, Division of Surgery,
Anaesthetics and Intensive Care, Imperial College School
of Medicine, St Mary's Hospital, London, UK

PLANES André, M.D.,
Orthopedic Surgeon, Department of Orthepic Surgery,
Clinique du Mail, La Rochelle, France

POTRON Gérard, M.D.
Professor, Central Laboratory of Hematology
Centre Hospitalier Robert-Debré, Reims, France

PRANDONI Paolo, M.D., Ph.D.
Professor, Institute of Medical Semeiotics, University
of Padua, Padova, Italy

SAMAMA Charles Marc, M.D.
Department of Anesthesia, Pitié-Salpetrière, Paris, France

SAMAMA Michel M., M.D..
Professor, Central Laboratory of Hematology,
Hôtel-Dieu, Paris, France

SARRET Monique, Ph.D.
Scientific Advisor, Medical Thrombosis Unit, Sanofi,
Paris, France

SETTEMBRINI Pier Giorgio, M.D.
Professor, Department of Vascular Surgery, San Carlo
Borromeo Hospital, University of Milano, Milano, Italy

TOULEMONDE Francis, M.D.
Senior Clinical Research, Bailly, France

TURPIE Alexander G., M.B., F.R.C.P., F.A.C.P.,F.A.C.C.,
H.G.H.-McMaster Clinic Hamilton General Hospital,
Hamilton, Ontario, Canada

WALLENTIN Lars, M.D., Ph.D.
Professor, Department of Internal Medicine, Cardiology,
Uppsala, Sweden

1

Marketed
low molecular weight heparins

The various indications described in this review may have been approved or not
by local health authorities and may vary from product to product. Please consult prescribing information
for each LMWH.

**Marketed
low molecular weight
heparins**

INTERNATIONAL NON PROPRIETARY NAME	CODE NUMBER	TRADE NAMES	CORPORATIONS
ARDEPARIN sodium	RD11885	Normiflo®	Wyeth-Ayerst (United States)
CERTOPARIN sodium	CH8140	Embolex® NM Mono Embolex® Sandoparine® Troparin® Alphaparin®	Novartis (Switzerland) Sandoz AG (Germany)
DALTEPARIN sodium	KABI2125 FR86 (Japan)	Fragmin® Low Liquemine® Boxol® Fragmine®	Pharmacia & Upjohn (Sweden and USA)
ENOXAPARIN sodium	PK10169	Lovenox® Clexane® Klexane® Decipar® Trombenox® Plaucina®	Rhône Poulenc Rorer (France and USA)
NADROPARIN calcium	CY216	Fraxiparin® Fraxiparine® Fraxiparina® Seleparina® Ultraparina®	Sanofi Winthrop (France)
PARNAPARIN sodium	OP2123 Alfa LMWH1	Fluxum® Minidalton® Lowepa® Lowhepa® Tromboparin®	Alfa-Wasserman (Italy)
REVIPARIN sodium	LU47311	Clivarin® Clivarine®	Knoll (Germany) BASF Pharma (Germany)
TINZAPARIN sodium	LNH1	Innohep® Logiparin®	Novo-Nordisk (Denmark) Leo Pharmaceuticals (Denmark)

Corporation	**WYETH-AYERST (United States)**
Manufacturer	WYETH-AYERST (United States)

Code number

RD11885

Trade name   **NORMIFLO®**

Sodium salt of low molecular mass heparin obtained by peroxidative cleavage of porcine intestinal mucosa at elevated temperature

Mass-average molecular mass	≈ 6500
Characteristic value	≈ 5300
Degree of sulfation per disaccharidic unit	not reported

In vitro activity   Anti Xa: 120±25 IU/mg

Anti IIa ≈ 60±15 IU/mg

Anti-factor Xa/IIa ratio ≈ 2

Data from literature

CERTOPARIN
sodium

Corporations	**NOVARTIS (Switzerland)** **SANDOZ AG (Germany)**
Licensee	ALPHA THERAPEUTIC (United Kingdom)
Manufacturer	BIOCHEMIE (Austria)

Code number

CH8140

Trade names	**EMBOLEX® NM / MONO-EMBOLEX® / SANDOPARINE® / TROPARIN® / ALPHAPARIN®**

Sodium salt of low molecular mass heparin obtained by isoamylnitrite depolymerization from porcine intestinal mucosa

Mass-average molecular mass range	4200-6200
Characteristic value	3800
Degree of sulfation per disaccharidic unit	not reported

In vitro activity	Anti Xa:	80-120 IU/mg
	Anti IIa ≈	30- 35 IU/mg

Anti-factor Xa/IIa ratio ≈ 1.5-2.5

European Pharmacopeia 1995

Corporation	**PHARMACIA & UPJOHN (Sweden)**
Licensees	KISSEI PHARMACEUTICALS (Japan)
	PIERREL (Italy)
	ROCHE (Switzerland)
	ROVI (Spain)
Manufacturer	PHARMACIA (Sweden)

Code number
KABI 2165
FR860 (Japan)

Trade names **FRAGMIN® / LOW-LIQUEMINE® / BOXOL® / FRAGMINE®**

Sodium salt of a low molecular mass heparin obtained by nitrous acid depolymerization of heparin from porcine intestinal mucosa

Mass-average molecular mass range	5600-6400	In vitro activity	Anti Xa:	110-210 IU/mg
			Anti IIa ≈	60 IU/mg
Characteristic value	≈ 6000		Anti-factor Xa/IIa ratio ≈ 1.9-3.2	
Degree of sulfation per disaccharidic unit	2.0 to 2.5		*European Pharmacopeia 1997*	

ENOXAPARIN
sodium

Corporation	**RHÔNE POULENC RORER (France and USA)**
Licensees	ITALFARMACO (Spain)
	MENARINI (Italy)
	TECNOBIO (Spain)
Manufacturer	PHARMUKA (France)

Code number

PK10169

Trade names	**LOVENOX® / CLEXANE® / KLEXANE® / DECIPAR® / TROMBENOX® / PLAUCINA®**

Sodium salt of a low molecular mass heparin obtained by alkaline depolymerization of the benzylester derivative of heparin from porcine intestinal mucosa

Mass-average molecular mass range	3500-5500
Characteristic value	4500
Degree of sulfation per disaccharidic unit	≈ 2

In vitro activity	Anti Xa:	90-135 IU/mg
	Anti IIa $\approx$	25-30 IU/mg
	Anti-factor Xa/IIa ratio $\approx$ 3.3-5.3	

European Pharmacopeia 1997

Corporations	**SANOFI WINTHROP (France)**
Licensees	ITALFARMACO (Italy)
	NEO-FARMOFER (Portugal)
Manufacturer	SANOFI WINTHROP INDUSTRIES (France)

Code number

CY216

Trade names	**FRAXIPARIN® / FRAXIPARINE® / FRAXIPARINA® / SELEPARINA® / ULTRAPARINA®**

Calcium salt of a low molecular mass heparin obtained by nitrous acid depolymerization of heparin from porcine intestinal mucosa, followed by fractionation to eliminate selectively most of the chains with a molecular mass lower than 2000

Mass-average molecular mass range	3600-5000
Characteristic value	≈ 4300
Degree of sulfation per disaccharidic unit	≈ 2

In vitro activity	Anti Xa:	95-130 IU/mg
	Anti IIa ≈	25- 30 IU/mg
	Anti-factor Xa/IIa ratio ≈ 2.5-4.0	

European Pharmacopeia 1997

PARNAPARIN

sodium

Corporation	**ALFA WASSERMAN (Italy)**
Licensees	SCHWARZ PHARMA (Italy)
	SHIMITZU (Japan)
Manufacturer	OPOCRIN (Italy)

Code number

OP 2123

LMWH 21-23

ALFA LMWH 1

Trade names   **FLUXUM® / MINIDALTON® / LOWEPA® / LOWHEPA® / TROMBOPARIN®**

Sodium salt of a low molecular mass heparin obtained by radical-catalyzed depolymerization, with hydrogen peroxide and with a cupric salt of heparin from bovine or porcine intestinal mucosa

Mass-average molecular mass range	4000-6000	In vitro activity	Anti Xa:	75-110 IU/mg
			Anti IIa:	< 30 IU/mg
Characteristic value	5000		Anti-factor Xa/IIa ratio ≈ 1.5-3.0	
Degree of sulfation per disaccharidic unit	2.0-2.6	*European Pharmacopeia 1997*		

REVIPARIN
sodium

Corporations	**KNOLL AG (Germany)**
	BASF PHARMA (Germany)
Licensees	MITSUI (Japan)
	HMR (Argentina)
Manufacturers	NORDMARK (Germany)
	IMMUNO (Germany)

Code number

LU47311

Trade names **CLIVARIN® / CLIVARINE®**

Depolymerization by chemical process: sodium salt of low molecular mass heparin obtained by nitrous acid depolymerization of heparin from porcine intestinal mucosa

Average relative molecular mass ≈ 3900

Degree of sulfation per disaccharidic unit ≈ 2.2

WHO Drug Information 1990

In vitro activity Anti Xa: 130 IU/mg
Anti IIa ≈ 40 IU/mg

Anti-factor Xa/IIa ratio > 3

Data from literature

TINZAPARIN
sodium

Corporations	**NOVO NORDISK (Denmark)**
	LEO PHARMACEUTICALS (Denmark)
Licensees	BRAUN (Germany)
	FORMENTI (Italy)
Manufacturer	LEO PHARMACEUTICALS (Denmark)

Code number

LNH1

Trade name	**INNOHEP® / LOGIPARIN®**

Sodium salt of a low molecular mass heparin obtained by controlled enzymatic depolymerization of heparin from porcine intestinal mucosa using heparinase from Flavobacterium heparinum

Mass-average molecular mass range	5600-7500	In vitro activity	Anti Xa: 70-120 IU/mg
			Anti IIa ≈ 45 IU/mg
Characteristic value	6500		Anti-factor Xa/IIa ratio ≈ 1.5-2.5
Degree of sulfation per disaccharidic unit	1.8-2.5		*European Pharmacopeia 1997*

2

Low molecular weight heparins

chemical
and biological properties

Biochemical and biological key points
MONIQUE SARRET

Natural occurrence

Heparins and heparin derivatives such as low molecular weight heparins (LMWHs) are polydisperse heterogeneous mixtures of sulfated polysaccharide chains belonging to the wide glycosaminoglycan (GAG) family and are naturally present in the granules of mast cells of several mammalian tissues such as lung, skin, ileum, lymph nodes, and thymus. The absolute contents of heparin in tissues varied among different species or organs (no heparin could be detected in brain tissue).

Although lower vertebrates generally contain less heparin than mammals, heparin has also been found in some invertebrates (mollusc) and it is interesting to point out that there is no direct evidence that endogenous heparin plays a role in maintaining blood flow through the vasculature.

Commercial heparins are extracted from natural sources and are obtained from intestinal mucosa -mostly of pigs- in Europe, South America, China or from bovine lung in the U.S.A. and Hungary.

As a result of the recent problems related to viral risk contamination causing bovine spongiform encephalopathy (BSE), heparin crude material is presently obtained from porcine mucosa only (Fig.1).

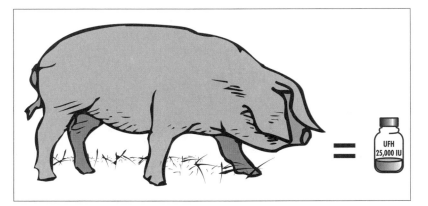

Figure 1: *25,000 IU of unfractionated heparin, corresponding to about a daily dose for the initial treatment of DVT, necessitate the whole intestinal mucus of a pig.*

The basic approach to prepare the drug form of heparin involves proteolytic treatment, extraction and complexing with ion pairing reagents followed by fractional precipitation treatment with base to remove the residual protein and /or bleaching of crude material.

The major criterion for batch-to-batch standardization remains their biological in vitro anticoagulant activity expressed in international units per milligram of dry substance according to Pharmacopeial assays (see section "measurement of potency").

Chemical structure

The chemical structure of LMWH is related to that of parent drug heparin, also named unfractionated heparins (UFH).

Although heparin has been used clinically for 60 years, its precise structure is not totally described due to the several levels of the structural complexity of this polydisperse heterogeneous mixture.

The polysaccharide chains of mammalian heparin molecules may be considered structurally as linear anionic polyelectrolytes of various lengths consisting mainly of regular sequences of a trisulfated disaccharide, a copolymer formed by combination of a uronic acid and a hexosamine (disaccharide unit). The major constituents of the glycosaminoglycan chains are the acid L-iduronic 2- O-sulfate and the amino sugar D-glucosamine N-6,-O-disulfate, linked 1-4 (Fig.2).

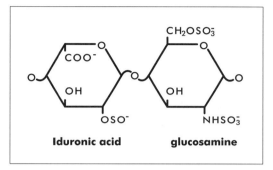

Figure 2: *Regular sequence of a disaccharide unit*

This regular repeated sequence is interrupted at intervals along its length, and it is replaced by irregular disaccharides.

Among these irregular segments, as the site has been identified which enables UFH or LMWH to bind to antithrombin III (ATIII) and modulates its biological (anticoagulant) activity. This specific site or "pentasaccharide sequence" included an atypical glucosamine N-6 trisulfate (Fig.3).

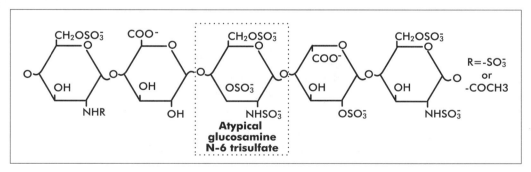

Figure 3: *ATIII-binding pentasaccharidic sequence*

Heparin molecules have a strongly anionic nature due to their sulfate and carboxyl groups. The degree of sulfation is about 2 to 2.5 per disaccharide unit.

The strength of the interaction between these polyanionic molecules, and cationic compounds is inversely related to their degree of polymerization and sulfation. Consequently, because of their low and homogeneous MW, LMWHs have limited non-specific interactions with basic cell constituents and plasma proteins. For this reason, they have a high bioavailability and predictable and sustained pharmacokinetics after subcutaneous administration.

Mean molecular weight - Depolymerization processes

LMWHs are obtained from "classical" or unfractionated heparins (parent drug) by physical, chemical or biological depolymerization processes.

LMWHs may be either fractions or fragments with a mean molecular weight (MW) - or mean molecular mass - range between 4000 and 6000 daltons. These values are inferior to the mean MW of the parent drug (15,000 daltons) (Fig.4).

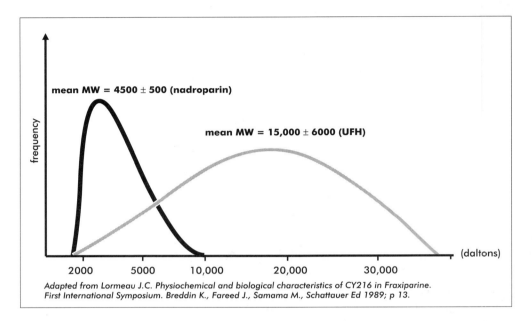

Figure 4: *Schematic MW (molecular weight) distribution of a LMWH (nadroparin) and UFH according to an HPLC elution profile*

During the depolymerization process, desulfation, deamination and other chemical modifications occur beside a reduction in the molecular weight. The structural characteristics of fragments formed also differ in these products and are largely dependent on the type of chemical processes used. For example, several LMWHs are produced by nitrous acid depolymerization (dalteparin, nadroparin, reviparin), one by enzymatic degradation using a heparinase -Flavobacterium heparinum- (tinzaparin), one by benzylation followed by alkaline hydrolysis (enoxaparin). Chemical and enzymatic degradation of heparin molecules produces specific changes or end-residues of fragments. The relative functional significance of these modifications is unknown at this time.

It has been suggested that the depolymerization process may also affect the pharmacokinetic and ex vivo biological properties of LMWH depending on the presence of a negatively charged sulfamino group at the reducing end of the molecule.

Although heparin fragments may have a similar mean MW, they may present different biological characteristics due to the distribution of their constituting molecular chains.

Heparin fractions represent material already present in naturally occurring GAGs and can be obtained by gel filtration or solvent extraction. Fragments are obtained from UFH (parent drug) by various depolymerization processes (Fig.5).

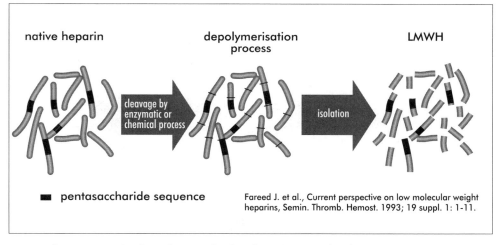

Figure 5: *Production of LMWH by depolymerization of unfractionated heparin*

Mechanism of anticoagulant/antithrombotic action

Heparin and heparin fragments are not direct anticoagulants but exert their antithrombotic effect principally by catalyzing the action of an endogenous plasmatic coagulation inhibitor, antithrombin III (ATIII) on factor Xa and thrombin (factor IIa). Not all heparin molecules have the capacity to interfere with ATIII. For LMWHs, only 20-25 % of the chains constituting the heparin molecules possess the particular structure -a pentasaccharide structure ($\approx$ 1800 daltons)- required to bind to ATIII. As for UFH, these chains are defined as "high affinity" (HA) heparin oligosaccharides. It cannot be excluded that the other chains with low affinity also contribute to the antithrombotic properties of the molecule.

When these HA heparin chains bind to ATIII they convert this natural anticoagulant protease from a slow inhibitor to a very rapid one.

The complex pentasaccharide-ATIII is sufficient to inhibit the activation of factor X. To inhibit factor IIa (thrombin), the pentasaccharide moiety must be included onto a chain of adequate length of at least octadecasaccharide units (MW > 6000).

Heparin chains of less than 6000 daltons maintain their inhibitory property against factor Xa, but with increasing length chains gain a stronger inhibitory capacity against thrombin (Fig.6).

The unexpected discovery that heparins of low molecular weight prolong the clotting time moderately (indicating mild thrombin inhibition) but are still capable of potentiating the inhibition of factor Xa, raised the hope of dissociating the antithrombotic property (attributed to anti-factor Xa) from the anticoagulant property (attributed to inhibition of thrombin), which might reduce the hemorrhage inducing effect of UFH.

In the mid seventies, fractionation and/or fragmentation was proposed as a mean of obtaining safer and more efficient antithrombotic agents with more specific chemical and biological characteristics than those of UFH. It was argued that heparin fragments might exert an antithrombotic effect by virtue of their undiminished anti-Xa function while their decreased influence on overall coagulation would lead to fewer hemorrhagic complications; this later expected point has not totally been verified in clinical situations.

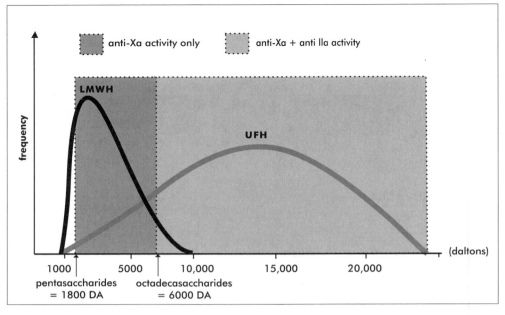

Figure 6: *Biological activities (for high affinity chains) according to MW distribution*

Measurement of potency

Since UFH and LMWHs are extractive drugs, the in vitro measurement of their "potency" is essential for manufacturers. It is also important that such measurements be properly standardized.

Potency is the measurement of the biological activity of the drug in a well defined assay system usually against a reference standard, comparing dose-response lines of the test preparation and the standard. The in vitro assays should measure a biologically relevant effect, but they are intended as a statement of the active principle present in determined gravimetric units (mg of dry substance) and are not a measurement of clinical efficacy which can only be determined by clinical trials.

Assay methods for low molecular weight heparins

One of the major characteristics of the anticoagulant activities of LMWHs is that when compared to UFH, their anti-Xa activity is higher than their activity measured with APTT or anti-IIa assays. Therefore, it is essential to test each batch of every LMWH by at least one method from each of these two groups of assays, and the ratio of anti-Xa/anti-IIa activity can be regarded as a "fingerprint" for each product which should remain within narrowly defined limits.

Anti-Xa methods

The measurement of anti-Xa activity can be carried out using both clotting or amidolydic (chromogenic) methods. In addition, this latter assay may be performed using either plasma or ATIII alone (purified or isolated system).

Obviously, the expression of potency may be different according to the testing system, the anti-Xa clotting assays giving higher potency than the anti-Xa chromogenic method with plasma, which in turn may indicate titer higher than the anti-Xa chromogenic in an isolated system.

Recent European Pharmacopeial directives have formulated the measurement of anti-Xa activity in an isolated system by using a chromogenic substrate and ATIII excluding plasma.

These different methodological approaches for standardization may have raised some questions for clinicians. The case of nadroparin is representative: this first LMWH was launched for prophylaxis of DVT in general surgery with syringes of 0.3ml containing 7500 AXa units tested at that time against the IVth Standard of UFH with a clotting assay and named Institut Choay units (ICU). Later on, when this drug was assayed against the First LMWH Standard (WHO 85/600) in plasma system, these 7500 AXa ICU became approximately 3000 international units. With the recent European Pharmacopeial directives (dosage in an isolated system without plasma), these 3000 IU decrease down to about 2850 IU despite the same amount of dry substance. Similar modifications were also observed for parnaparin.

In conclusion, because of uncertainty about the relevance of current in vitro assays to events in vivo, it is strongly suggested that comparison between LMWHs on the basis of in vitro assays against the LMWH standard could be misleading.

Pharmacokinetics

The study of the kinetic properties of both UFH and LMWHs is peculiar because the composite structure of the molecules makes the determination of their direct plasma concentration impossible. Therefore, the assessment of their pharmacokinetic profile is based on their biological activity on the coagulation cascade (inhibition of serine proteases).

These properties measured ex-vivo reflect only the activity of those molecular chains containing the binding site of heparin molecules to AT III.

Different biological markers can be used to determine the anticoagulant/antithrombotic properties of heparins such as activated partial thromboplastin time (APTT), thrombin clotting time (TCT), Heptest, anti-thrombin (anti-IIa) and anti-Xa activity. It is unknown which marker (if any) is best correlated with clinical efficacy. However, for LMWHs, the most significant and most widely used parameter for the evaluation of pharmacokinetic profile is the anti-Xa activity using a chromogenic substrate. Different methods can be used for the determination of this activity but the two main types of anti-Xa tests assess residual factor Xa.

An alternative approach has recently been offered, applying a more sensitive test or plasma thrombin neutralization assay (PTNA) (Agnelli et al 1995) for evaluating anti-factor IIa activity, but this method is not commonly used in current practice.

To avoid the presentation of complex tables, the main published pharmacokinetics studies carried out with each marketed LMWH are reported in the references of this chapter and only some relevant aspects are summarized hereafter.

Absorption and plasma concentration

The rate of absorption of LMWH is mainly determined by using the rate of appearance of anti-Xa activity in plasma.

Following sc administration, plasma AXa levels are dose-dependent, the maximum AXa activity being found within 3-4 hours. Depending on the LMWH preparation, dose and test used, plasma AXa levels may still be detected after 18 hours or even later.

After iv injection of LMWH, maximum AXa and AIIa activities are dose-dependent and are quickly detected ($\approx$ 5 minutes). Depending on the dose applied, AXa levels can be detected during 5-8 hours following administration; AIIa levels disappear faster (2-4 hours).

Distribution and metabolism

Heparins are removed from the blood via two mechanisms, saturable and non saturable. The reticulo-endothelial system and endothelial cells represent the saturable mechanism, while renal elimination represents the non-saturable and linear removal mechanism.

The LMWHs, which bind much less than UFH to endothelial cells, have elimination mainly via the renal (non-saturable) mechanism.

The area under the plasma concentration versus time curve (AUC) increases with rising doses as well as with repeated dosages.

The elimination half-lives of LMWHs after IV administration are double in comparison with UFH.

Following subcutaneous administration, elimination half-lives on the basis of AXa activity are slightly different for the various LMWHs and range between 3 and 4 hours. For prophylactic doses of UFH (5000 IU), the half-life does not exceed 90 min.

The metabolism and elimination of UFH and LMWH involve depolymerization and desulfation. They are partially desulfated in the liver, and eliminated by the kidneys, often in forms retaining some biological activity (mainly anti-Xa activity). The clearance of plasma AXa and AIIa activities is reduced in patients with severe renal insufficiency treated with high doses of LMWHs.

Bioavailability

The bioavailability of sc UFH is dose-dependent, and with prophylactic doses (5000-10,000 IU) is usually low (10-30 %). The poor biovailability of UFH has been explained by the lower absorption of its high molecular weight molecules. On the contrary, the shorter chains of LMWHs are readily absorbed from the subcutaneous injection site, and their biovailability is considerably higher than that of UFH. Based on plasma anti-Xa activity, the bioavailability of LMWHs is about 90 %. The bioavailability of LMWH is higher than that of UFH, also when calculated based on the measurement of anti-IIa activity.

The better bioavailability and the persistence of anti-factor Xa activity in the circulation following sc administration of LMWHs is probably pivotal to the efficacy of these compounds and may be an essential difference between the parent drug UFH and its fragments/fractions.

Bioequivalence

All LMWH suppliers have documented efficacy of their drug in clinical studies on thromboprophylaxis and treatment of thromboembolic disorders and established their own dose regimens. Since LMWH have different molecular weight distribution and are used in different doses on a molar basis, it is difficult to claim their bioequivalence as based on kinetic parameters alone. Little information regarding a direct comparison of the efficacy of LMWH using recommended doses has been available until now. All LMWH preparations have documented their efficacy in clinical studies and established their own dose regimens, although their biological activity reported in units gravimetric or in international units might be different.

Conclusion

Clinical practice has justified not only the once daily administration of LMWHs (at least in European practice), but also the doses used for each individual LMWH. Their kinetic profile is complex, and not necessarily fully applicable to the logic of their clinical use. Their clinical efficacy and safety are not based on kinetic parameters, and do not correlate completely with their pharmacodynamic profile.

REFERENCES

Overview

BONEU B., CARANOBE C., SIE P. Pharmacokinetics of heparin and low molecular weight heparin in Baillière's Clinical Haematology. International practice and research 1990; Vol 3/ (3) : 531-544. Antithrombotic Therapy. J. Hirsh Editor. Baillière Tindall London.

FRYDMAN A.M. Low molecular weight heparins: an overview of the pharmacodynamics, pharmacokinetics and metabolism in humans. Haemostasis 1996; 26 (Suppl.2) : 24-38

Ardeparin

OZAWA T., DOMAGALSKI J., MAMMEN E.F., Determination of low molecular weight heparin by heptest on the automated coagulation laboratory system. Am. J. Clin. Pathol. 1993; 99 : 157-162

TROY S., FRUNCILLO R., OZAWA T. et al. The dose proportionality of the pharmacokinetics of ardeparin or low molecular weight heparin in healthy volunteers. J. Clin. Pharmacol. 1995; 35 : 1194-1199

KESSLER C.M., ESPARRAGUERA I.M., JACOBS H.M. Monitoring the anticoagulant effects of a low molecular weight heparin preparation. Correlation of assays in orthopedic surgery patients receiving ardeparin sodium for prophylaxis of deep venous thrombosis. Am. J. Clin. Pathol. 1995; 103 : 642-648

TROY S., FRUNCILLO R., OZAWA T. et al. Absolute and comparative subcutaneous bioavailability of ardeparin sodium, a low molecular weight heparin. Thromb. Haemostasis 1997; 78 : 871-875

Certoparin

HARENBERG J., GIESE CH., DEMPFLE C.E. Biological activity and safety of low molecular weight heparin for 8 days in human volunteers. Thromb. Haemostasis 1989; 61 : 357-362

FASANELLE T., HOPPENSTEAD D.A., FAREED J. et al. Intravenous and subcutaneous pharmacokinetics of a low molecular weight heparin (certoparin) in man. Blood 1995; 86 (Suppl.1) 915 (Abstract)

Dalteparin

BRATT G., TÖRNEBOHM E., LOCKNER D. et al. A human pharmacological study comparing conventional heparin and a low molecular weight heparin fragment. Thromb. Haemostasis 1985; 53 : 208-211

LOCKNER D., BRATT G., TÖRNEBOHM E. et al. Pharmacokinetics of intravenously and subcutaneously administered Fragmin in healthy volunteers. Haemostasis 1986; 16 (Suppl.2) : 8-10

SIMONNEAU G., BERGMANN J.F., KHER A. et al. Pharmacokinetics of a low molecular weight heparin (Fragmin ®) in young and elderly subjects. Thromb. Res. 1992; 66 : 603-607

Enoxaparin

FRYDMAN A., BARA L., LE ROUX Y. et al. The antithrombotic activity and pharmacokinetic of enoxaparin a low molecular weight heparin in human given single subcutaneous doses of 20 to 80mg. J. Clin. Pharmacol. 1988; 28 : 609-618

BENDETOWICZ A.V,. BEGUIN S., CAPLAIN H., HEMKER H.C. Pharmacokinetics and pharmacodynamics of a low molecular weight heparin (enoxaparin) after subcutaneous injection - comparison with unfractionated heparin -. A three way cross over study in human volunteers. Thromb. Haemostasis 1994: 71 : 305-313

Nadroparin

HARENBERG J., WÜRZNER B., ZIMMERMANN R. et al. Bioavailability and antagonization of the low molecular weight heparin CY216 in man. Thromb. Res. 1986: 44 : 549-554

DAWES J., PROWSE C.V., PEPPER D.S. Absorption of heparin, LMW heparin and SP54 after subcutaneous injection assessed by competitive binding assay. Thromb. Res. 1986; 44: 683-693

ROSTIN M., MONTASTRUC J.L., HOUIN G. et al. Pharmacodynamics of CY216 in healthy volunteers: inter-individual variations. Fundam. Clin. Pharmacol. 1990; 4 : 17-23

FREEDMAN M.D., LEESE P., PRASAD R. et al. An evaluation of the biological response to Fraxiparine (a low molecular weight heparin) in healthy individuals. J. Clin. Phamacol. 1990; 30 : 720-727

MISMETTI P., PERPOINT B., LAPORTE-SIMILSIDIS et al. Prophylactic dose of a low molecular weight heparin (nadroparin): chronopharmacological study after subcutaneous administration to healthy volunteers. (Fr). Therapie 1992; 47 : 557-560

Parnaparin

DETTORI G., TAGLIAFERRI A., DALL'AGLIO E. Clinical pharmacology of a new molecular weight heparin Alfa LMWH- Fluxum. Inter. Angio. 1988; 7 (Suppl.3) : 7-18

VERARDI S., CASCIANI C.V., BABBINI M. et al. Comparative dynamics of the effects of two salts of a low molecular weight heparin in surgical patients. J. Drug. Dev. 1988; 1: 87-91

Reviparin

ANDRASSY K., ESCHENFELDER V., KODERISCH J. et al. Pharmacokinetics of clivarin a new low molecular weight heparin in healthy volunteers. Thromb. Res. 1994; 73 : 95-108

DESNOYERS P.C., SAMAMA M.M. Pharmacokinetics and metabolism of reviparin. Drugs of today 1995; 31 (Suppl.D) : 61-72

PINDUR G., KÖLHER M., WENZEL E. Study of a new low molecular weight heparin LU47311 administered to healthy volunteers. Folia Haematol. 1989: 6 : 859-866

Tinzaparin

MÄTZCH T., BERGQVIST D., HEDNER U. et al. Effects of an enzymatically depolymerized heparin as compared with conventional heparin in healthy volunteers. Thromb. Haemostasis 1987; 57 : 97-101

PEDERSEN P.C., OSTERGAARD P.B., HEDNER U. et al. Pharmacokinetics of a low molecular weight heparin logiparin, after intravenous and subcutaneous administration to healthy volunteers. Thromb. Res. 1991; 61 : 477-487

Drug comparisons

ERIKSSON B.I., SOEDERBERG K., WIDLUND L. A comparative study of three low molecular weight heparins LMWH and unfractionated heparin in healthy volunteers. Thromb. Haemostasis 1995; 73 : 398-401 *(enoxaparin/ dalteparin/ tinzaparin)*

COLLIGNON F., FRYDMAN A., CAPLAIN H. et al. Comparison of the pharmacokinetic profiles of three low molecular mass heparins - dalteparin, enoxaparin and nadroparin- administered subcutaneously in healthy volunteers (doses for prevention of thromboembolism). Thromb. Haemostasis 1995; 73 : 630-640

AZIZI M., VEYSSIER-BELOR C., ALHENC GELAS et al. Comparison of biological activities of two low molecular weight heparins in 10 healthy volunteers. Br. J. Clin. Pharmacol. 1995; 40 : 577-584 *(enoxaparin/ reviparin)*

AGNELLI G.C., LORIO A., RANGE C. et al.   Prolonged antithrombin activity of low molecular weight heparins: clinical implications for the treatment of thromboembolic diseases. Circulation 1995; 92 : 2819-2824 *(enoxaparin/ nadroparin)*

BRIEGER D., DAWES J. Production method affects the pharmacokinetics and ex vivo biological properties of low molecular weight heparins. Thromb. Haemostasis 1997; 77: 317-322 *(enoxaparin/ dalteparin/ tinzaparin)*

Mode of action of low molecular weight heparins

COENRAAD H. HEMKER, SUZETTE BÉGUIN

LMWHs accelerate the interaction between antithrombin (AT), previously called antithrombin III, and thrombin. By this action less free thrombin becomes available in the body to exert prothrombotic actions and consequently the tendency to develop thrombosis diminishes. In this respect there is no difference between LMWH and unfractionated heparin.

This leaves the question of what distinguishes LMWH from unfractionated heparin. Our answer is that, firstly LMWH have a higher bioavailability after subcutaneous injection and secondly LMWHs do not contain a hemorrhagic component present in unfractionated heparin.

In contrast to prevalent thought in the field we hold that the role of the higher anti-factor Xa activity (AXa) of LMWHs is negligible.

This view is based upon two kinds of evidence.

In the first place, the amount of anti-factor Xa activity that accompanies the anti-thrombin activity in common LMWH preparations is usually insufficient to sufficiently inhibit factor Xa in plasma and to obtain inhibition of thrombin production in vivo (1-4). Ten times as much anti-Xa activity is required than anti-thrombin activity to achieve inhibition of the APTT, of thrombin generation and of experimental thrombosis (1,2,5). It is indeed readily possible to inhibit coagulation and thrombus formation by attacking factor Xa, but the high concentrations that are required are not usually attained after injection of the current types of LMWH (5-10). Doses of synthetic pentasaccharide that are reported to have an antithrombotic action will inhibit thrombin generation by about 20%. We could show that inhibition of prothrombin conversion does not contribute to the anticoagulant action of preventive and therapeutic doses of unfractio-nated heparin and at the most contributes marginally to that of some (not even all) LMWH preparations (1,2,4). It has been claimed but never demonstrated that this inhibition has an advantage over inhibiting thrombin directly (11, 12).

In the second place there are reasons to believe that it is not the presence of very low molecular material in LMWHs that makes the difference with unfractionated heparin but rather the absence of material of very high molecular weight. In order to develop this thought further we need to first dwell on the heterogeneity of heparins.

On the heterogeneity of heparins.

In any heparin preparation only a fraction of the molecules contains the pentasaccharide sequence that is required for their effect on the AT mediated inactivation of clotting factors (6). This percentage ranges from about 40 in unfractionated heparin to 10 in some types of LMWH. This fraction we call the high affinity material (HAM). The remaining low affinity material is not completely devoid of biological effects but does not significantly inhibit thrombosis and can be ignored for the purpose of this article (13-16).

Within the HAM fraction three classes are to be recognized (fig.1). Molecules with a size of between 5 and 17 sugar units (1.7–5.4 KD), are effective catalysts of the inactivation of factor Xa but will not influence the inactivation of thrombin (17,18). As exposed above, such molecules are necessarily inefficient inhibitors of the clotting process. Molecules with more than 17 sugar units (always including the AT-binding pentasaccharide) are capable of fostering the AT-dependent inhibition of both factor Xa and thrombin. Their effect on thrombin makes them powerful inhibitors of the amount of free thrombin appearing in clotting plasma, not only because they catch thrombin into the AT-trap, but also because, as a secondary effect, less thrombin is available for the feedback activation of factor VIII and blood platelets (3,4,10,19,20). (The feedback activation of factor V is not affected probably because it is brought about by heparin-insensitive, membrane-bound meizothrombin). Because 17 sugars is the critical chain length required for the anti-thrombin action we called active heparin-molecules that are smaller Below Critical Length Material or BCLM. Active heparin molecules that catalyze both thrombin and factor Xa inactivation we call Above Critical Length Material or ACLM.

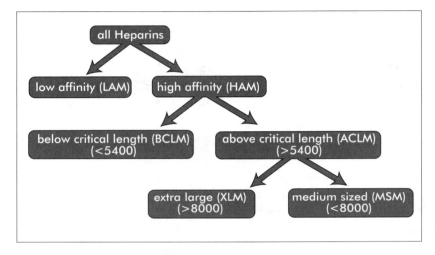

Figure 1: *The subdivision of heparin species*

Active heparins longer than about 30 sugar units require special attention. We call them extra large material or XLM, which is a subspecies of ACLM. The fraction of ACLM that is not XLM, i.e. the active heparins between 17 and 30 sugars we will call medium sized material, MSM.

It is important to note that, for all practical purposes, unfractionated heparin can be thought of as to exist of a mixture of MSM and XLM, BCLM hardly being present. In LMWH there is hardly any XLM and the active material consists of a mixture of MSM and BCLM.

Unlike BCLM and MSM, the XLM fraction requires Ca^{++}-ions for their full anti-factor Xa activity. The international standard is an unfractionated heparin, so it contains XLM and is dependent upon the presence of Ca^{++}. The usual anti-factor Xa measurements are carried out in the absence of Ca^{++}. So when a LMWH is compared to the standard, the latter is handicapped and the sample is not. The anti-Xa activity of LMWHs is for that reason always overestimated (22); this mistake is carried on when the standard for LMWH is used, because the activity of that standard is itself tested against the original (high molecular weight) heparin standard.

In order to unravel the complicated pharmacology of LMWHs, we established methods to determine the molar concentration of ACLM and BCLM in a plasma sample from its AXa and AIIa activities (23, 24). In this way we are no longer dependent upon comparison with a standard or by the complications that arise when impure preparations of different molecular weight composition are to be compared upon a weight basis.

We determined the course of ACLM and BCLM after injection of normal unfractionated heparin and of a LMWH preparation in healthy volunteers. After injection of unfractionated heparin no BCLM was found, because this fraction is not contained in unfractionated heparin and the ACLM rose to moderate levels. After injection of LMWH, high concentrations of BCLM were found but the concentrations of ACLM were also up to 7 times higher than those seen after injection of conventional heparin. The impressive concentrations of BCLM did not significantly inhibit the coagulation system (fig. 2). We could show that the inhibition of thrombin generation is a function of the ACLM level, independent of whether this was brought by unfractionated heparin or LMWH. The main difference between unfractionated heparin and LMWHs is in the fact that higher levels of ACLM are obtained from subcutaneous LMWH injections.

If this were the only difference, then the same effect as that of LMWH should be obtained by injecting six times as much unfractionated heparin. This hypothesis could not be tested however because of the risks involved. The normal dose of unfractionated heparin, 5000 IU twice daily, is the result of many years of clinical experience and represents a reasonable compromise between risk of induced bleeding and risk of thromboses prevented (25). Increasing the dose sevenfold would in all probability increase the bleeding tendency beyond acceptable limits. This means that the same dose of circulating ACLM obtained after an injection of unfractionated heparin is more hemorrhagic than after an injection of LMWH.

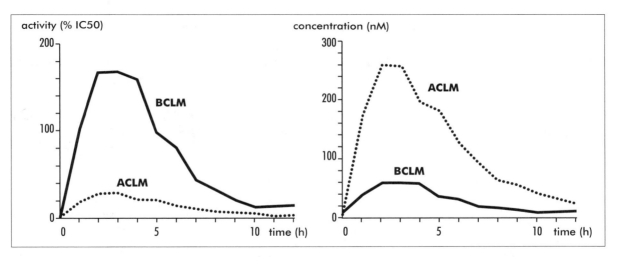

Figure 2: *Levels of ACLM and BCLM after injection of 1 mg/kg of a LMWH.*
Left frame: Expressed as activity (% of the IC50); Right frame: Expressed as concentration.

Thus we correlate the presence of XLM in unfractionated heparin and its absence in LMWH and we surmise that, in fact, the XLM fraction is responsible for the induction of bleeding.

After intravenous injection of a bolus of unfractionated heparin, there is a very rapid drop of activity, followed by a phase in which the disappearance is much slower (26). However, after subcutaneous injection, the apparent half-life of the ACLM from both types of heparin, is comparable (23). The XLM fraction might disappear quickly from the circulation, bind to the vessel wall and exert a hemorrhagic effect there. The remaining, circulating ACLM may not be very different between unfractionated heparin and LMWH.

In the presence of platelets there is one more advantage of LMWHs over unfractionated heparin: they are less readily adsorbed by platelet factor 4, so they remain more active and are less immunogenic.

From the above it will be clear that the anti-Xa activity in a plasma sample is of limited use to judge the pharmacological situation because it does not distinguish between ACLM and BCLM, which are molecules with a quite different anticoagulant power. This would not be serious if the ratio of ACLM to BCLM would always be the same. It is, however, different for different LMWHs and, more important, also changes after injection of a LMWH because the half-life time depends upon the chain-length (9, 27).

The time-honored method to study the heparin effect, the APTT, shows a large experimental variation and is strongly method and machine dependent. More important, the same amount of heparin activity produces very variable prolongation of the APTT in different individuals (28-30). Most important: the APTT is insensitive to the moderate inhibition of thrombin generation that already has an antithrombotic effect but raises sharply as soon as inhibitions approach the 80% level. Its relation to the level of anticoagulation is strongly non-linear and hence prolongation of the APTT can be used as a primitive warning signal of overdose but not for the control of therapy.

There are good reasons to believe that the current practice could be improved significantly if AXa or AIIa measurements were carried out for the determination of drug levels and if a method measuring thrombin generation (31-33) would replace the APTT.

Summary and conclusions

The current LMWHs, like unfractionated heparin, act mainly by accelerating the inhibition of thrombin by AT. The anti-Xa action of these heparins hardly contributes to their anticoagulant effect. Anyhow, the AXa activity of LMWHs is about two times overestimated. The favorable difference between LMWH and unfractionated heparin is explained by more favorable pharmacokinetic properties and by the absence of hemorrhagic components of very high molecular weight.

The current methods for heparin estimation and the determination of the heparin effect are inadequate. The future will show whether heparin prophylaxis and treatment can be ameliorated by applying more adequate methods.

REFERENCES

In the context of this article we cannot give complete reference to all the relevant literature. For a more complete review see e.g.: ref.9.

(1) BÉGUIN S, WIELDERS S, LORMEAU JC, HEMKER HC. The mode of action of CY 216 and CY 222 in plasma. Thromb. Haemost. 67: 33-41 1992

(2) BÉGUIN S., MARDIGUIAN J., LINDHOUT T., HEMKER HC. The Mode of Action of Low Molecular Weight Heparin Preparation (PK10169) and two of its Major Components on Thrombin Generation in Plasma. Thromb. Haemost., 61(1): 30-34 1989

(3) BÉGUIN S., LINDHOUT T, HEMKER HC. The Mode of Action of Heparin in Plasma. Thromb. Haemost., 60(3): 457-462 1988

(4) HEMKER HC. The Mode of Action of Heparin in Plasma. In: Thrombosis and Haemostasis. Eds. M. Verstraete, J. Vermylen, H.R. Lijnen, J. Arnout, University Press, Leuven. pp. 17-36 1987

(5) WALENGA J, PETITOU M, LORMEAU JC, SAMAMA M, FAREED J, CHOAY J. Antithrombotic activity of a synthetic heparin pentasaccharide in a rabbit stasis thrombosis model using different thrombogenic challenges. Thromb.Res. 46: 187-198 1987.

(6) CHOAY J, PETITOU M, LORMEAU JC, SINAY P, CASU B, GATTI G. Structure - activity relationships in heparin. A synthetic pentasaccharide with high affinity for antithrombin III and eliciting high anti-factor Xa activity. Biochem. Biophys. Res. Commun. 116: 492-497 1983

(7) BÉGUIN S., CHOAY J., HEMKER HC. The Action of a Synthetic Pentasaccharide on Thrombin Generation in Whole Plasma. Thromb. Haemost. 61: 379-401 1989

(8) THOMAS DP., MERTON RE., GRAY E., BARROWCLIFFE TW. The Relative Antithrombotic Effectiveness of Heparin, a Low Molecular Weight Heparin, and a Pentasaccharide Fragment in an Animal Model. Thromb. Haemost., 61(2): 204-207 1989

(9) BARROWCLIFFE T W, JOHNSON E A, THOMAS DP. Low molecular weight heparin. John Wiley & Sons, Chichester, 1992

(10) BÉGUIN S., DOL F., HEMKER HC. Factor IXa Inhibition Contributes to the Heparin Effect. Thromb. Haemost., 66: 306309 1991.

(11) YIN ET., WESSLER S., STOLL PJ. Biological Properties of the Naturally Occurring Plasma Inhibitor to Activated Factor X. J. Biol.Chem., 246(11): 3703-3711 1971

(12) YIN ET., WESSLER S., STOLL PJ. Identity of Plasma-Activated Factor X Inhibitor with Antithrombin III and Heparin Cofactor. J. Biol.Chem., 246(11): 3712-3719 1971

(13) MERTON,R.E. THOMAS DP. HAVERCROFT SJ. BARROWCLIFFE TW. LINDAHL U. High and Low Affinity Heparin Compared with Unfractioned Heparin as Antithrombotic Drugs. Thromb. Haemost. 51(2):254-256 1984

(14) OCKELFORD PA. CARTER CJ. CERSKUS A. SMITH CA. HIRSH J. Comparison of the In Vivo Hemorrhagic and Antithrombotic Effects of a Low Antithrombin-III Affinity Heparin Fraction Thromb.Res. 27:679-690 1982

(15) ZAMMIT A., DAWES J. Low-Affinity Material Does not Contribute to the Antithrombotic Activity of Orgaran (Org 10172) in Human Plasma. Thromb. Haemost., 71(6): 759-767 1994

(16) BARROWCLIFFE TW., MERTON RE., HAVERCROFT SJ., THUNBERG L., LINDAHL U., THOMAS DP. Low-Affinity Heparin Potentiates the Action of High-Affinity Heparin Oligosaccharides. Thromb.Res., 34: 125-134 1984

(17) LANE DA., DENTON J., FLYNN AM., THUNBERG L., LINDAHL U. Anticoagulant Activities of Heparin Oligosaccharides and their Neutralisation by Platelet Factor 4.Biochem.J., 218: 725-732 1984

(18) LANE DA., MACGREGOR IR, VANROSS M., CELLA G, KAKKAR VV. Molecular Weight Dependence of the Anticoagulant Properties of Heparin: Intravenous and Subcutaneous Administration of Fractionated Heparins to Man. Thromb.Res., 16: 651-662 1979

(19) OFOSU F.A., SIE P, MODIG J, FERNANDEZ F, BUCHANAN MR, BLAJCHMAN MA, BONEU B, HIRSH J.The Inhibition of Thrombin-dependent Positive-feedback Reactions is Critical to the Expression of the Anticoagulant Effect of Heparin. Thromb. Haemost. 65: 6 Abs 2183 1991

(20) BÉGUIN S, LINDHOUT T, HEMKER HC. The Effect of Trace Amounts of Tissue Factor on Thrombin Generation in Platelet Rich Plasma: its Inhibition by Heparin.Thromb.Haemost., 61(1): 25-29 1989

(21) HEMKER HC, BÈGUIN S, KAKKAR VV. Can the haemorrhagic component of heparin be identified? Or an attempt at clean thinking on a dirty drug. Haemostasis 26: 117-26 1996.

(22) HEMKER HC, BÉGUIN S.The Activity of Heparin in the Presence and Absence of Ca2+ Ions; why the Anti-Xa Activity of LMW Heparins Is about two Times Overestimated.Thromb.Haemost., 70(4): 717-718 1993

(23) BENDETOWICZ AV, BÉGUIN S, CAPLAIN H, HEMKER HC. Pharmacokinetics and Pharmacodynamics of a Low Molecular Weight Heparin (Enoxaparin) after Subcutaneous Injection, Comparison with Unfractionated Heparin. A Three Way Cross Over Study in Human Volunteers. Thromb.Haemost., 71: 305-313 1994

(24) HEMKER HC, BÉGUIN S. Standard and Method Independent Units for Heparin Anticoagulant Activities. Thromb.Haemost.70, 724728 1993.

(25) KAKKAR VV, COHEN AT, EDMONSON RA, PHILLIPS MJ, COOPER DJ. DAS SK, MAHER KT, SANDERSON RM, WARD VP, KAKKAR S. Low molecular weight versus standard heparin for prevention of venous thromboembolism after major abdominal surgery LANCET. 341/8840 (259-265) 1993

(26) SWART DE CAM, NIJMEYER B, ANDERSSON L, HOLMER E, VERSCHOOR L, BOUMA BN, SIXMA JJ. Elimination of high affinity heparin fractions, their anticoagulant and lipase activity. Blood 6: 836-842 1984.

(27) BONEU B, BUCHANAN MR, CARANOBE C, GABAIG AM, DUPOUY D, SIE P, HIRSH J. The Disappearance of a Low Molecular Weight Heparin Fraction (CY 216) Differs from Standard Heparin in Rabbits.Thromb.Res., 46: 845-853 1987

(28) POLLER L, THOMSON J M, YEE K F. Heparin and partial thromboplastin time, an international survey. Brit.J.Haematol. 44: 161-165 1980.

(29) BESSELAAR Van DEN AMHP, MEEUWISSE-BRAUN J, BERTINA R M. Monitoring heparin therapy: Relationship between the activated partial thromboplastin time and heparin assays based on ex-vivo heparin samples. Thromb.Haemost. 63: 16-23 1990.

(30) Van PUTTEN JJ, Van de RUIT M, BEUNIS M, HEMKER HC. Interindividual variation in relationship between plasma heparin concentration and the results of five heparin assays. Clin Chim Acta 122: 261-270 1982

(31) HEMKER HC, WIELDERS S, BÉGUIN S. The Thrombin Potential. A Parameter to Assess the Effect of Antithrombotic Drugs on Thrombin Generation.In: Fraxiparine, Second International Symposium Recent Pharmacological and Clinical Data. Eds. H.Bounameaux, M. Samama and J.W. ten Cate, pp.89-101, Schattauer, Stuttgart-New York 1990

(32) HEMKER HC, WIELDERS S, KESSELS H, BÉGUIN S. Continuous Registration of Thrombin Generation in Plasma, Its Use for the Determination of the Thrombin Potential. Thromb.Haemost., 70: 617624 1993.

(33) WIELDERS S, MUKHERJEE M, MICHIELS J, RIJKERS DTS, CAMBUS J-P, KNEBEL RWC, KAKKAR V, HEMKER HC, BÉGUIN S. The routine determination of the Endogenous Thrombin Potential in different forms of hyper- and hypocoagulability. Thromb.Haemost. 77(4) 629-636 1997

Abbreviations used throughout text and tables

ACT	activated clotting time
AMI	acute myocardial infarction
anti Xa or AXa	anti factor Xa
anti II a or AIIa	anti factor IIa
APTT	activated prothrombin time
ASA	aspirin
b.i.d.	twice-a-day
BW	body weight
CABG	coronary artery bypass graft
CT	computerized tomographic
D	day
DVT	deep vein thrombosis
ECG	electrocardiographic changes
FUT	fibrinogen uptake test
ICU	Institut Choay unit
INR	international normalized ratio
ITT	intention-to-treat
IU	international unit
iv	intravenous (route)
LMWH	low molecular weight heparin
MI	myocardial infarction
N	number
NS	not significant
OAC	oral anticoagulant
o.d.	once-a-day
p	95% of probability
PE	pulmonary embolism
preop	preoperative
postop	postoperative
PTCA	percutaneous transluminal coronary angioplasty
PTT	prothrombin time
sc	subcutaneous (route)
t.i.d.	three-time-a-day
TIMI	thrombolysis in myocardial infarction (classification)
UFH	unfractionated heparin
VQ	ventilation/perfusion (lung scan)

3

Low molecular weight heparins
Prophylaxis
of venous thromboembolism

Abbreviations used throughout text and tables

ACT	activated clotting time
AMI	acute myocardial infarction
anti Xa or **AXa**	anti factor Xa
anti II a or **AIIa**	anti factor IIa
APTT	activated prothrombin time
ASA	aspirin
b.i.d.	twice-a-day
BW	body weight
CABG	coronary artery bypass graft
CT	computerized tomographic
D	day
DVT	deep vein thrombosis
ECG	electrocardiographic changes
FUT	fibrinogen uptake test
ICU	Institut Choay unit
INR	international normalized ratio
ITT	intention-to-treat
IU	international unit
iv	intravenous (route)
LMWH	low molecular weight heparin
MI	myocardial infarction
N	number
NS	not significant
OAC	oral anticoagulant
o.d.	once-a-day
p	95% of probability
PE	pulmonary embolism
preop	preoperative
postop	postoperative
PTCA	percutaneous transluminal coronary angioplasty
PTT	prothrombin time
sc	subcutaneous (route)
t.i.d.	three-time-a-day
TIMI	thrombolysis in myocardial infarction (classification)
UFH	unfractionated heparin
VQ	ventilation/perfusion (lung scan)

3.1

Prophylaxis
of venous thromboembolism
in general, oncological, gynecological
and neurological surgery

Prevention of thromboembolism
with low-molecular weight heparin in abdominal surgery
(German)

AUTHORS	ADOLF J., KNEE H., RODER J.D. et al.
REF	Dtsch. Med. Wschr. 1989; 114: 48-53

STUDY	Randomized, double-blind
CENTERS *(n)*	2
COUNTRY	Germany
PATIENTS *(n)*	*included* 410
	evaluated 404 (ITT)
	390 with prophylaxis

TYPE OF SURGERY
General: colectomy 33%,
gastrectomy 23%, cholecystectomy 15%,
others

ANESTHESIA
General

STUDY DRUG   **Certoparin**   sc daily dose: 1500 APTT U o.d.

first injection: 2h preop

treatment duration: at least 7 days

REFERENCE DRUG   **UFH**   sc daily dose 5000 IU t.i.d.

first injection: 2h preop

treatment duration: at least 7 days

ASSESSMENTS
- ❏ Isotopic DVT; if positive, phlebography and lung scan.
- ❏ Bleeding complications.

ADOLF J. et al. 1989

	Certoparin 1500 APTT U x 1		UFH 5000 IU x 3		p
Treated patients	202		202		
Complete prophylaxis	195		195		
DVT total (FUT)	21	10.8%	23	11.4%	NS
Clinical DVT	4		3		
PE (positive lung scan) in patients with complete prophylaxis	0		0		
Bleeding complications					
wound hematomas	14	6.9%	19	9.4%	NS
hematomas at injection site	33	16.3%	58	28.7%	< 0.004

COMMENTS

❑ This single daily dose of certoparin 1500 APTT units provided effective prophylaxis in general surgery (this dosage cannot be related to classical AXa IU).

❑ A second study using certoparin 3000 AXa IU has been published by Koppenhagen K. et al in 1992 (see after).

Low molecular weight heparin and prevention of postoperative thrombosis in abdominal surgery

AUTHORS	KOPPENHAGEN K., ADOLF J., MATTHES M. et al.
REF	Thromb. Haemostasis 1992; 67: 627-630

			TYPE OF SURGERY
STUDY	Multicenter, randomized, double-blind		Elective abdominal surgery, 65% of patients with malignant diseases
CENTERS (n)	3		
COUNTRY	Germany		**ANESTHESIA**
			General
PATIENTS (n)	*included*	673	
	evaluated	653	

STUDY DRUG	**Certoparin**	sc daily dose: 3000 AXa IU o.d.
		first injection: 2h preop
		+ 2 placebo injections
		treatment duration: not stated
REFERENCE DRUG	**UFH**	sc daily doses: 5000 IU t.i.d.
		first injection: 2h preop
		treatment duration: not stated

ASSESSMENTS

- ❑ Isotopic DVT (FUT): if positive, venography.
- ❑ Bleeding events.
- ❑ PE: assessment not stated.
- ❑ Death.

KOPPENHAGEN K. et al. 1992

	Certoparin 3000 AXa IU x 1		UFH 5000 IU x 3		p
Patients	323		330		
Total DVT (FUT/venography)	24	7.4%	26	7.9%	NS
Clinical DVT	3		4		
Non fatal PE	0		2		
Fatal PE	0		1		
Wound hematomas	2		0		
Hematomas at the injection site	16		21		
Death	2 (1 cardiac failure) (1 malignancy)		3 (1 PE) (1 pulmonary insufficiency) (1 malignancy)		

COMMENTS

❑ These two prophylactic regimens were equivalent for efficacy and safety.

❑ Age older than 60 years was a clear risk factor as well as gastric and colon/rectum surgery.

❑ No hemorrhagic complications in patients (n=36) with an epidural catheter for anesthetics administration over a period of 1 to 2 days.

Low-dose-heparin versus low-molecular-weight heparin as thrombosis prophylaxis in gynecological oncology

AUTHORS	HEILMANN L., von TEMPELHOFF G.F., HERRLE B. et al.
REF	Geburtshilfe Frauenheilkd. 1997; 57: 1-6

STUDY	Randomized, double-blind
CENTERS (n)	1
COUNTRY	Germany
PATIENTS (n)	*included* 330
	evaluated 324

TYPE OF SURGERY
Gynecological for malignancy (mastectomy, hysterectomy, pelvic lymphodectomy)

ANESTHESIA
general

STUDY DRUG	**Certoparin**	sc daily dose: 3000 AXa IU o.d. + 2 placebo injections
		first injection: 2h preop
		treatment duration: 7 days
REFERENCE DRUG	**UFH**	sc daily doses: 5000 IU t.i.d.
		first injection: 2h preop
		treatment duration: 7 days

ASSESSMENTS
- ❏ DVT: impedance plethysmography (IPG) and venography.
- ❏ PE: lung scan.
- ❏ Bleeding complications.

HEILMANN L. et al. 1997

	Certoparin 3000 AXa IU x 1		UFH 5000 IU x 3		p
Patients	160		164		
Total DVT	10	6.3%	10	6.1%	NS
Proximal DVT	4	2.5%	7	4.2%	NS
PE	7	4.3%	4	2.4%	NS
	(1 fatal)				
Perioperative bleeding complications	15		23		
Patients requiring transfusions	21		29		
Wound hematomas	26	17.0%	47	28.7%	0.01
Death	5	3.1%	3	1.8%	NS

COMMENTS
- A prophylactic treatment with certoparin was as effective and safe as UFH regimen given t.i.d.
- The incidence of DVT was higher in women undergoing pelvic lymphodectomy (15-18%) (results not shown).
- An other interesting study "Blood coagulation and thrombosis in patients with ovarian malignancy" published by von Tempelhoff G.F. et al in Thromb. Haemostasis 1997; 77: 446-461, showed that:
  1 - only D-dimer and fibrinogen levels were correlated with malignancy (FIGO) stage;
  2 - DVT incidence was 6.7% up to the 7th day after surgery (prophylaxis with LMWH or UFH) and 10.6% during successive chemotherapy;
  3- after a median of 26-month follow-up, 21.4% of LMWH-treated patients and 37.5% of UFH-treated patients died of cancer (p=0.26).

Low molecular weight heparin once daily compared with conventional low-dose heparin twice daily. A prospective double-blind multicentre trial on prevention of post-operative thrombosis

AUTHORS	BERGQVIST D., BURMARK U.S., FRISELL J. et al.
REF	Br. J. Surg. 1986; 73: 204-208

STUDY	Multicenter, randomized, double-blind	TYPE OF SURGERY	Elective general abdominal (colonic, rectal, biliary, other) 45% for malignancy
CENTERS (n)	4		
COUNTRY	Sweden		
PATIENTS (n)	included 468 evaluated 432	ANESTHESIA	Not stated

STUDY DRUG	**Dalteparin**	sc daily dose: 5000 AXa IU o.d. + 1 placebo injection
		first injection: 2h preop
		second injection: placebo 12h postop (D0)
		treatment duration: 5-7 days

REFERENCE DRUG	**UFH**	sc daily dose: 5000 IU b.i.d.
		first injection: 2h preop
		second injection: 12h postop (D0)
		treatment duration: 5-7 days

ASSESSMENTS
- ❏ Isotopic DVT (FUT): preoperatively and at D1, 3, 5, 7 postop.
- ❏ Bleeding complications.
- ❏ Laboratory tests.
- ❏ 30-day follow-up for complications.

BERGQVIST D. et al. 1986

	Dalteparin 5000 AXa IU x 1		UFH 5000 IU x 2		p
Total patients	215		217		
Patients with correct prophylaxis	190		192		
Total DVT (FUT)	13	6.4%	9	4.3%	NS
DVT with correct prophylaxis	—	4.3%	—	5.4%	NS
Major hemorrhage					
excessive perioperative bleeding	25	11.6%	10	4.7%	<0.01
reoperation due to bleeding	10		2		
AXa IU/ml (mean x ± SD) at D4 *	0.7±0.2		0.1±0.2		<0.01
APTT sec (mean ± SD) at					
D0 (preop)	30±3		30±3		NS
D4*	34±4		32±5		NS

* 4h after injection.

COMMENTS
- Same efficacy but more hemorrhagic complications in patients treated with dalteparin than in UFH-treated patients.
- Most of these hemorrhagic complications occurred early after surgery in the dalteparin group.
  This studied prophylactic dose may have been administered too close to surgery and/or was too high as a preoperative dose.
- Significant delay in the onset of DVT in the dalteparin group.
- Patients with malignancy did not develop more DVT.
- Of the 10 patients who died, no death was due to PE (data not shown).

Low molecular weight heparin (Kabi 2165) as thromboprophylaxis in elective visceral surgery. A randomized, double-blind study versus unfractionated heparin

AUTHORS	KOLLER M., SCHOCH U., BUCHMANN P. et al.
REF	Thromb. Haemostasis 1986; 56: 243-246

STUDY	Two randomized, double-blind, studies
CENTERS (n)	1
COUNTRY	Switzerland
PATIENTS (n)	*included* 46 + 150
	evaluated 43 + 146

TYPE OF SURGERY
Thoracic and abdominal, lung resection, colon resection, cholecystectomy, herniotomy, other

ANESTHESIA
Not stated (general ?)

STUDY DRUG **Dalteparin** sc daily dose: • first study: 7500 AXa IU o.d.+ 1 placebo injection
• second study: 2500 AXa IU o.d. + 1 placebo injection
first injection: 1h preop
second injection: placebo 12h postop
treatment duration: at least 5 days

REFERENCE DRUG **UFH** sc daily dose: 5000 IU b.i.d.
first injection: 2h preop
second injection: 12h postop
treatment duration: at least 5 days

ASSESSMENTS
❏ Perioperative blood loss.
❏ Isotopic DVT (FUT) every day; if positive, venography.
❏ Lung scan if clinical PE suspected.
❏ Laboratory tests.

KOLLER M. et al. 1986

	First study		Second study	
	Dalteparin	**UFH**	**Dalteparin**	**UFH**
Patients	7500 AXa IU x 1 23	5000 IU x 2 20	2500 AXa IU x1 70	5000 IU x 2 68
Excessive perioperative bleeding	11	2	5	2
Thromboembolic events	Study discontinued early		2 2.9% (0 PE)	2 2.9% (1 PE)
AXa IU/ml mean ± SD at D1** APTT (sec) mean ± SD at D0/D1**	0.48±0.12* 25±3/32±3	0.01±0.02 27±3/31±4	0.11±0.05* 25±2/28±3	0.007±0.02 25±2/27.5±3

* $p < 0.01$ vs UFH.
** 4h after injection.

COMMENTS
- ❑ Interesting study because it is one of the first where the relationship between laboratory parameters (APTT and AXa values) and safety has been investigated.
- ❑ Dalteparin 7500 AXa IU o.d. was associated with an unacceptably high number of hemorrhagic complications although the APTT values were in the normal range.
- ❑ In the two studies, no laboratory test discriminated between patients with and without bleeding complications.
- ❑ Dalteparin 2500 AXa IU o.d. was as safe and as effective as UFH 5000 IU b.i.d.

**Efficacy and safety of two regimens
of low molecular weight heparin fragment (Fragmin) in preventing
postoperative venous thromboembolism**

AUTHORS	KAKKAR V.V., KAKKAR S., SANDERSON R.M. et al.
REF	Haemostasis. 1986; 16, suppl: 19-24

STUDY	Open-label, non randomized
CENTERS *(n)*	1
COUNTRY	United Kingdom
PATIENTS *(n)*	*included* 220
	evaluated 206

TYPE OF SURGERY	abdominal (45% for malignancy)
ANESTHESIA	Not stated

STUDY DRUG   **Dalteparin**   sc daily dose: two regimens

- 2500 AXa IU o.d. or
- 2500 AXa IU b.i.d.

first injection: 2h preop

second injection at D1

treatment duration: at least 6 days

REFERENCE DRUG   **None**

ASSESSMENTS

- ❑ Isotopic DVT (FUT), confirmed by venography if positive.
- ❑ PE: clinical observation; if suspicion, lung scan.
- ❑ Bleeding complications.

KAKKAR V.V. et al. 1986

	Dalteparin 2500 AXa IU x 1		Dalteparin 2500 AXa IU x 2		p
Patients	94		112		
Total DVT	7	7.4%	3	2.6%	NS
PE	1	(at D1)	0		NS
Excessive postoperative blood loss	4		10		NS
Prophylaxis discontinued	1		4		NS
Wound hematomas	0		2		NS

COMMENTS

❏ No significant difference in efficacy between the two regimens.

❏ In cancer patients, the incidence of DVT was 16.6% (7/42) in the first group and 6.3% (3/47) in the second group (NS). The number of patients was too small to show any significant difference.

❏ Safety appeared to be better with the dalteparin o.d. regimen but without statistical significant difference.

**Low molecular weight heparin
given the evening before surgery compared with conventional
low dose heparin in prevention of thrombosis**

AUTHORS	BERGQVIST D., MÄTZSCH T., BURMARK U.S. et al.
REF	Br. J. Surg. 1988; 75: 888-891

STUDY	Multicenter, randomized, double-blind
CENTERS (n)	7
COUNTRY	Sweden
PATIENTS (n)	*randomized* 1040
	evaluated 1002

TYPE OF SURGERY

Major elective abdominal surgery
(colonic, rectal, gastric, biliary, other)
63% for malignancy

ANESTHESIA

Not stated

STUDY DRUG	**Dalteparin**	sc daily dose: 5000 AXa IU o.d. + 1 placebo injection
		first injection: evening before surgery (10 p.m.)
		second injection: 2h preop (placebo)
		then, every evening
		treatment duration: 5-8 days
REFERENCE DRUG	**UFH**	sc daily dose: 5000 IU b.i.d.
		first injection: evening before surgery (10 p.m.)
		second injection: 2h preop
		treatment duration: 5-8 days

ASSESSMENTS

❑ Isotopic DVT (FUT) every day for 7 days. If positive, venography.
❑ Hemorrhagic complications, wound hematomas.

BERGQVIST D. et al. 1988

	Dalteparin 5000 AXa IU x 1		UFH 5000 IU x 2		p
Patients	505		497		
Total DVT (FUT)	28	5.5%	41	8.3%	NS
DVT with correct prophylaxis	21/421	5.0%	38/405	9.2%	0.02
PE	0		4 (1 fatal)		
Perioperative hemorrhagic complications	30	5.9%	15	3.0%	0.03
diffuse bleeding	25		10		0.01
surgical bleeding	4		4		
Hematomas at injection site	36	7.1%	47	9.5%	NS
Local pain	23	4.6%	59	11.9%	0.01
Death within 30 days *	10		9 (+ 1 fatal PE)		

* of fatal cases, 13 were operated on for malignancy.

COMMENTS

❑ Frequency of DVT significantly reduced among patients receiving dalteparin 5000 IU o.d.

❑ More diffuse bleeding in dalteparin group but no difference in the reoperation rate or in transfusion requirement.

❑ Contrary to previous studies, this "high" dose of dalteparin was safe when administered the evening before surgery.

❑ Local pain at injection site significantly reduced among patients given dalteparin.

Comparison of low molecular weight heparin vs unfractionated heparin in gynecological surgery

AUTHORS	BORSTAD E., URDAL K., HANDELAND G. and ABILDGAARD U.
REF	Acta. Obstet. Gynecol. Scand. 1988; 67: 99-103

STUDY	Double-blind, randomized, UFH-controlled
CENTERS (n)	1
COUNTRY	Sweden
PATIENTS (n)	included 215
	evaluated 215

TYPE OF SURGERY
Major gynecological (laparotomy, colposuspension, vaginal repair, hysterectomy)

ANESTHESIA
General

STUDY DRUG	Dalteparin	sc daily dose: 5000 AXa IU o.d. + 1 placebo
		first injection: 1h preop
		treatment duration: 7 days

REFERENCE DRUG	UFH	sc daily doses: 5000 IU b.i.d.
		first injection: 1h preop
		treatment duration: 7 days

ASSESSMENTS

- DVT: clinical observation and plethysmography on D3 and 7; if positive findings, venography.
- PE: clinical observation.
- Bleeding complications.
- Laboratory tests.

BORSTAD E. et al. 1988

	Dalteparin 5000 AXa IU x 1		UFH 5000 IU x 2		p
Patients	105		110		
Total DVT	0		0		
PE	0		0		
Total bleeding complications:	61	58%	55	50%	NS
blood transfusions	27		11		0.02
pelvic hematomas	10		11		
wound hematomas	26		15		0.02
reoperation	1		1		
prophylaxis stopped	4		1		
AXa activity IU/ml at D3 2h after injection (mean ± SD)	0.34 ± 0.04		0.13 ± 0.09		

COMMENTS

❏ Venography performed in 7 patients on clinical and/or plethysmographic indications.

❏ In gynecological surgery, this dalteparin regimen (5000 AXa IU) was not well tolerated in perioperative period as regard to safety, even though bleeding complications were not related to AXa levels.

❏ Was the first injection (preop) of 5000 IU too high to be administered just one hour before surgery?

Low dose heparin versus low molecular weight heparin (Kabi 2165, Fragmin) in the prophylaxis of thromboembolic complications of abdominal oncological surgery

AUTHORS	FRICKER J.P., VERGNES Y., SCHACH R. et al.
REF	Eur. J. Clin. Invest. 1988; 18: 561-567

STUDY	Open-label, randomized
CENTERS (n)	1
COUNTRY	France
PATIENTS (n)	*included* 80
	evaluated 80

TYPE OF SURGERY
Digestive 75%, gynecological 7%
all for malignancy

ANESTHESIA
General

STUDY DRUG	**Dalteparin**	sc daily dose: 5000 IU o.d. + 2 placebo injections
		first injection: 2h preop (2500 AXa IU) and 2500 AXa IU for
		first postop injection (12h postop), then 5000 AXa IU/day
		treatment duration: 10 days
REFERENCE DRUG	**UFH**	sc daily dose: 5000 IU t.i.d.
		first injection: 2h preop
		second injection: the next day postop
		treatment duration: 10 days

ASSESSMENTS
❑ Isotopic DVT (FUT) confirmed by venography.
❑ For clinically suspected PE, lung scan.
❑ Perioperative blood loss.
❑ Clinical follow-up for 4 weeks.

FRICKER J.P. et al. 1988

	Dalteparin 5000 AXa IU x 1	UFH 5000 IU x 3	p
Patients	40	40	
Total DVT (FUT)	2*	0	NS
PE	0	2 (non fatal)	NS
Severe postoperative bleeding (treatment cessation)	2	1	NS
Moderate postoperative bleeding	2	11	0.006
AXa activity IU/ml (peak) at			
D1	0.49	0.03	
D10	0.54	0.06	
Follow-up: late DVT/PE	2 (DVT)	4 (1 DVT/3PE)	
death	4 late deaths (treated-groups not reported)		

* Not confirmed by venography.

COMMENTS

❏ In this study, very low rate of DVT even though these patients underwent general surgery for malignancy.

❏ Despite the rather high AXa plasma level (almost 0.5 IU/ml) few severe hemorrhagic complications occurred contrary to what was observed in Borstad's study where AXa activity was about 0.25 AXa IU/ml (at 2 hours).

A randomized double-blind study between a low molecular weight heparin Kabi 2165 and standard heparin in the prevention of deep vein thrombosis in general surgery. A French Multicenter Trial

AUTHORS	CAEN J.P.
REF	Thromb. Haemostasis 1988; 59: 216-220

STUDY	Multicenter, randomized, double-blind
CENTERS (n)	5
COUNTRY	France
PATIENTS (n)	*included* 391
	evaluated 385

TYPE OF SURGERY
Major abdominal (cholecystectomy, colostomy, eventration, hysterectomy, others) about 30% for malignancy

ANESTHESIA
General

STUDY DRUG	**Dalteparin**	sc daily dose: 2500 AXa IU o.d. + 1 placebo injection
		first injection: 2h preop
		second injection: placebo 12h postop
		treatment duration: 7 days
REFERENCE DRUG	**UFH**	sc daily dose: 5000 IU b.i.d.
		first injection: 2h preop
		treatment duration: 7 days

ASSESSMENTS
- ❏ Isotopic DVT: FUT on D1 up to D7.
- ❏ PE clinical observation; if suspicion, lung scan.
- ❏ 30-day follow-up.

CAEN J.P. 1988

	Dalteparin 2500 AXa IU x 1		UFH 5000 IU x 2		p
Patients	195		190		
Total DVT	6	3.1%	7	3.7%	NS
PE	0		0		
Major hemorrhage	0		0		
Wound hematomas*	4	2.1%	3	1.6%	NS
AXa IU/ml (mean ± SE)**	0.15 ± 0.09		0.03 ± 0.05		
Thirty-day follow-up:					
thromboembolic events	0		2		
death	2		3		

* none required evacuation.
** 4 hours after injection.

COMMENTS

❏ Same efficacy and safety with these two prophylactic regimens in patients with moderate risk undergoing general surgery.

❏ AXa activity was greater in dalteparin-treated patients than in heparin group - varying between 0,12-0,18 IU/ml; the level of FXa inhibition was not related to hemorrhagic risk.

❏ No thrombocytopenia in both groups.

A double-blind randomized placebo controlled trial of thromboprophylaxis in major elective general surgery using once daily injections of a low molecular weight heparin fragment (Fragmin)

AUTHORS	OCKELFORD P.A., PATTERSON J., JOHNS A.S. et al.
REF	Thromb. Haemostasis 1989; 62: 1046-1049

STUDY	Randomized, double-blind, placebo-controlled
CENTERS (n)	1
COUNTRY	New Zealand
PATIENTS (n)	*included* 197
	evaluated 183

TYPE OF SURGERY	Major abdominal (≈ 43% for malignancy)
ANESTHESIA	General + epidural: ≈ 87% or with intercostal block: ≈ 13%

STUDY DRUG	**Dalteparin**	sc daily dose: 2500 AXa IU o.d.
		first injection: 2h preop
		second injection postop: morning day 1
		treatment duration: 5-9 days
REFERENCE DRUG	**Placebo**	first injection: 2h preop
		second injection postop: morning day 1
		treatment duration: 5-9 days

ASSESSMENTS
- Isotopic DVT (FUT).
- Major/minor hemorrhagic events.
- Clinical 6-week follow-up.

OCKELFORD P.A. et al. 1989

	Dalteparin 2500 AXA IU x 1		Placebo 0.2 ml x 1		p
Patients	95		88		
Total DVT (FUT)	4	4.2%	14	15.9%	0.008
DVT in malignant patients	3	7.1%	10	27.0%	< 0.001
DVT in non malignant patients	1	1.8%	4	7.8%	0.18
PE	0		2		
Major bleeding* (therapy discontinued)	4	2.2%	4	2.2%	NS
Minor bleeding*	6	3.3%	0	0.0%	0.03
Death	0		2 (D10)		

* All in malignancy.

COMMENTS

❏   Dalteparin 2500 AXa IU o.d. significantly reduced the incidence of DVT in cancer patients. A positive trend was observed in non-cancer patients.

❏   Thrombotic events occurred predominantly in cancer patients.

❏   No difference in major bleeding complications was observed between dalteparin and placebo groups.

Prophylaxis of thromboembolism in general surgery: comparison between standard heparin and Fragmin

AUTHORS	HARTL P., BRÜCKE P., DIENSTL E. and VINAZZER H.
REF	Thromb. Res. 1990; 57: 577-584

STUDY	Double-blind, randomized, controlled
CENTERS (n)	1
COUNTRY	Austria
PATIENTS (n)	included 250
	evaluated 227

TYPE OF SURGERY
Elective abdominal: (stomach, gall-bladder, colon, other)
(no appendectomy or herniotomy)

ANESTHESIA
not stated

STUDY DRUG	**Dalteparin**	sc daily dose: 2500 AXa IU o.d. + 1 placebo injection
		first injection: 2h preop
		second injection: placebo 12h postop, D0
		treatment duration: at least 7 days

REFERENCE DRUG	**UFH**	sc daily dose: 5000 IU b.i.d.
		first injection: 2h preop
		second injection: placebo 12h postop, D0
		treatment duration: at least 7 days

ASSESSMENTS
❑ Isotopic DVT (FUT) confirmed by venography.
❑ Death and autopsy.

HARTL P. et al. 1990

	Dalteparin 2500 AXa IU x 1		**UFH** 5000 AXa IU x 2		**p**
Patients	112		115		
Calf DVT (venography)	5	4.5%	5	4.3%	NS
Thigh DVT (venography)	0		0		
PE (fatal)	1		1		
Total thrombotic events	6	5.3%	6	5.2%	NS
Blood units transfused (D1-D6)	6		37		<0.01
Wound hematomas	1		1		
Reoperation for bleeding	1		3		
Death (not thrombosis-related)	5		8		

COMMENTS
- ❑ Prophylaxis with dalteparin 2500 IU o.d. induced far fewer blood transfusions than UFH 5000 IU b.i.d. in the postoperative period.
- ❑ No significant difference in efficacy between the two regimens.

Low molecular weight heparin versus standard heparin for prevention of venous thromboembolism after major abdominal surgery

AUTHORS	KAKKAR V.V., COHEN A.T., EDMONSON R.A. et al.
REF	Lancet 1993; 341: 259-265

STUDY	Multicenter, double-blind, randomized
CENTERS (n)	19
COUNTRY	United Kingdom
PATIENTS (n)	included 3938
	evaluated 3809

TYPE OF SURGERY

Major abdominal:
mainly gynecological, cholecystectomy, colectomy; about 37% malignancies

ANESTHESIA

General

STUDY DRUG	**Dalteparin**	sc daily dose: 2500 AXa IU o.d. + 1 placebo injection
		first injection: 1-4h preop
		placebo in the evening DO
		treatment duration: at least 5 days

REFERENCE DRUG	**UFH**	sc daily dose: 5000 IU b.i.d.
		first injection: 1-4h preop
		second injection in the evening DO
		treatment duration: at least 5 days

ASSESSMENTS

- ❏ Clinical DVT confirmed by venography.
- ❏ Clinical PE confirmed by lung scan.
- ❏ Safety: major and minor bleeding.
- ❏ 6-week follow-up.

KAKKAR V.V. et al. 1993

	Dalteparin 2500 AXa IU x 1		UFH 5000 IU x 2		p
Patients	1894		1915		
Total thromboembolic events:	19	1.1%	22	1.1%	NS
total PE	13	0.7%	14	0.7%	
fatal PE	5	0.2%	3	0.2%	
total DVT	11	0.6%	11	0.6%	
proximal DVT	3		3		
Total major bleeding*:	69	3.6%	91	4.8%	NS
prophylaxis discontinued	36	1.9%	40	2.1%	NS
bleeding heparin-related	10	0.5%	12	0.6%	NS
wound hematomas	27	1.4%	52	2.7%	0.007
reoperations	20	1.0%	38	1.7%	0.05
Severe bleeding**	18	1.0%	36	1.9%	0.02
Total mortality	63	3.3%	47	2.5%	NS
Six-week follow-up					
Total thromboembolic events	15	0.9%	10	0.6%	NS
PE	9	0.5%	5	0.3%	
DVT	8	0.5%	6	0.4%	
Death	10	0.6%	9	0.5%	
PE (fatal)	2		1		

* For major bleeding events, several items may have been observed in the same patient.
** With at least 2 described items.

COMMENTS

❑ Low incidence of clinical thromboembolic complications in both groups. 61% of these events occurred in patients operated for malignancy.

❑ Frequency of major bleeding was slightly (but not significantly) reduced in dalteparin group (by 23%).

❑ No report of thrombocytopenia.

Unexpectedly high rate of phlebographic deep venous thrombosis following elective general abdominal surgery among patients given prophylaxis with low molecular weight heparin

AUTHORS	BOUNAMEAUX H., HUBER O., KHABIRI E. et al.
REF	Arch. Surg. 1993; 128: 326-328

STUDY	Randomized, single-blind, comparing two approved LMWH regimens
CENTERS (n)	2
COUNTRY	Switzerland
PATIENTS (n)	*included* 194
	evaluated 185

TYPE OF SURGERY

Elective general abdominal in very high risk patients: 47% with malignancy, duration of operation > 4h in 40% of patients

ANESTHESIA

Not stated

STUDY DRUGS **Dalteparin** sc daily dose: 2500 AXa IU o.d. (0.2ml)

versus

Nadroparin sc daily dose: 2850 AXa IU o.d. (0.3ml)
first injection: 2h preop
treatment duration: about 9 days

+ *Elastic compression stockings*

ASSESSMENTS

❑ DVT:
- liquid contact thermography preoperatively and every second day following surgery,
- bilateral venography at D9 or at hospital discharge.

❑ PE, clinical symptoms confirmed by lung scan.

BOUNAMEAUX H. et al. 1993

	Dalteparin 2500 AXa IU x 1		Nadroparin 2850 AXa IU x 1		p
Patients with venography	93		92		
Total DVT	30	32.2%	15	16.3%	< 0.02
Proximal DVT	9	9.7%	5	5.4%	NS

COMMENTS

❏ As announced in the title, "unexpectedly" high DVT incidence was reported in both treated-groups. It should be emphasized that the patients included in this study were at very high risk: DVT was present in about 58% of patients with cancer.

❏ These DVT were asymptomatic in most cases; PE was confirmed by lung scan in 3 cases.

❏ This study was the first in general surgery in which cases of DVT were documented solely by venography (and not by FUT, confirmed -in some trials- by venography).

Low molecular weight heparin started before surgery as prophylaxis against deep vein thrombosis: 2500 versus 5000 AXa units in 2070 patients

AUTHORS	BERGQVIST D., BURMARK U.S., FLORDAL P.A. et al.
REF	Br. J. Surg. 1995; 82: 496-501

STUDY Multicenter, randomized, double-blind dosage comparison

CENTERS (n) 7
COUNTRY Sweden

PATIENTS (n)
included 2097
evaluated 2070
(1957 for DVT)

TYPE OF SURGERY
Elective general surgery, mainly colonic, rectal and gastric (66% for malignant disorders). No urogenital surgery

ANESTHESIA
General, supplementary epidural block in 30%

STUDY DRUG **Dalteparin**
- sc daily dose: 2500 AXa IU o.d.
  first injection: evening before surgery mainly 8-16h preop
  treatment duration: 8 days
  versus
- sc daily dose: 5000 AXa IU o.d.
  first injection: evening before surgery mainly 8-16h preop
  treatment duration: 8 days

ASSESSMENTS
- ❑ DVT: FUT daily up to D7; if positive, venography when possible.
- ❑ PE: clinical observation confirmed by lung scan.
- ❑ Bleeding complications.
- ❑ Death: autopsy whenever possible.

BERGQVIST D. et al. 1995

	Dalteparin 2500 AXa IU x 1		Dalteparin 5000 AXa IU x 1		p
Patients	1034	696 (with cancer)	1036	679 (with cancer)	
Patients available for analysis	976		981		
Patients with correct prophylaxis	868		864		
Total DVT (ITT)*	124	12.7%	65	6.6%	< 0.001
Total DVT with correct prophylaxis	114	13.1%	59	6.8%	< 0.001
Total DVT in malignancy (ITT)*	104	14.9%	58	8.5%	< 0.001
PE (confirmed by lung scan)	6 (1 fatal)		4 (1 fatal)		
Total hemorrhagic complications	28	2.7%	49	4.7%	0.02
Major bleeding	3 (1 fatal)		13		
Reoperation for bleeding	2		13		
Hemorrhage in malignancy	—	3.6%	—	4.6%	NS
Hemorrhage in benign condition	—	0.9%	—	5.0%	0.01
Discontinuation of prophylaxis	9		21		
Death within 30 days	35		32		

* ITT= intention-to-treat.

COMMENTS

❑ Dalteparin 5000 AXa IU was more effective than 2500 IU at the cost of a small bleeding risk.

❑ In patients with malignancy, dalteparin 5000 AXa IU did not increase risk of bleeding.

❑ In patients operated on for benign disease, dalteparin 2500 AXa IU (low regimen) was sufficient for prophylaxis and was associated with a very low risk of bleeding.

Low molecular weight heparin compared with unfractionated heparin in prevention of postoperative thrombosis

AUTHORS	SAMAMA M.M., BERNARD P., BONNARDOT J.P. et al. (for GENOX multicentric trial)
REF	Br. J. Surg. 1988; 75: 128-131

STUDY	Dose-finding, 3 consecutive open label, multicenter, randomized studies
CENTERS (n)	11
COUNTRY	France
PATIENTS (n)	*included* 885
	evaluated 803

TYPE OF SURGERY
General: abdominal, gynecological, thoracic, urological

ANESTHESIA
General

STUDY DRUG	**Enoxaparin**	sc daily doses, three groups:
		• group I 60mg o.d.
		• group II 40mg o.d.
		• group III 20mg o.d.
		first injection: 2h preop
		treatment duration: 7 days
REFERENCE DRUG	**UFH**	sc daily dose: 5000 IU t.i.d.
		first injection: 2h preop
		treatment duration: 7 days

ASSESSMENTS
- ❏ Isotopic DVT (FUT) daily up to D7.
- ❏ PE: lung scan or angiography if clinical suspicion.
- ❏ Major/minor hemorrhage.
- ❏ Other adverse effects.

SAMAMA M. et al. 1988

	Total DVT (FUT) (number/total patients) %		Major hemorrhage (n)		Prophylaxis discontinued (n)	
	Enox.	**UFH** 5000 IU x 3	**Enox.**	**UFH**	**Enox.**	**UFH**
I • **Enox** 60mg x 1	(4/137) 2.9%	(5/133) 3.8%	4*	3	4	1
II • **Enox** 40mg x 1	(3/106) 2.8%	(3/110) 2.7%	2	2	0	1
III • **Enox** 20mg x 1	(6/159) 3.8%	(12/158) 7.6%	3	4	1	3

* reoperation was required in one of these 4 patients.

COMMENTS

❑ Results of this dose-finding study did not clarify which is the best regimen; the recommended sc dosage for moderate risk of thrombosis was 20mg.

❑ Group III patients were very different compared to those in Groups I and II: mainly urological surgery (36%), no thoracic surgery (more than 50% of gynecological surgery in groups I and II).

❑ No PE occurred in any group.

**Enoxaparin in the prevention
of deep venous thrombosis after major surgery;
multicentric study**

AUTHORS	GAZZANIGA G.M., ANGELINI G., PASTORINO G. et al.
REF	Int. Surg. 1993; 78: 271-275

STUDY	Open-label, multicenter, randomized
CENTERS *(n)*	40
COUNTRY	Italy
PATIENTS *(n)*	*included* 1122 (with negative Doppler or IPG at entry)
	evaluated 1122

TYPE OF SURGERY

Major general (≈ 94%) vascular (≈ 6%)
about 50% with malignancy

ANESTHESIA

General

STUDY DRUG	Enoxaparin	sc daily dose: 20mg o.d.
		first injection: 2h preop
		treatment duration: 7-10 days

REFERENCE DRUG	UFH	sc dose: 5000 IU b.i.d.
		first injection: 2h preop
		treatment duration: 7-10 days

ASSESSMENTS

❑ DVT: Doppler, impedance plethysmography (IPG) between D7-D10.

❑ PE clinical symptoms: lung scan/angiography if clinical suspicion.

❑ Hemorrhages, local tolerability.

❑ Clinical follow-up during 6 weeks (death).

GAZZANIGA G.M. et al. 1993

	Enoxaparin 20mg x 1		UFH 5000 IU x 2	
Patients	561		561	
Total DVT	2	0.53%	6	1.06%
PE non fatal	2	0.36%	1	0.18%
fatal	1	0.18%	3	0.53%
Hemorrhage and wound hematomas	29	5.20%	34	6.10%
Treatment discontinued due to bleeding	13	2.30%	14	2.50%
Local hematomas at injection site	88	16.10%	139	25.30%
Death (6-week follow-up)	3	0.53%	9	1.60%

COMMENTS

❏ Surprisingly low incidence of DVT despite the "low" prophylactic dosage and the high number of cancer patients:

 • was this diagnosis method not sensitive enough?

 • was it a consequence of the unusual previous elimination of patients with a history of DVT?

Antithromboembolic efficacy and safety of enoxaparin in general surgery: German multicentre trial

AUTHORS	HAAS S., FLOSBACH C.W.
REF	Eur. J. Surg. 1994; 571: 37-43

STUDY	Open-label, multicenter
CENTERS (n)	197
COUNTRY	Germany
PATIENTS (n)	*included* 9919
	evaluated 9919

TYPE OF SURGERY

Major elective general surgery (abdominal, gynecological, urological) at medium risk

ANESTHESIA

General ≈ 80%, locoregional ≈ 20%

STUDY DRUG	**Enoxaparin**	sc daily dose: 20mg o.d.
		first injection: not stated
		treatment duration: 7 days
REFERENCE DRUG	**None**	

ASSESSMENTS

❑ DVT - PE: clinical symptoms, if suspicion, venography or lung scan.

❑ Hemorrhage.

❑ Other adverse drug reactions (thrombocytopenia).

HAAS S. et al. 1994.

| | **Enoxaparin** 20mg x 1 | | | |
	Number	DVT	PE	Fatal PE
Type of operations:				
Gastrointestinal	1299	1	3	
Cholecystectomy	1812	5	11	1
Herniotomy	2421	1	1	
Laparotomy	221	1	1	1
Hysterectomy	2030	2	5	1
Nephrectomy	154	0	0	
Transurethral resection	691	0	0	
Others	1291	1	3	
Total	9919	11 0.1%	24 0.24%	3 0.03%
Major bleeding (reinterventions)	51 0.5%			

COMMENTS

❏ Very low incidence of clinical DVT but without control group, no comparison is possible.

❏ In this large study based on clinical symptoms, it clearly appears that the number of PE was higher than the number of DVT and more frequent in females than in males. The cholecystectomy group appears to be at higher risk.

❏ No case of thrombocytopenia despite the large number of treated patients.

❏ No hemorrhagic complication was observed in the 1899 cases of spinal anesthesia.

A comparative trial of a low molecular weight heparin (enoxaparin) versus standard heparin for the prophylaxis of postoperative deep vein thrombosis in general surgery

AUTHORS	NURMOHAMED M.T., VERHAEGHE R., HAAS S. et al.
REF	Am. J. Surg. 1995; 169: 567-571

STUDY	Multicenter, randomized, double-blind
CENTERS (n)	20
COUNTRIES	Belgium, Germany, The Netherlands, Spain, United Kingdom, New Zealand
PATIENTS (n)	*included* 1471
	evaluated 1427

TYPE OF SURGERY
General: colon 30%,
cholecystectomy 23%, gastric 12%,
gynecological 13%,
one third with malignancy

ANESTHESIA
General

STUDY DRUG	**Enoxaparin**	sc daily dose: 20mg o.d. + 2 placebo injections
		first injection: 2h preop
		treatment duration: 10 days
REFERENCE DRUG	**UFH**	sc daily dose: 5000 IU t.i.d.
		first injection: 2h preop
		treatment duration: 10 days

ASSESSMENTS

- ❑ DVT: daily clinical and isotopic FUT up to D10 or discharge; if positive findings, venography when possible.
- ❑ Clinical PE confirmed by lung scan or angiography.
- ❑ Total thromboembolic events at D10 ± 1.
- ❑ Major/minor hemorrhage.
- ❑ Death.
- ❑ Side effects: thrombocytopenia.

NURMOHAMED M.T. et al. 1995

	Enoxaparin 20mg x 1		UFH 5000 IU x 3		p
Patients	718		709		
Total DVT	54	7.5%	37	5.2%	NS
Clinical DVT	2	0.3%	3	0.4%	NS
Clinical suspicion of PE	2	0.3%	5	0.7%	NS
Total thromboembolic events	58	8.1%	45	6.3%	NS
Major hemorrhage	11	1.5%	18	2.5%	NS
Minor hemorrhage	100	13.8%	117	16.3%	NS
Death (PE/major hemorrhage)	4	(1/1)	6	(0/2)	NS
Thrombocytopenia (platelets < 100 x 10^9/L)	11	1.5%	20	2.8%	NS

COMMENTS

❑ In this study, the enoxaparin regimen (20mg o.d.) was similar for efficacy and safety to UFH 5000 IU t.i.d.

❑ Relevant incidence of thrombocytopenia even though the majority of the cases did not necessitate cessation of treatment.

Efficacy and safety of enoxaparin versus unfractionated heparin for prevention of deep vein thrombosis in elective cancer surgery: a double-blind randomized multicenter trial with venographic assessment

AUTHORS	BERGQVIST D. for ENOXACAN study group
REF	Brit. J. Surg. 1997; 84: 1099-1103

STUDY	Double-blind, randomized, multicenter
CENTERS (n)	34
COUNTRIES	10: Europe, United States, Israel, Australia
PATIENTS (n)	*randomized* 1116
	evaluated 631

TYPE OF SURGERY
Major elective surgery for abdominal or pelvic malignancy

ANESTHESIA
general

STUDY DRUG	**Enoxaparin**	sc daily dose: 40mg o.d. + 2 placebo injections
		first injection: 2h preop
		treatment duration: 8-12 days

REFERENCE DRUG	**UFH**	sc daily doses: 5000 IU t.i.d.
		first injection: 2h preop
		treatment duration: 8-12 days

ASSESSMENTS

❏ DVT: bilateral venography on day 8-12; unilateral venography if clinical symptoms of DVT developed before the end of treatment.

❏ PE: if clinical suspicion, lung scan or angiography.

❏ Major/minor hemorrhage.

❏ Adverse events.

❏ Three-month follow-up.

BERGQVIST D. et al. 1997

	Enoxaparin 40 mg x 1		UFH 5000 IU x 3		p
Treated patients	556		560		
Evaluable venographies	312	56.0%	319	57.0%	
DVT	45	14.4%	56	17.6%	NS
PE + DVT	0	0.0%	2*	0.6%	
Major bleeding	23	4.1%	16	2.9%	
Discontinuation of prophylaxis	18	3.2%	12	2.1%	NS
Thrombocytopenia**	1		3 (1 severe on D8)		
Death (thrombosis-related)	2	0.6%	0	0	
Three-month follow-up :					
Total death	26 (3 thrombosis-related)		34 (4 thrombosis-related)		NS

* PE with clinical symptoms.
** Platelet count below 70,000/ml.

COMMENTS

❑ Large study carried out exclusively in cancer patients with vein thromboses documented by bilateral venography (41.2% of inadequate venograms).

❑ This diagnostic method indicated an higher frequency of total DVT than that observed with FUT in other studies. The distribution of DVT was mainly distal.

❑ No significant difference in efficacy and safety was observed between the two prophylactic treatments.

Enoxaparin plus compression stocking compared with compression stockings alone in the prevention of venous thromboembolism after elective neurosurgery

AUTHORS	AGNELLI G., PIOVELLA F., BUONCRISTIANI P. et al.
REF	N.E.J. Med. 1998; 339: 80-85

STUDY	Multicenter, randomized, double-blind
CENTERS (n)	7
COUNTRY	Italy
PATIENTS (n)	*randomized* 307
	evaluated 260

TYPE OF SURGERY
Cranial or spinal surgery

ANESTHESIA
General

STUDY DRUG	**Enoxaparin**	sc daily dose: 40mg
		first injection: within 24h after surgery
		treatment duration: at least 7 days
	+ Elastic compression stockings	
REFERENCE DRUG	**Placebo**	sc daily dose 0.4ml
		first injection: within 24h after surgery
		treatment duration: at least 7 days
	+ Elastic compression stockings	

ASSESSMENTS

❑ Symptomatic documented venous thromboembolism or DVT detected by venography at D8±1 (blind lecture).

❑ PE symptomatic confirmed by VQ lung scan, angiography, autopsy.

❑ Major, minor bleeding.

AGNELLI G. et al. 1998

	Enoxaparin 40mg x 1 + Elastic stockings		Placebo + Elastic stockings		p
Patients	153		154		
Evaluable venography (D8±1)	130		129		
Thromboembolic events	22	17%	43	33%	0.004
Total DVT	22	17%	42	32%	0.004
Proximal DVT	7	5%	17	13%	0.04
PE	0		1 (fatal at D9)		
Total bleeding	18	12%	11	7%	NS
Major bleeding	4	3%	4	3%	
Intracranial bleeding	3		4		
Minor bleeding (wound hematoma)	8		2		
Death (D0-D10)	2		2		

COMMENTS

❑ In neurosurgery, the prophylaxis of venous thromboembolism is better when a LMWH (enoxaparin 40mg) is associated with compression stockings than with compression stockings alone.

❑ The risk of major bleeding is not increased with enoxaparin.

Efficacy and safety of low molecular weight heparin (CY216) in preventing postoperative venous thromboembolism: a cooperative study
(first part)

AUTHORS	KAKKAR V.V., MURRAY W.J.G.
REF	Br. J. Surg. 1985; 72: 786-791

STUDY	Double-blind, multicenter, randomized
CENTERS *(n)*	5
COUNTRY	United Kingdom
PATIENTS *(n)*	*included* 400
	evaluated 395

TYPE OF SURGERY

General: gynecological 30%, abdominal 20%, cholecystectomy 20%, about one third with malignant disease

ANESTHESIA

General

STUDY DRUG	**Nadroparin (CY216)**	sc daily dose: 7500 AXa ICU (2850 AXa IU) = 0.3ml o.d. + 1 placebo injection first injection: 2h preop treatment duration: ≥ 7 days
REFERENCE DRUG	**UFH**	sc daily doses: 5000 IU b.i.d. first injection: 2h preop treatment duration: ≥ 7 days

ASSESSMENTS

❑ Isotopic DVT (FUT) confirmed by venography when possible.
❑ Clinical PE confirmed by lung scan.
❑ Hemorrhage (postoperative), wound hematomas.
❑ Death (autopsy).

KAKKAR V.V. et al. 1985

	Nadroparin 0.3ml x 1		UFH 5000 IU x 2		p
Patients	196		199		
Total DVT (FUT)	5	2.5%	14	7.5%	<0.05
PE	0		1 (fatal)*		
Excessive postop blood loss	10	5.3%	7	3.5%	NS
Wound hematomas	11	5.6%	14	7.0%	NS
Prophylaxis discontinued	3	1.5%	6	3.0%	NS
Death	5		5 (2 AMI)		

* Patient with disseminated carcinoma.

COMMENTS

❏ In this pioneering trial, the efficacy of a LMWH administered o.d. by sc injection was better than UFH b.i.d. Safety in terms of hemorrhage was similar.

❏ Of the 25 patients who developed wound hematomas, 20 (80%) had undergone gynecological surgery.

❏ For the first time, it was shown that a single daily sc injection was satisfactory for DVT prophylaxis.

Efficacy and safety of low molecular weight heparin (CY216) in preventing postoperative venous thromboembolism: a co-operative study
(second part)

AUTHORS	KAKKAR V.V., MURRAY W.J.G.
REF	Br. J. Surg. 1985; 72: 786-791

STUDY	Open-label	**TYPE OF SURGERY**	
		General: gynecological (hysterectomy)	
CENTERS (n)	5	cholecystectomy/urological, other.	
COUNTRY	United Kingdom	About one third with malignancy	
PATIENTS (n)	*included* 1007	**ANESTHESIA**	
	evaluated 910	General	

STUDY DRUG	**Nadroparin (CY216)**	sc daily dose: 7500 AXa ICU (2850 AXa IU) = 0.3ml o.d.
		first injection: 2h preop
		treatment duration: ≈ 9 days

REFERENCE DRUG	**None**

ASSESSMENTS

❏ Isotopic DVT (FUT) confirmed by venography when possible.
❏ Clinical PE confirmed by lung scan.
❏ Hemorrhage (postoperative), wound hematomas.

KAKKAR V.V. et al. 1985

	Nadroparin 0.3ml x 1		p
Patients	910		
Total DVT (FUT)			
• In intention-to-treat	31	3.4%	
• In patients effectively treated	27	2.9%	
under 60 years old (n=464)	10	2.2%	NS
over 60 years old (n=444)	21	4.7%	
malignant disease (n=310)	21	6.7%	<0.01
benign disease (n=597)	10	1.6%	
Excessive postop hemorrhage	29	3.2%	
Therapy discontinued	17	1.8%	
Wound hematomas	36	3.9%	
under 60 years old	27	5.8%	<0.01
over 60 years old	9	2.0%	
Three-week follow-up			
Death	19	2.2%	

COMMENTS

❏ The validity of this nadroparin prophylactic dosage (0.3ml) was confirmed in a large open-label trial.

❏ Malignancy was a clear risk factor for DVT.

❏ Age was a clear risk factor for hemorrhage.

❏ Gynecologic surgery was a clear risk for wound hematomas.

Comparison of a low molecular weight heparin and unfractionated heparin for the prevention of deep vein thrombosis in patients undergoing abdominal surgery

AUTHORS	The European Fraxiparine Study (EFS) Group
REF	Br. J. Surg. 1988; 75: 1058-1063

STUDY	Randomized, double-blind	
CENTERS (n)	2	
COUNTRY	Germany	
PATIENTS (n)	*included*	410
	evaluated	404 (ITT)
		390 with prophylaxis

TYPE OF SURGERY

General: gastric/biliary/colon/rectum. Malignancy in more than 50% of the cases

ANESTHESIA

General

STUDY DRUG	**Nadroparin**	sc daily dose: 7500 AXa ICU (2850 AXa IU) = 0.3ml o.d.
		first injection: 2h preop
		second injection: 8h postop D0
		treatment duration: 7 days
REFERENCE DRUG	**UFH**	sc daily doses: 5000 IU t.i.d.
		first injection: 2h preop
		treatment duration: 7 days

+ Elastic compression stockings in both groups

ASSESSMENTS

- ❏ Isotopic DVT (FUT) daily up to D7 confirmed by venography if positive.
- ❏ Clinical PE confirmed by lung scan or angiography.
- ❏ Hemorrhage, wound hematomas.
- ❏ Death, autopsy when possible.

The EFS Group, 1988

	Nadroparin 0.3ml x 1		UFH 5000 IU x 3		p
Evaluated patients	960		936		
DVT total	27	2.8%	42	4.5%	<0.05
Proximal DVT	4	0.4%	13	1.4%	<0.05
With clinical symptoms	3	0.3%	9	1.0%	
Patients with cancer	355		349		
Total DVT	15	4.2%	19	5.4%	
Postoperative transfusions	106	30.0%	107	31.0%	
Patients without cancer	605		587		
Total DVT	12	2.0%	23	3.9%	
Postoperative transfusions	44	7.3%	37	6.3%	
PE	2	0.2%	5*	0.5%	
Hemorrhage	No difference between the 2 groups				

* 1 fatal.

COMMENTS

❑ Nadroparin o.d. (0.3ml) was at least as effective as UFH 5000 IU t.i.d. in preventing DVT after general surgery.

❑ In both groups, about 70% of DVT occurred between the day of surgery and D3.

❑ The incidence of DVT and blood transfusions was higher in cancer patients than in non cancer patients

❑ A clear relationship appeared between incidence of DVT and centers.

Prophylaxis of fatal pulmonary embolism in general surgery using low molecular weight heparin CY216: a multicentre, double-blind, randomized, controlled clinical trial versus placebo (STEP)

AUTHORS	PEZZUOLI G., NERI SERNERI G.G., SETTEMBRINI P. et al.
REF	Int. Surg. 1989; 71: 205-210

STUDY	Multicenter, double-blind, randomized, placebo-controlled
CENTERS (n)	18
COUNTRY	Italy
PATIENTS (n)	*included* 4498 with moderate risk for overall mortality and/or for thromboembolism
	evaluated 4498

TYPE OF SURGERY

General (abdominal/thoracic/others).
One third with malignancy

ANESTHESIA

General

STUDY DRUG	**Nadroparin (CY216)**	sc daily dose: 7500 AXa ICU (2850 AXa IU)= 0.3ml o.d. first injection: 2h preop treatment duration: at least 7 days (8.9±1.9 injections)
REFERENCE DRUG	**Placebo**	sc daily dose: 0.3 ml o.d. first injection: 2h preop teatment duration: at least 7 days (9.0±1.2 injections)

ASSESSMENTS

- ❏ Fatal PE (autopsy).
- ❏ Other thromboembolic mortality.
- ❏ General mortality (autopsy in 85% of deaths).
- ❏ Major hemorrhage.

PEZZUOLI G. et al. 1989

	Nadroparin 0.3ml x 1		Placebo 0.3ml x 1		p
Patients	2247		2251		
Fatal PE	2	0.09%	4	0.18%	NS
Thromboembolic mortality	2	0.09%	8	0.36%	<0.05
Total mortality	8	0.36%	18	0.80%	<0.05
Intraoperative bleeding (considerably increased)	48	2.10%	24	1.10%	<0.01
Wound hematomas (medium + large)	119	5.30%	44	1.90%	<0.01
Injection site hematomas	230	10.20%	149	6.60%	<0.01
Bleeding episodes	173	7.70%	69	3.10%	<0.01
Treatment discontinued	56/173	32.40%	18/69	26.10%	NS
Patients with platelets <100,000/mm3 (D8)	13	0.60%	10	0.40%	NS

COMMENTS

❑ Very low mortality in the two groups. Was it due to the exclusion of patients with potentially high risk?

❑ Both thromboembolic and total mortality were significantly reduced in nadroparin-treated patients.

❑ Interesting trial regarding tolerance since placebo-controlled: while operative bleeding was only slightly increased, postoperative bleeding was more pronounced in nadroparin-treated patients.

❑ However, the clinical significance of these events was limited (no death was related to hemorrhage).

Unexpectedly high rate of phlebographic deep venous thrombosis following elective general abdominal surgery among patients given prophylaxis with low molecular weight heparin

AUTHORS	BOUNAMEAUX H., HUBER O., KHABIRI E. et al.
REF	Arch. Surg.1993; 128: 326-328

STUDY	Randomized, single-blind, comparing two approved LMWH regimens
CENTERS (n)	2
COUNTRY	Switzerland
PATIENTS (n)	*included* 197
	evaluated 185

TYPE OF SURGERY

Elective general abdominal in very high risk patients: 47% with malignancy, duration of operation > 4h in 40% of patients

ANESTHESIA

Not stated (general probably)

STUDY DRUGS

Nadroparin sc daily dose: 2850 AXa IU o.d. (0.3ml)
first injection: 2h preop
treatment duration: about 9 days

versus

Dalteparin sc daily dose: 2500 AXa IU o.d. (0.2ml)
first injection: 2h preop

+ Elastic compression stockings

ASSESSMENTS

❑ DVT:
  • liquid contact thermography preoperatively and every second day following surgery,
  • bilateral venography at D9 or at hospital discharge.
  PE, clinical symptoms confirmed by lung scan.

BOUNAMEAUX H. et al. 1993

	Dalteparin 2500 AXa IU x 1		**Nadroparin** 2850 AXa IU x 1		**p**
Patients with venography	93		92		
Total DVT	30	32.2%	15	16.3%	<0.02
Proximal DVT	9	9.7%	5	5.4%	

COMMENTS *(see also p. 56)*

❑ As announced in the title, "unexpectedly" high DVT incidence was reported in both treated-groups. It should be emphasized that the patients included in this study were at high risk: DVT was present in about 58% of patients with cancer.

❑ Nadroparin regimen — slightly higher dose than the dalteparin one — appeared to be more effective.

❑ These DVT were asymptomatic in most cases; PE was confirmed by lung scan in 3 cases.

❑ This study was the first in general surgery in which cases of DVT were documented solely by venography (and not by FUT, confirmed in some trials by venography).

Prevention of post-operative deep vein thrombosis in cancer patients.
A randomized trial with low molecular weight heparin (CY216)

AUTHORS	MARASSI A., BALZANO G., MARI G. et al.
REF	Int. Surg.1993; 78: 166-170

		TYPE OF SURGERY
STUDY	Open-label, randomized parallel-group	Major abdominal for malignancy surgery
CENTERS (n)	1	**ANESTHESIA**
COUNTRY	Italy	General
PATIENTS (n)	*randomized* 64	
	evaluated 61	

STUDY DRUG	**Nadroparin**	sc daily dose: 7500 AXa ICU (2850 AXa IU) = 0,3ml
		first injection: not clearly stated
		second injection: 12h postop
		treatment duration: ≥ 7 days
REFERENCE DRUG	**None**	(no prophylaxis)

ASSESSMENTS

- ❏ Isotopic DVT: daily FUT up to D7 confirmed by venography if positive.
- ❏ Bleeding complications.
- ❏ Side effects.
- ❏ Laboratory data.

MARASSI A. et al. 1993

	Nadroparin 0.3ml x 1		Control no prophylaxis		p
Patients	30		31		
Total DVT	2	7%	11	35%	<0.01
Proximal DVT	0		1		
Patients with blood transfusion	14		13		NS
Wound hematomas	0		1		NS
Local hematomas at injection site	4		0		
Mean AXa level* IU/ml at:					
D1	0.38		—		
D3	0.25				

* Time not stated.

COMMENTS

❑ This study clearly shows the high incidence of DVT without prophylaxis in oncological surgery.

❑ The administered prophylactic regimen, i.e. two injections the day of surgery followed thereafter by one daily injection, significantly decreased the incidence of DVT without increased risk of hemorrhagic complications.

❑ Interestingly, the two patients who developed DVT in the group given prophylaxis had postoperative AXa activity lower than 0.25 IU/ml the first day.

Efficiency and tolerance of Fraxiparine (CY216) for the prevention of postoperative deep vein thrombosis in patients undergoing general surgery under epidural anesthesia *(French)*

AUTHORS	EURIN B.
REF	Ann. Fr. Reanim. 1994; 13: 311-317

STUDY	Open-label, multicenter, randomized	**TYPE OF SURGERY** General/pelvic
CENTERS (n)	78	**ANESTHESIA**
COUNTRY	France	Epidural 30%, spinal 70%
PATIENTS (n)	*included* 480 *evaluated* 479	

STUDY DRUG	**Nadroparin**	sc daily dose: 7500 AXa ICU (2850 AXa IU) = 0.3ml first injection: 2h postop treatment duration: 7 days
REFERENCE DRUG	**UFH**	sc daily doses: 5000 IU t.i.d. first injection: 2h postop treatment duration: 7 days

ASSESSMENTS

❏ DVT - Doppler, echo-Doppler, rheoplethysmography — if abnormal findings, bilateral venography.

❏ PE: clinical symptoms.

❏ Bleeding complications.

EURIN B. 1994

	Nadroparin 0,3ml x 1		UFH 5000 IU x 3	
Patients	240		239	
DVT	1	0.4%	0	0%
PE	0		0	
Major hemorrhage	1		0	
Minor hemorrhage	39	16.2%	37	15.5%

COMMENTS

❑ These two anticoagulant treatments, started early after surgery, did not cause any spinal hemorrhage complications.

❑ In this study, the incidence of DVT was very low in the two treated groups. This is likely due to the low sensitivity of the Doppler method in asymptomatic postoperative patients.

**Clinical tolerance of CY216 (Fraxiparine®)
for thromboembolic prophylaxis after neurosurgery**
(French)

AUTHORS	PAOLETTI C., MAUBEC E. RAGGUENEAU et al.
REF	Agress. 1989; 30: 363-366

STUDY	Open-label
CENTERS (n)	2
COUNTRY	France
PATIENTS (n)	*included* 99
	evaluated 97

INCLUSION CRITERIA
Patients undergoing craniotomy mainly for intracerebral tumoral malformations (66%).

STUDY DRUG	**Nadroparin**	sc daily dose: 7500 AXa ICU o.d. (2850 AXa IU) = 0.3ml
		first injection: postop, not later than D3
		treatment duration: 8 days
REFERENCE DRUG	**None**	

ASSESSMENTS
- ❏ Daily Glasgow coma score outcome.
- ❏ CT scan: just postop, at D1 and D7±1 (Fischer's scale).
- ❏ DVT: clinical symptoms confirmed by Doppler and venography.
- ❏ PE; clinical symptoms; if suspicion, pulmonary angiography.

PAOLETTI C. et al. 1989

	Nadroparin 0.3ml x 1
Patients	97
Percent of patients	
• without cerebral hemorrhage (CH) at D1 and D8	58.8%
• with CH at D1 but without at D8	21.6%
• with CH at D1 and same Glascow score at D8	11.4%
• with CH at D1 and Glascow score worsened at D8	8.2%*
Thromboembolic events	0

* No reoperation was necessary and the clinical state of these patients improved.

COMMENTS

❏ Interesting study with two postop CT scans in order to assess the potential cerebral hemorrhagic effect of a LMWH. In this trial, nadroparin 0.3ml did not cause any dramatic hemorrhagic event. Unfortunately, no control group.

Low molecular weight heparin and compression stockings in the prevention of venous thromboembolism in neurosurgery

AUTHORS	NURMOHAMED M.T., VAN RIEL A.M., HENKENS M.A. et al.
REF	Thromb. Haemostasis 1996; 75: 233-238

STUDY	Multicenter, randomized, double-blind, placebo-controlled
CENTERS (n)	4
COUNTRIES	The Netherlands, Canada
PATIENTS (n)	*included* 485
	evaluated 345
	(with venography)

TYPE OF SURGERY
Neurosurgery (craniotomy, spinal surgery)

ANESTHESIA
Not stated

STUDY DRUG **Nadroparin** sc daily dose: 7500 AXa ICU (2850 AXa IU) = 0.3ml
first injection:18-24h postop
treatment duration: ≥ 10 days

REFERENCE DRUG Placebo daily dose: 0.3ml (saline)
first injection: 18-24h postop
treatment duration: ≥ 10 days

+ Elastic compression stockings in both groups

ASSESSMENTS

- ❏ DVT: B-mode compression ultrasonography on D6, 8 and 10; if abnormal findings, bilateral venography.
- ❏ Bilateral venography at D10 or at hospital discharge blindly assessed for all patients.
- ❏ PE: clinical symptoms; lung scan/angiography if clinical suspicion.
- ❏ Major, minor hemorrhage.
- ❏ Two-month follow-up.

NURMOHAMED M.T. et al. 1996

	Nadroparin 0.3ml x 1 + Elastic stockings		Placebo + Elastic stockings		p
Patients	241		244		
Evaluable venography	166	68.9%	179	73.4%	
Total DVT (D0-D10)	31	18.7%	47	26.3%	0.05
Proximal DVT	12*	6.9%	21*	11.5%	NS
Major bleeding (D0-D10)	6	2.5%	2	0.8%	NS
All bleeding complications	10	4.1%	3	1.2%	0.047
56-day follow-up:					
Total DVT (D0-D56)	33	13.7%	51	20.9%	0.02
Proximal DVT and PE (fatal PE)	14 (1)	5.8%	25 (2)	10.2%	0.03
Death (D0-D56)	22		10		

* None of the patients developed symptomatic PE.

COMMENTS
- This prophylactic regimen appeared to significantly reduce the incidence of DVT or thromboembolic events in neurosurgery at the cost of increased bleeding complications.
- None of the observed deaths can be attributed to the study drug according to the blind adjudication committee.

Controlled clinical study of the efficacy of a new low molecular weight heparin administered subcutaneously to prevent post-operative deep venous thrombosis

AUTHORS	VALLE I., SOLA G. ORIGONE A.
REF	Curr. Med. Res. Opin. 1988; 11: 80-86

STUDY	Randomized, double-blind, placebo-controlled
CENTERS (n)	1
COUNTRY	Italy
PATIENTS (n)	included 100

TYPE OF SURGERY
General (hernioplasty, cholecystectomy, colic resections, others)
≈ 20% with malignancy

ANESTHESIA
General

STUDY DRUG	Parnaparin	sc daily dose: 7500 AXa U o.d. first injection: 2h preop treatment duration: 7 days
REFERENCE DRUG	Placebo	sc saline 0.3ml first injection: 2h preop treatment duration: 7 days

ASSESSMENTS

- ❑ DVT: clinical examination, Doppler sonography; if suspicion, venography.
- ❑ PE: clinical symptoms confirmed by lung scan.
- ❑ Perioperative blood transfusions.
- ❑ Laboratory test: AXa activity.

VALLE I. et al. 1988

	Parnaparin 7500 AXa U x 1	Placebo 0.3ml x 1
Patients	50	50
Total DVT	0 0%	3 6% (D1, D3, D4)
PE	0	0
Blood transfusions	no difference	
Mean AXa activity at peak (U/ml)* at • D1	0.10	
• D3	0.18	
• D7	0.22	

* Evaluated from figure.

COMMENTS

❑ Despite the reduced number of patients, the results suggested that parnaparin 7500 AXa U had
prophylactic activity. It must be noted that these initial units were expressed as coagulometric units;
in chromogenic assay, they correspond to about 3000-3200 AXa IU.

A new low molecular weight heparin for deep vein thrombosis prevention: effectiveness in postoperative patients

AUTHORS	SALCUNI P.F., AZZARONE M., PALAZZINI E.
REF	Curr. Therap. Res. 1988; 43: 824-831

STUDY	Open-label, randomized, controlled
CENTERS (n)	1
COUNTRY	Italy
PATIENTS (n)	*selected* 141
	evaluated 73

TYPE OF SURGERY
general abdominal
50% for malignancy

ANESTHESIA
general

STUDY DRUG	**Parnaparin**	sc daily dose: 15,000 AXa U o.d. (6400 AXa IU) first injection: 2h preop treatment duration: 7 days
REFERENCE DRUG	**UFH**	sc daily doses: 5000 IU t.i.d. first injection: 24h preop treatment duration: 7 days

ASSESSMENTS

- ❏ DVT: clinical symptoms and Doppler ultrasonography.
- ❏ PE: clinical symptoms, chest X-rays.
- ❏ Perioperative blood loss.
- ❏ AXa activity.

SALCUNI P.F. et al. 1988

	Parnaparin 15,000 AXa U x 1	UFH 5000 IU x 3	p
Patients	37	36	
Total DVT	4 5.5%	10 14.7%	0.01
PE	1 (D6)	2 (D1 and D9)	
AXa activity (U/ml ± SD) D4 at peak	0.26±0.04	0.09±0.01	<0.01
Patients with transfusions (D0-D10)	45.1%	61.7%	
Wound hematomas	6.8%	11.7%	NS

COMMENTS

❑ Statistical difference in favor of parnaparin 15,000 AXa U o.d. compared with UFH 5000 IU t.i.d. This LMWH dosage corresponding to approximatively 6400 IU is higher than the usual LMWH dosages (2500-4000 IU) administered for prophylaxis of DVT after general surgery.

A multicenter study
on LMW-heparin effectiveness in preventing
post surgical thrombosis

AUTHORS	VERARDI S., CASCIANI C.U., NICORA E. et al.
REF	Intern. Angio. 1988; 7- Suppl n°3: 19-24

STUDY	Open-label, multicenter, comparative
CENTERS *(n)*	6
COUNTRY	Italy
PATIENTS *(n)*	*included* 610
	evaluated 511

TYPE OF SURGERY
General (cholecystectomy, colectomy, others)
≈ 30% of patients with malignancy

ANESTHESIA
Not stated

STUDY DRUG	Parnaparin	sc daily dose (as reported on the publication): 4000 AXa IU or 8000 AXa IU o.d.
		first injection: 2h preop
		treatment duration: 7 days

REFERENCE DRUG	UFH	sc daily doses: 5000 IU b.i.d. or 5000 IU t.i.d.
		first injection: 2h preop
		treatment duration: 7 days

ASSESSMENTS

- ❏ DVT: FUT test; if positive, confirmed with Doppler ultrasonography or plethysmography, or venography.
- ❏ PE: clinical; if suspicion, lung scan.
- ❏ Biological tests: basal and 4h after morning injection: APTT, AXa levels.

VERARDI S. et al. 1988

	Parnaparin		UFH	
	4000 AXa IU x 1	8000 AXa IU x 1	5000 IU x 2	5000 IU x 3
Patients (distribution %)	250 (41.0%)	58 (9.5%)	134 (22.0%)	168 (27.5%)
DVT	9 3.6%	1 1.7%	7 5.2%	12 7.1%
PE (non fatal)	1 0.4%	0 —	0 —	3 1.8%
Excessive perioperative blood loss	2	1	4	7
Wound hematomas	5 2.0%	1 1.7%	7 5.2%	16 9.5%
APTT (sec ± SD)	27.4±2.9	35.1±3.9*	35.5±5.1*	38.3±6.0*
AXa (IU/ml ±SD) at D7, 4h post-injection	0.12±0.05	0.29±0.09*	0.05±0.03*	0.08±0.05*

* $p < 0.05$ vs basal values (in the publication: 0.286±0.87 probably typing error for SD).

COMMENTS

❏ Parnaparin both regimens appeared to be at least as effective and safe as UFH 5000 IU b.i.d. or t.i.d.
❏ The optimal dosage remains to be defined.
❏ With the higher dosage of parnaparin, APTT values were significantly increased.
❏ No correlation between AXa level and hemorrhagic events.

Effectiveness of thrombosis prevention with a low molecular weight heparin preparation in gynaecological patients undergoing surgery: an open study

AUTHORS	TARTAGLIA P., PEROLO F., D'ALES A.
REF	Curr. Med. Res. Opin. 1989; 11 : 360-365

STUDY	Open-label
CENTERS _(n)_	_1_
COUNTRY	Italy
PATIENTS _(n)_	_included_ 92

TYPE OF SURGERY

Hysterosalpingo-oophorectomy, total hysterectomy, hysterosalpingo plus lymphadenectomy

ANESTHESIA

not stated

STUDY DRUG   **Parnaparin**   sc daily dose: 7500 AXa U o.d. or
15,000 AXa U o.d. according to the risk factors for developing DVT

first injection: 2h preop
second injection: postop D1

REFERENCE DRUG   **None**

Note: These dosages are expressed with UFH as reference curve. Using the first standard for LMWH and a chromogenic assay, they correspond to 3200, 6400 AXa IU respectively.

ASSESSMENTS

❑ DVT: daily physical evaluation confirmed by venography if clinical suspicion.

❑ PE: confirmed by chest X-ray.

❑ Hemorrhagic complications.

❑ Laboratory test: AXa activity.

TARTAGLIA P. et al. 1989

	Parnaparin	
	7500 AXa IU x 1	15,000 AXa IU x 1
Patients at: low risk high risk	48 52%	44 48%
DVT PE	1 0	2 0
Blood transfusions, wound hematomas or hematoma at injection site	no difference between treated groups no excessive bleeding nor blood transfusions	
AXa activity (U/ml ± SD) 3h after injection at • D1 • D7	0.21±0.04 (no discrimination between 0.25±0.04 the two regimens)	

COMMENTS

❑ This study has been reported to illustrate the safety of LMWH in gynecological surgery known to be at high hemorrhagic risk.

Post-surgical deep vein thrombosis prevention: evaluation of the risk/benefit ratio of fractionated and unfractionated heparin

AUTHORS	GARCEA D., MARTUZZI F., SANTELMO N. et al.
REF	Curr. Med. Res. 1992; 12: 572-583

STUDY	Open-label, randomized, controlled
CENTERS (n)	1
COUNTRY	Italy
PATIENTS (n)	*included* 90
	evaluated 85

TYPE OF SURGERY
General
48% for gastric and intestinal malignancies

ANESTHESIA
Not stated

STUDY DRUG	**Parnaparin**	sc daily dose: 7500 AXa U o.d.
		first injection: 2h preop
		treatment duration: 7 days
REFERENCE DRUG	**UFH**	sc daily doses: 5000 IU t.i.d.
		first injection: 2h preop
		treatment duration: 7 days

ASSESSMENTS

- ❏ DVT: daily FUT, Doppler ultrasonography and venography if positive findings.
- ❏ PE: clinically confirmed with lung scan.
- ❏ Bleeding complications.
- ❏ Laboratory tests.
- ❏ Qualitative evaluation of the usefulness of the two treatments.

GARCEA D. et al. 1992

	Parnaparin 7500 AXa U x 1	UFH 5000 IU x 3
Patients	45	45
DVT according to:		
FUT	0	1
Doppler	0	0
venography	0	1
clinical symptoms	3	6
Hemorrhagic complications	0	5
PE	0	0

COMMENTS

❑ Despite the limited number of the patients, illustration of the discrepancy observed between the various diagnostic procedures used for DVT assessment. Surprisingly, in this study, the frequency of DVT with clinical symptoms was more marked than with the other diagnostic methods.

❑ The qualitative evaluation by Italian physicians of benefit/risk ratio and cost/benefit ratio indicated a greater usefulness for the LMWH.

Dose-effect relationship in the prevention of post-surgical thromboembolism by a low molecular weight heparin

AUTHORS	BECCHI G., BONOMO G.M., SCATARELLA M. et al.
REF	Act. Therap. 1993; 19: 163-179

STUDY	Open-label, randomized, multicenter, comparing three dosages	**TYPE OF SURGERY**	General
CENTERS *(n)*	3	**ANESTHESIA**	
COUNTRY	Italy	Not stated	
PATIENTS *(n)*	*evaluated* 195		

STUDY DRUG **Parnaparin** sc daily dose:

- 2500 AXa U o.d.
- 7500 AXa U o.d.
- 15,000 AXa U o.d.

first injection: 2h before surgery

treatment duration: 7 days

Note: These dosages are expressed with UFH as reference curve. Using the first standard for LMWH and a chromogenic assay, they correspond to 1100, 3200, 6400 AXa IU respectively.

ASSESSMENTS
- ❏ DVT: plethysmography.
- ❏ Bleeding complications.

BECCHI G. et al. 1993

	Parnaparin			p
	2500 AXa U x 1	7500 AXa U x 1	15,000 AXa U x 1	
Patients	61	69	65	
Thromboembolic events	8 13%	3 5%	1 3%	chi 2 <0.01
All hematomas	3	7	19	
Mean number of blood units transfused	20	22	39	

COMMENTS
- ❏ Relative relationship between dose and efficacy for preventing DVT.
- ❏ The best effective dose seemed to be ranging between 7500 and 15,000 AXa U, but the safer doses appeared to be less than 15,000 AXa U.

Prospective randomized clinical study in general surgery comparing a new low molecular weight heparin with unfractionated heparin in the prevention of thrombosis

AUTHORS	LIMMER J., ELLBRUCK D., MULLER H. et al.
REF	Clin. Investig. 1994; 72: 913-919

STUDY   Randomized, controlled

CENTERS *(n)*

COUNTRY   Germany

PATIENTS *(n)*   *included*   230
                    evaluated   203

TYPE OF SURGERY
General, 45-55% of patients
with malignancy

ANESTHESIA
General
about 40% of patients were receiving
hydroxyethyl starch (HES)

STUDY DRUG   **Parnaparin**   sc daily dose: 2500 AXa U o.d.
first injections: 12h and 2h preop then
                                          24h postop
treatment duration: 7 days

REFERENCE DRUG   **UFH**   sc daily doses: 5000 IU t.i.d.
first injections: 12h and 2h preop then
                                          24h postop
Elastic compression stockings for both groups
Early ambulation   treatment duration: 7 days

ASSESSMENTS

❏ Daily clinical observation for any adverse events.

❏ DVT: FUT; if positive findings, phlebography.

❏ Bleeding complications.

❏ Hematological investigations.

LIMMER J. et al. 1994

	Parnaparin 2500 AXa U x 1		UFH 5000 IU x 3	
Patients	103		100	
DVT (FUT)	4	3.9%	5	5.0%
Clinical DVT	0		0	
PE	0		0	
Severe hemorrhage	0		0	
Hematomas at injection site	39	38.0%	46	46.0%
AXa activity (IU/ml ± SE)* at				
• D0 (preop)	0.06±0.1		0.07±0.06	
• D3	0.12±0.1		0.05±0.08	
• D7	0.16±0.1		0.05±0.04	<0.01**

* Time not stated.
** vs parnaparin.

COMMENTS

❑ No significant difference between the two treatments regarding efficacy.

❑ The additive administration of HES did not significantly influence either the rate of DVT or bleeding complications (results not shown).

Efficacy and safety of low molecular weight heparin and standard unfractionated heparin for prophylactic of postoperative venous thromboembolism: European multicenter trial

AUTHORS	KAKKAR V.V., BOECKL O., BONEU B. et al.
REF	World. J. Surg. 1997; 21: 2-9

STUDY	Multicenter, randomized, double-blind, controlled
CENTERS (n)	15
COUNTRIES	Austria, France, Germany, Italy, United Kingdom
PATIENTS (n)	*included* 1351
	evaluated 1342
	(1311 for efficacy)

TYPE OF SURGERY

General or gynecological, more than half for malignancies

ANESTHESIA

General (95%)

STUDY DRUG	**Reviparin**	sc daily dose: 1750 AXa IU o.d.
		first injection: 2h preop, second injection 8h postop
		treatment duration: 5 days at least
REFERENCE DRUG	**UFH**	sc daily doses: 5000 IU b.i.d.
		first injection: 2h preop, second injection 8h postop
		treatment duration: 5 days at least

ASSESSMENTS

- ❏ Isotopic DVT (FUT), if positive, venography.
- ❏ PE, if clinical symptoms, lung scan and/or angiography.
- ❏ Bleeding complications, adverse events.
- ❏ Laboratory tests.

KAKKAR V.V. et al. 1997

	Reviparin 1750 AXa IU x 1	UFH 5000 IU x 2	p
Patients with evaluable venogr.	648	663	
Total DVT	30 4.6%	28 4.2%	NS
PE	1 (fatal)	3 (2 fatal)	
Hemorrhagic complications	55 8.5%	80 13.3%	0.03
Major hemorrhage with discontinuation of therapy	9	15	
Wound hematomas	29	52	
AXa levels IU/ml mean value (range)*	0.1 (0.03-0.17)	0.04 (0.0-0.12)	
Death	3	5	

* Time not stated.

COMMENTS

❑ The relative "low dose" used in this indication (1750 AXa IU) was as effective as UFH twice daily. The safety and tolerability were better.

❑ Despite the large number of patients with malignancy, this publication did not report the incidence of DVT on patients with or without cancer according to their treatment group.

❑ The first publication of this study appeared in Blood Coag. Fibrinolysis 1993; 4 (Suppl 1) 521-522.

Prevention of perioperative deep vein thrombosis in general surgery: a multicentre double-blind study comparing two doses of Logiparin and standard heparin

AUTHORS	LEIZOROVICZ A., PICOLET H., PEYRIEUX J.C., BOISSEL J.P.
REF	Br. J. Surg. 1991; 78 : 412-416

STUDY	Multicenter, randomized, double-blind
CENTERS (n)	23
COUNTRIES	France, United Kingdom
PATIENTS (n)	*randomized* 1290
	evaluated 1290
	(as intention-to-treat)

TYPE OF SURGERY

General surgery: patients undergoing abdominal/gynecological/urological or thoracic surgery

ANESTHESIA

General

STUDY DRUG	**Tinzaparin**	sc daily dose + 1 placebo injection:
		• 2500 AXa IU o.d. or
		• 3500 AXa IU o.d.
		first injection: 2h preop
REFERENCE DRUG	**UFH**	sc daily doses: 5000 IU b.i.d.
		first injection: 2h preop
		treatment duration: 7-10 days

ASSESSMENTS

❏ Isotopic DVT: daily FUT from D2 to D7/D8 confirmed by venography if positive.

❏ Major clinical events, hemorrhage, wound hematomas, surgical reinterventions.

❏ PE: clinical symptoms.

❏ One-month follow-up.

LEIZOROVICZ A. et al. 1991

	Tinzaparin (AXa IU)				UFH		p
	2500 x 1		3500 x 1		5000 IU x 2		
Patients	431		430		429		
Total DVT at D7							chi 2 test
• Positive or doubtful FUT	34	7.9%	16	3.7%	18	4.2%	0.01
• Venography: superficial and DVT	24	5.6%	10	2.3%	13	3.0%	0.03
DVT (only)	16	3.7%	7	1.6%	7	1.6%	NS
PE (non fatal)	4		1		2		
Wound hematomas	5		21		28		<0.001
Severe hemorrhage and reinterventions	No statistical difference between the 3 groups						
Thrombocytopenia (treatment stopped)	0		1 (D5)		1 (D8)		
Death	10		10		9		
One-month follow-up Total thromboses	26	6.0%	11	2.6%	15	3.5%	

COMMENTS

❑ The lower daily dose of tinzaparin 2500 IU appeared to be less effective than 3500 IU daily and than UFH in prevention of DVT after general surgery.

❑ The efficacy and safety of tinzaparin 3500 IU o.d. and UFH 5000 IU b.i.d. were similar.

❑ It is interesting to note that the incidence of total venous thromboses (superficial and deep) was not greatly modified after one-month follow-up (the diagnostic method used was not clearly stated).

Correlation between anti Xa and occurrence of thrombosis and haemorrhage in post-surgical patients treated with either Logiparin® (LMWH), or unfractionated heparin

AUTHORS	BARA L., LEIZOROVICZ A. PICOLET H., SAMAMA M.
REF	Thromb. Research 1992; 65 : 641-650

STUDY	Randomized, multicenter, double-blind (same study published by Leizorovicz et al. 1991)
CENTERS (n)	23
COUNTRIES	France, United Kingdom
PATIENTS (n)	*evaluated* 1158

TYPE OF SURGERY
Abdominal/gynecological/urological or thoracic surgery.

ASSAYS
Coagulation tests blindly performed in a core laboratory using the First International LMWH and the IVth International Heparin Standard

STUDY DRUG	**Tinzaparin**	• 2500 uAXa IU x 1 or • 3500 uAXa IU x 1 first injection: 2h preop
REFERENCE DRUG	**UFH**	sc daily dose: 5000 IU b.i.d. first injection: 2h preop treatment duration: 7-10 days

ASSESSMENTS

❑ Measurement of AXa amidolytic activity in treated patients at D3, D5 and at discharge, 3-4 hours after injection (used test: CBS 3139).

❑ Correlation with incidence of DVT.

❑ Correlation with hemorrhage.

BARA L. et al. 1992

	Tinzaparin		UFH
	2500 AXa IU x 1	3500 AXa IU x 1	5000 IU x 2
Patients	394	381	383
Mean AXa levels (IU/ml ± SE*) at			
• D3	0.097±0.003	0.151±0.004	0.034±0.003
• D5	0.111±0.003	0.161±0.004	0.032±0.003
Hospital discharge	0.082±0.005	0.148±0.006	0.024±0.003
Positive FUT	7.9%	3.7%	4.2%
Positive venogram	5.6%	3.0%	3.3%
Severe hemorrhage	9/431 2.1%	13/430 3.0%	14/429 3.3%

* 3-4h after injection.

COMMENTS

❑ Interesting support to the previous study published by Leizorovicz et al. in B.J. Surg. 1991 regarding the large systematic measurement of AXa activity:
- significant correlation was observed between AXa levels and tinzaparin injected doses;
- AXa activities were higher in both tinzaparin groups than in UFH group;
- no correlation between AXa levels and DVT incidence;
- no correlation between AXa activity and bleeding events;
- only weak corrrelation between AXa levels and body weight which accounts for only 16% in the interindividual variability of AXa activity.

Thromboprophylaxis with a low molecular weight heparin (tinzaparin) in emergency abdominal surgery. A double-blind multicenter trial

AUTHORS	BERGQVIST D., FLORDAL P.A., FRIBERG B. et al.
REF	Vasa. 1996; 25: 156-160

STUDY	Multicenter, randomized, double-blind, placebo-controlled
CENTERS (n)	3
COUNTRY	Sweden
PATIENTS (n)	included 80
	evaluated 80

TYPE OF SURGERY

Emergency abdominal surgery (gastric, biliary, colorectal, other)

ANESTHESIA

Not stated

STUDY DRUG	Tinzaparin	sc daily dose: 3500 AXa IU o.d.
		first injection: 24h or less postop
		second injection: 12-24h later
		treatment duration: at least 5 days

REFERENCE DRUG	Placebo	sc route one daily injection of saline
		treatment duration: at least 5 days

ASSESSMENTS

❏ Isotopic DVT (FUT): daily measurement for one week; when positive, venography.

❏ Major bleeding complications.

❏ Death.

BERGQVIST D. et al. 1996

	Tinzaparin 3500 AXa IU x 1		Placebo		p
Patients	39		41		
DVT					
Intention-to-treat	3	7.7%	9	22.0%	NS
Correct prophylaxis	NR*	8.3%	NR*	21.1%	
PE	0		1 (non fatal)		
Major bleeding	1		0		
Death	0	0%	2	2.5%	

* NR = not reported.

COMMENTS

❑ This study had to be terminated prematurely because of interrupted delivery of radiolabelled fibrinogen.

❑ Although not significant, there was a clear trend toward a prophylactic effect of LMWH in emergency general surgery.

Experts comments

HENRI BOUNAMEAUX. *Prophylaxis in general surgery*

In this section devoted to general surgery (including gynecologic surgery and neurosurgery), the editors of this guide have identified and carefully analyzed 38 studies that compared new prophylactic regimens using seven low molecular weight heparin (LMWH) brands with either placebo, another LMWH scheme, or different dosages of unfractionated heparin (UFH). The studies were published over a 15-year period (1982-1996).

Most studies were randomized but a minority had a double-blinded design, and some were open-labeled. The sample size ranged from 80 patients to 3938 (randomized, controlled trial) and even 9919 (open study without control group). The evaluation was not always based on an intention-to-treat analysis.

The end points included deep vein thrombosis (DVT) and/or pulmonary embolism (PE), but diagnosis could be established by several means: fibrinogen-uptake test or plethysmographic examination (in both cases, abnormal results were usually confirmed by venography), systematic venography and/or lung scintigraphy. In addition, one study addressed mortality as its principal end point, two other trials were focusing primarily on safety, and one aimed mainly at establishing the performances of a novel diagnostic tool for asymptomatic DVT.

The characteristics of patient populations also were highly variable. They consisted either of unselected, consecutive patients undergoing surgery or of patients who were selected because they were at (very) high risk of experiencing thromboembolic complications or because they were at low hemorrhagic risk. Even the type of anesthesia differed among the trials but was not described in several studies.

As could have been anticipated, this extreme heterogeneity of LMWH regimens, study designs, end points, sample sizes, and patient populations parallels extremely variable results. Thus, the prevalence of postoperative DVT ranged in the patients given LMWH from 0 (in a study in which patients undergoing gynecologic surgery were evaluated clinically) to 32.2% (in a study in which systematic venography was performed in general surgery patients with a high prevalence of maligancy).

These observations deserve a few comments:

   • First, obviously, if you do not look for a postoperative DVT, it is very unlikely that you'll find it, which means that experts should provide guidelines to investigators with respect to the appropriate diagnostic tool to screen for asymptomatic, postoperative DVT in patients undergoing general surgery.

   • Second, most trials listed in this section used the fibrinogen uptake test (FUT) followed, whenever possible, by confirmatory venography when FUT was abnormal; this screening procedure supposes that FUT is highly sensitive to the presence of DVT. Unfortunately, a systematic review of the performances of leg scanning led to the conclusion that the method is insensitive for the screening of postoperative venous thrombosis in orthopedic patients and that the data in general surgery populations are insufficient, the usually reported 100% sensitivity being based on a series of 8 patients (!) published in 1971 and in whom the diagnosis had been made on a clinical basis (1). Fortunately, FUT became obsolete in the meantime because of safety considerations (potential risk of transmission of viral particles by the human fibrinogen).

   • Third, venography, which was used systematically in a trial that found a very high prevalence of postoperative DVT, is not devoid of disadvantages, the first, unexpected one being an only fair interobserver agreement, at least in the setting of asymptomatic patients in thromboprophylactic trials (2). Nonetheless, venography is likely to be more sensitive to the presence of postoperative DVT than other diagnostic tools. This should allow, at least in phase 2 or early phase 3 clinical trials, study designs with fewer patients, especially if they are at high risk of thromboembolic complications.

• Fourth, direct comparisons of LMWH regimens are now needed because equivalence between them is far from established.

In spite of these shortcomings, in most trials, the prevalence of postoperative DVT and PE, as well as the frequency of bleeding, were consistently slightly higher in the corresponding control groups. This observation was confirmed by two meta-analyses in 1992 which concluded that LMWH was at least as efficacious and safe as UFH (3), or even significantly more efficacious than UFH (4). An almost miraculous conclusion after reading the critical analysis of the individual trials!

Anyway, the crucial advantage of LMWHs over UFH for prevention of DVT following general surgery does not derive from results of clinical trials nor from meta-analyses but rather from the improved bioavailability and prolonged half-life of the novel compounds with its practical consequence: once daily injection instead of twice or three times daily. If you're not convinced of this advantage, ask the patient and the nurse!

REFERENCES

(1) LENSING A.W.A., HIRSH J. 125 I-fibrinogen leg scanning: reassessment of its role for the diagnosis of venous thrombosis in postoperative patients. Thromb. Haemostasis 1993; 69 : 2-7

(2) COUSON F., BOUNAMEAUX C., DIDIER D. et al. Influence of variability of interpretation of contrast venography for screening of postoperative deep venous thrombosis on the results of a thromboprophylactic study. Thromb. Haemostasis 1993; 70 : 573-575

(3) LEIZOROVICZ A., HAUGH M.C., CHAPUIS F.R., SAMAMA M.M., BOISSEL J.P. Low molecular wieght heparin in prevention of perioperative thrombosis. BMJ 1992; 305 : 13-20

(4) NURMOHAMED M.T., ROSENDAAL F.R., BULLER H.R. et al. Low molecular weight heparin versus standard heparin in general and orthopaedic surgery: a meta-analysis. Lancet 1992; 340 : 152-156

SYLVIA HAAS. *Prophylaxis in general surgery*

Low molecular weight heparins have been well established as routine prophylaxis in general surgical patients, since numerous clinical trials, review articles and meta-analyses have provided evidence that these compounds seem to be at least equivalent when compared to unfractioned heparin (1-4). However, the performance of meta-analysis implies that all LMWH preparations are comparable with respect to their pharmacologic profiles, their antithrombotic efficacy and safety. Preclinical studies have shown that the commercially available LMWHs differ in various biochemical, biophysical and pharmacological properties. They are prepared by different techniques, have variable molecular-weight distributions and are therefore likely to have different pharmacodynamic characteristics, which have significant clinical implications. In addition, differing dosing schedules have been used in various trials. Thus, there are some substantial concerns that the effectiveness and safety of LMWHs can be properly assessed by meta-analysis. This, however, also proves true for assessing the efficacy and safety of unfractionated heparin (UFH) when given as low dose heparin (LDH) prophylaxis for the control groups. LDH means a fixed dosage of a 10,000 - 15,000 IU/day; however, the dosing schedules may contribute significantly to the wide range of clinical results. Since the dosage- and substance-related differences of UFH and LMWH-prophylaxis do not support the assessment of efficacy by meta-analysis, this method may only allow for global orientation. Thus, the objective data tabulation prepared by the editors is a timely and conceptually important approach to provide clinicians, pharmacists and any other researchers interested in the field of LMWH with invaluable information on how to assess and to compare the efficacy and safety of different products and dosing schedules.

Today, an individual risk assessment of the patient, including the risk due to type and duration of surgery and the patient's predisposing risk profile, plays an important role with regard to the use of prophylaxis and to which dosage to choose. The majority of the studies comparing UFH- and LMWH-prophylaxis does not allow for firm conclusions about how the patient's risk had been assessed by the investigators, since there are trials comparing higher doses of UFH with lower doses of LMWH and lower doses of UFH with higher doses of LMWH. This information can only be obtained by source data analysis as it is provided in this book.

Furthermore, the test for diagnosis of DVT, the time of dosing, the duration of prophylaxis, and the type of anesthesia may be important for the result of any thrombosis study. In most of the studies, patients undergoing general surgery were screened for asymptomatic DVT by means of the radiolabeled fibrinogen uptake test, but also clinical symptoms of venous thromboembolism verified by objective tests had been defined as primary endpoints. LMWH was given either two or twelve hours preoperatively, sometimes the start of prophylaxis was even postponed to the postoperative period. Prophylaxis was only given to hospitalized patients, but the entire duration of prophylaxis varied from study to study. The patients were operated under intubation or spinal or epidural anesthesia respectively, and in most of the studies the patients have not been stratified according to the type of anesthesia. All these heterogeneities may also influence the outcome of pooled data analysis. Therefore, the detailed compilation of study results provided by the editors of this clinical trials review offers a unique opportunity to an impression of the strengths and the weaknesses of various compounds and dosing schedules. Furthermore, this objective data tabulation allows for a discrimination of studies with extremely small patient numbers and will help the clinician in his decision making on which type of prophylaxis to use.

REFERENCES

(1) HAAS S, HAAS P: Efficacy of low molecular weight heparins : An overview. Semin Thromb Hemost 1993 ; (Suppl 1) ; 101-105

(2) LASSEN M, BORRIS L, CHRISTIANSEN et al.: Clinical trials with low molecular weight heparins in the prevention of postoperative thromboembolic complications : A meta-analysis. Semin Thromb Hemost 1991 ; 17 (Suppl 3) : 284-290

(3) LEIZOROVICZ A, HAUGH M, CHAPUIS F, BOISSEL J: Low molecular weight heparins in the prevention of perioperative thrombosis. BMJ 1992 ; 305 : 913-920

(4) NURMOHAMED MT, ROSENDAAL FR, BÜLLER HR et al. : Low molecular weight heparin in general and orthopaedic surgery : A meta-analysis. Lancet 1991 ; 340 : 152-156

AJAY K. KAKKAR. *Low molecular weight heparins in cancer*

The advent of low molecular weight heparins (LMWHs), with their efficacy and safety now well proven in prospective clinical trials involving thousands of patients, offer novel and exciting antithrombotic agents for use in those with cancer. It is well recognized that cancer in itself predisposes to the development of thrombosis and that any intervention in the cancer patient - operation, chemotherapy, use of central venous lines - is also associated with enhanced thrombotic risk (reviewed in ref 1). The hypercoagulable state of malignancy which results from tumor procoagulant elaboration (tissue factor) with subsequent coagulation pathway activation (primarily extrinsic) and excess thrombin generation (2) is most likely responsible for this. The most commonly available antithrombotic agents -unfractionated heparin (UFH) and oral anticoagulants (OAC) - have serious limitations when used in cancer patients. Despite its well proven efficacy in the primary prevention of fatal postoperative venous thromboembolism (3) including those patients undergoing cancer surgery, UFH needs to be given 2 or 3 times a day and the rates of deep vein thrombosis (DVT) are still around 12-15%. Heparin, although effective in the initial treatment of DVT, including that associated with cancer, is associated with the phenomenon of heparin resistance which is thought to be more common in those with malignancy (4). OAC used routinely for secondary prevention after initial treatment of DVT or pulmonary embolism (PE) are associated with nearly twice the risk of recurrent venous thromboembolism (VTE) in the cancer patient than in a non cancer subject (5).

Chemotherapy given over prolonged periods on an outpatient basis requires a thromboprophylactic agent that can be given once daily without need for regular laboratory monitoring for up to six months, neither UFH nor warfarin fulfill these criteria. LMWHs have the potential for overcoming these limitations in the cancer patient.

Prophylaxis of venous thromboembolism

Numerous studies and meta-analyses have now confirmed that LMWH and UFH are equally effective in DVT prevention after major abdominal surgery and the large outcome study by Kakkar (6) confirmed the two agents to be equally effective in preventing perioperative death after in hospital therapy with either LMWH 2500 units once daily or UFH 5000 units twice daily. Recently, the study by Bergqvist (7) demonstrated a reduction in postoperative DVT rates from 14.9% in cancer patients receiving 2500 units of LMWH to 8.6% in those receiving 5000 units with no increase in bleeding. LMWH is also effective in reducing central line associated thrombosis in cancer patients (8) but studies are needed to determine which patients will benefit from routing central line thromboprophylaxis and how cost effective such therapy may prove to be. Although it appears LMWHs may be effective and ideally suited for prevention of VTE associated with chemotherapy no such studies have been undertaken. The few studies that have evaluated the ability of LMWHs for thromboprophylaxis in "medical patients" have included small numbers of cancer patients. Thrombosis is common in the bedridden cancer patient but further studies targeted specifically at this population are required before any firm recommendations can be made.

DVT/PE teatment

LMWHs are now well established in the initial treatment of DVT (9). The studies which confirmed the equal efficacy of intravenous UFH and subcutaneous LMWH in this indication included cancer patients and it is on this basis that the out of hospital unmonitored treatment of DVT is advocated in those with cancer. Although such outpatient therapy is a major advance in terms of quality of life for a cancer patient there remains concern that such patients, with gross hemostatic derangement due to an underlying cancer, can all be safely treated this way.

An exciting novel use of LMWHs has been in the secondary prevention of recurrent venous thromboembolism. Two studies (10,11) comparing LMWH to warfarin have shown both agents to be equally effective in preventing recurrent VTE with LMWH having the advantage of fixed dose administration without the need for laboratory monitoring and substantially lower rates of hemorrhagic complications. In the cancer patient where recurrent venous thromboembolism is more common, the use of LMWH is worthy of investigation.

LMWH and cancer mortality

Studies evaluating either UFH or LMWH for the initial treatment of deep vein thrombosis have demonstrated a striking 65% reduction in 60-90 days mortality rates in those cancer patients who received the LMWH (12). The biological explanation for this clinical effect, that has continued to be reported in subsequent DVT treatment studies, has yet to be elucidated. This novel use of LMWHs is the subject of a prospective randomized placebo controlled study in patients with advanced malignant disease (1).

Summary

LMWHs are already proven as the agents of choice in the prevention of postoperative venous thromboembolism in high risk patients such as those with cancer. They are effective in DVT treatment. They offer the opportunity to provide routine thromboprophylaxis in patients receiving chemo or hormonal anti-cancer therapy and to improve secondary prophylaxis against recurrent VTE. They may help to prolong survival in patients with advanced malignancy.

REFERENCES

(1) KAKKAR A.K. and WILLIAMSON R.C.N. Haemostasis 1997; 27 : 32-39

(2) KAKKAR et al. Lancet 1995; 48 : 288-290

(3) International Multicentre Trial. Lancet 1975; 2 : 45-51

(4) LEVINE M.N. et al. Thrombosis and Haemostasis 1997; 78 : 133-136

(5) PRANDONI P. et al. Arch. Int. med. 1996

(6) KAKKAR V.V. et al. Lancet 1993; 341 : 259-265

(7) BERGQVIST D. et al. Br. J. Surg. 1995; 82 : 496-501

(8) MONREAL M. et al. Thrombosis and Haemostasis 1996; 75 : 231-253

(9) SIRAGUSA S. et al. Am. J. Med. 1996; 100 : 269-277

(10) DAS S.K. et al. World J. Surg. 1996; 20 (5) : 521-526

(11) PINI M. et al. Thrombosis and Haemostasis 1994; 72 : 191-197

(12) GREEN D. et al. Lancet 1992; 339 : 1476

ANNIE BOREL-DERLON. *Thromboembolic complications in neurosurgery*

The incidence of postoperative deep vein thrombosis (DVT) in neurosurgery demonstrated by radiolabelled method ranges between 29 and 43%, according to data from the literature, and warrants the use of antithrombotic therapy (1).

Clinical context determines the risk of thrombosis: a higher or lower rate, depending on location of a brain tumor and on duration of surgery, and the very high incidence of thrombosis in patients with trauma to the spine and spinal cord, in contrast to the very low risk of thrombosis following surgery for a herniated intervertebral disk.

Different methods for prevention of thrombosis have been recommended and used. But, apart from the efficacy of such methods, the neurosurgeon, more than anyone else, is concerned with the prevention of any intracerebral bleeding complication.

The number of clinical studies which have been conducted on this subject is low, and, outside of one, have involved small numbers of patients. One double blind, placebo-controlled study conducted on a series of patients, two-thirds of whom underwent serious intracranial neurosurgery, has demonstrated the relative efficacy and acceptable safety of combined use of low molecular weight heparin and elastic compression stockings (2).

In the setting of the most recent Consensus Conference held by the American College of Chest Physicians in 1995 (3), external pneumatic compression with or without graduated compression, was recommended as a prophylactic method in intracranial surgery. Combined use of external pneumatic compression and low dose standard heparin therapy can be recommended in high risk patients. Although studies previously conducted have demonstrated a reduction in the risk of thrombosis in neurosurgery by mechanical methods possibly in combination with low dose heparin therapy, the place of low molecular weight heparins in intracranial neurosurgery remains to be defined, taking into account the risk of bleeding.

REFERENCES

(1) DERLON A., KHER A. La prophylaxie des complications thromboemboliques en neurochirurgie. STV 1994; 6 : 41-46

(2) NURMOHAMED M.T. et al. Low molecular weight heparin and compression stockings in the prevention of venous thromboembolism in neurosurgery. Thromb. Haemostasis 1996; 75 : 233-238

(3) CLAGETT G., ANDERSON Jr A., HEIT J., LEVINE M., WHEELER H.B. Chest 1995 suppl; 108 : 2124S-324S

3.2
Prophylaxis
of venous thromboembolism
in orthopedic surgery

RD heparin compared with warfarin for prevention of venous thromboembolic disease following total hip or knee arthroplasty

AUTHORS	RD Heparin Arthroplasty Group
REF	J. Bone Joint Surg. 1994; 76-A: 1174-1185

STUDY
Open-label, multicenter, randomized, controlled comparison of two regimens

CENTERS (n) 20
COUNTRY United States

PATIENTS (n)
included 1207
evaluated 969

TYPE OF SURGERY
Elective total hip or knee arthroplasty (cemented or not)

ANESTHESIA
General ≈ 70%, regional ≈ 30%

STUDY DRUG **Ardeparin** sc daily dose:
- 50 AXa IU/kg b.i.d. or
- 90 AXa IU/kg o.d.

first injection: 50 AXa IU/kg postop (evening of operation) for both groups
treatment duration: ≈ 10 days (4-10)

REFERENCE DRUG **Warfarin** oral daily dose: 5mg
first dose: preop, second dose evening of operation, then PT-adjusted (x 1.2-1.5 control values)
treatment duration: ≈ 10 days

ASSESSMENTS
- ❑ DVT by non invasive tests: IPG, ultrasonography; if abnormal findings, unilateral or contra lateral venography; venography of the treated limb before discharge.
- ❑ Clinical PE, if suspicion lung scan and angiography.
- ❑ Bleeding complications, wound hematomas.
- ❑ Laboratory tests.

RD Heparin Arthroplasty Group. 1994

	Ardeparin (AXa IU/kg)				Warfarin	
	50 x 2		90 x 1			
	hip	knee	hip	knee	hip	knee
Patients	178	150	171	149	174	147
Total DVT	12 7%	37 25%*	22 13%	41 28%*	20 11%	60 41%
Proximal DVT	5 3%	9 6%	12 7%	7 5%	11 6%	15 10%
PE (non fatal)	0	0	0	1	0	1
Total thrombo-embolic events (DVT +PE)	14 8%	39 26%	24 14%	44 30%	24 14%	63 43%
Bleeding complications	No significant difference among the 3 treated groups and between patients with hip or knee arthroplasty					

* p ≤ 0.05 for total knee (o.d. or b.i.d. regimen) compared with warfarin.
  p non significant for total hip (once or twice daily) compared with warfarin.

COMMENTS

❑ In knee arthroplasty, the two regimens of ardeparin were significantly better than warfarin.

❑ Both regimens of ardeparin and OAC were equally safe; no correlation was observed between AXa or AIIa levels and bleeding events (results not shown).

❑ Apparent lack of efficacy with warfarin for distal thrombi in knee arthroplasty but not in hip arthroplasty.

Ardeparin (low molecular weight heparin) vs graduated compression stockings for the prevention of venous thromboembolism
A randomized trial in patients undergoing knee surgery

AUTHORS	LEVINE M., GENT M., HIRSH J. et al.
REF	Arch. Intern. Med. 1996; 156: 851-856

STUDY	Multicenter, randomized, double-blind, placebo-controlled	**TYPE OF SURGERY**	Knee replacement or tibial osteotomy cemented or not cemented prosthesis
CENTERS (n)	3		
COUNTRY	Canada	**ANESTHESIA**	General ≈ 90%, spinal ≈ 10%
PATIENTS (n)	*randomized* 246 *evaluated* 199		

STUDY DRUG	**Ardeparin**	sc daily doses: 50 AXa IU/kg b.i.d. first injection: 12- 24h postop treatment duration: 14 days or until discharge
REFERENCE DRUG	**Placebo**	sc daily dose: 0.05ml/ 10kg first injection:12- 24h postop treatment duration: 14 days or until discharge

+ Elastic compression stockings in both groups

ASSESSMENTS
- ❑ DVT: bilateral venography on D14 or before, at hospital discharge.
- ❑ PE: if clinical symptoms, lung scan or angiography.
- ❑ Bleeding complications.
- ❑ Death.

LEVINE M. et al. 1996

	Ardeparin 50 AXa IU x 2 + Elastic stockings		**Placebo** + Elastic stockings		**p**
Patients	122		124		
Evaluable venograms	96	78.7%	103	83.3%	
Total DVT	28	29.2%	60	58.2%	0.001
Proximal DVT	2	2.0%	16	15.5%	0.002
PE	1		1 (fatal)		
Major hemorrhage	3*	2.5%	3*	2.4%	NS
Minor hemorrhage	0		2		
Death	0		2 (1 PE at D5 and 1 stroke at D8)		

* Two patients with bleeding at the operative site in both groups.

COMMENTS
- ❏ The combination of ardeparin with compression stockings was associated with a significant reduction in both total and proximal DVT compared to graduated compression stockings only.
- ❏ It appears that graduated compression stockings have little effect in knee surgery.
- ❏ No difference for bleeding complications between ardeparin-treated patients and placebo group.
- ❏ Three patients in ardeparin group developed a platelet count less than 100,000/mm^3.
  For two of them, this count was low before initiating therapy. In these patients, the medication was continued and the platelet count rose.

Efficacy and safety of low molecular weight heparin (ardeparin sodium) compared to warfarin for the prevention of venous thromboembolism after total knee replacement surgery: a double-blind, dose-ranging study

AUTHORS	HEIT J.A., BERKOWITZ S.D., BONA R. et al.
REF	Thromb. Haemostasis 1997; 77: 32-38

STUDY	Multicenter, randomized, double-blind, dose-ranging parallel groups	
CENTERS (n)	27	
COUNTRY	United States	
PATIENTS (n)	*randomized*	860
	evaluated	833 for safety
		680 for efficacy

TYPE OF SURGERY
Total knee replacement (unilateral 80%, bilateral 10%, revision 10%)

ANESTHESIA
General ≈ 67%,
regional (epidural ≈ 18%, spinal ≈ 15%)

STUDY DRUG	**Ardeparin**	sc daily dose: 25- 35- 50 AXa IU/kg b.i.d.
		first injection: ≈ 12h postop
		treatment duration: 14 days
REFERENCE DRUG	**Warfarin**	oral daily dose: 4mg after surgery
		first dose: 6mg 18h and 3h preop,
		then adjusted to INR 2-3
		treatment duration: 14 days

ASSESSMENTS
- ❏ Incidence of DVT: unilateral or bilateral venography (for unilateral and bilateral knee replacements respectively) within 5 to 14 days after surgery.
- ❏ Clinical PE confirmed by lung scan or angiography.
- ❏ Hemorrhage - Thrombocytopenia.
- ❏ Death.

HEIT J.A. et al. 1997

	Ardeparin AXa IU/kg x 2			Warfarin
	25	35	50	
Patients	110	116	232	222
Total DVT	40 36%	32 28%	62 27%*	85 38%
Proximal DVT	not stated	not stated	15 6%	15 7%
PE	1	0	1	0
Death	0	2**	1**	0
Major hemorrhage (with cessation of treatment or reintervention)	2	2	9	1
Thrombocytopenia	1 (D3)	0	2 (D3) (1 interuption of treatment)	1 (D3)

* p value 0.019 vs warfarin.
** Not related to thromboembolism.

COMMENTS
❏ Ardeparin 35 AXa IU/kg b.i.d. may provide efficacy similar to ardeparin 50 AXa IU/kg b.i.d. but with reduced severe bleeding.
❏ Ardeparin 50 AXa IU/kg b.i.d. was significantly more effective than adjusted-dose warfarin at least for reducing total DVT.

Comparative efficacy and tolerance of Kabi 2165 and standard heparin in the prevention of deep vein thrombosis after total hip prosthesis

AUTHORS	BARRE J., PFISTER G., POTRON G. et al.
REF	J. Mal. Vasc. 1987; 12: 90-95

STUDY	Open-label, randomized	
CENTERS *(n)*	1	
COUNTRY	France	
PATIENTS *(n)*	*included*	80
	evaluated	80

TYPE OF SURGERY
Hip replacement

ANESTHESIA
Spinal

STUDY DRUG	**Dalteparin**	sc daily dose: 2500 AXa IU b.i.d.
		first injection: 2h preop
		second injection: 12h postop
		treatment duration: 10 days
REFERENCE DRUG	**UFH**	sc daily dose: 3750 IU t.i.d. at D1 then t.i.d.
		adjusted to APTT values (x 1.5-2)
		first injection: 2h preop
		treatment duration: 10 days

+ *Elastic compression stockings and early ambulation at D2 for all patients*

ASSESSMENTS
- ❏ Bilateral venography at D9 or D10.
- ❏ PE: clinical symptoms confirmed by lung scan.
- ❏ Bleeding complications.

BARRE J. et al. 1987

	Dalteparin 2500 AXa IU x 2		UFH 3750 IU x 3 (APTT-adjusted)		p
Patients	40		40		
Total DVT	7	17.5%	4	10.0%	NS
Proximal DVT	2	5.0%	2	5.0%	NS
PE	0		0		
Blood loss (ml) D0	517		606		NS
Transfusions (ml) D0	1191		1221		NS
Wound hematomas	4		3		NS

COMMENTS

❑ A fixed dose of dalteparin b.i.d. was as effective and safe as adjusted-dose of UFH t.i.d. in prophylaxis of DVT after hip surgery.

❑ To obtain the same target values for APTT, UFH dosages had to be increased from 12,000 IU at D1 up to more than 24,000 IU at D4.

Thrombosis prophylaxis with low molecular weight heparin in total hip replacement

AUTHORS	ERIKSSON B.I., ZACHRISSON B.E., TEGER-NILSSON A.C., RISBERG B.
REF	Br. J. Surg. 1988; 75: 1053-1057

STUDY	Open-label, randomized, comparative
CENTERS (n)	1
COUNTRY	Sweden
PATIENTS (n)	*included* 101
	evaluated 98

TYPE OF SURGERY
Total hip replacement

ANESTHESIA
Regional ≈ 85%, general ≈ 9%, combined 8%

STUDY DRUG	**Dalteparin**	sc daily doses: 2500 AXa IU b.i.d.
		first injection: 2h preop
		treatment duration: 7 days
REFERENCE DRUG	**Dextran 70**	iv dose: 500 ml during operation and within 6h postop
		500 ml at D1 and D3

ASSESSMENTS

- ❏ Isotopic DVT (FUT) on a daily basis for 2 weeks confirmed by venography if positive.
- ❏ Risk factors relationship.
- ❏ PE: if clinical suspicion, lung scan.
- ❏ Bleeding complications.
- ❏ Laboratory tests.

ERIKSSON B.I. et al. 1988

	Dalteparin 2500 AXa IU x 2		Dextran 70		p
Patients	49		49		
Total DVT	10	20%	22	45%	<0.01
Proximal DVT	0	0%	6	12%	<0.03
Non fatal PE	2	4%	2	4%	NS
Volume blood loss (x ± SD, ml)	1720 ± 650		2210 ± 1035		<0.01
Volume transfusions (x ± SD, ml)	1925 ± 910		2480 ± 1380		<0.02
Hospital stay (days ± SD)	18±5		19±5		NS

COMMENTS

❑ Dalteparin was significantly more effective and better tolerated than dextran.

❑ A significant delayed onset of DVT in the dalteparin group was reported: 6.2 D vs 3.5 D for dextran group.

❑ Age was a risk factor for DVT; no relationship between DVT and sex, type of anesthesia or type of prosthesis.

❑ AXa activity increased slightly from D0 up to D3 and reached a plateau at (0.2 IU/ml 4h after the morning injection) within 2 days of operation (data not shown).

Randomized trial of a low-molecular-weight heparin (Kabi 2165) versus adjusted-dose subcutaneous standard heparin in the prophylaxis of deep-vein thrombosis after elective hip surgery

AUTHORS	DECHAVANNE M., VILLE D., BERRUYER M. et al.
REF	Haemostasis. 1989; 1: 5-12

STUDY	Open-label, randomized, controlled dosage comparison
CENTERS (n)	2
COUNTRY	France
PATIENTS (n)	*included* 124
	evaluated 122

TYPE OF SURGERY

Hip replacement
Cemented (55%) and not cemented prosthesis

ANESTHESIA

General

STUDY DRUG	**Dalteparin**	sc daily doses:
		• 2500 AXa IU b.i.d. every 12h or
		• 2500 AXa IU b.i.d. from D0 to D2 then 5000 AXa IU o.d.
		first injection: 2h preop (2500 IU)
		treatment duration: 10-13 days
REFERENCE DRUG	**UFH**	sc daily doses: D1 and D2 5000 IU b.i.d. then APTT-adjusted
		first injection: 2h preop
		treatment duration: 10-13 days

ASSESSMENTS

❑ Isotopic DVT (FUT) daily screened for 10-13 D confirmed by bilateral venography if positive findings or between D10-D13 for negative FUT.

❑ Perioperative blood loss.

❑ Laboratory tests.

DECHAVANNE M. et al. 1989

	Dalteparin		UFH	p
	2500 AXa IU x 2	5000 AXa IU x 1	≈ 5000 IU x 2 (APTT-adjusted)	
Patients	41	41	40	
Total DVT (positive FUT)	2 4.9%	3 7.3%	4 10%	NS
Total DVT (venograms)	2/38	3/39	4/38	
Proximal DVT	1 2.4%	1 2.4%	3 7.5%	NS
Blood loss (ml)	1422	1318	1314	NS
Transfusions (ml)	2026	1714	2291	NS
AXa level IU/ml (mean ± SD) (at D0 2h after injection)	0.16±0.11	0.13±0.08	0.01±0.03	
Mean hospitalization stay (D±SD)	16.4±4.8	17.1±4.7	17.2±5.4	NS

COMMENTS

❏ A fixed-dose of dalteparin administered in one or two injections was as effective and safe as an adjusted-dose of UFH twice daily administered.

❏ Efficacy and safety were similar in both dalteparin groups.

❏ UFH dosage, APTT-adjusted, had to be increased from 10,000 U/d at D0 to almost 20,000 at D10.

Thromboprophylaxis
by low-molecular-weight heparin in elective hip surgery.
A placebo controlled study

AUTHORS	TØRHOLM C., BROENG L., JØRGENSEN P.S. et al.
REF	J. Bone and Joint Surg. 1991; 73: 434-438

STUDY	Double-blind, randomized, placebo-controlled
CENTERS (n)	1
COUNTRY	Denmark
PATIENTS (n)	*included* 120
	evaluated 112

TYPE OF SURGERY
Total hip replacement (primary and revision)

ANESTHESIA
General ≈ 85%, regional ≈ 15%

STUDY DRUG	**Dalteparin**	sc daily dose: 5000 AXa IU o.d.
		first injection: 2h preop (2500 AXa IU) D0
		second injection: 12h postop (2500 AXa IU) D0
		treatment duration: 6 days
REFERENCE DRUG	**Placebo**	sc daily dose: saline 0.2ml
		first injection: 2h preop
		treatment duration: 6 days

ASSESSMENTS
- ❏ Isotopic DVT (FUT, once daily until D10) confirmed by venography when positive and when possible.
- ❏ Perioperative blood loss.

TØRHOLM C. et al. 1991

	Dalteparin 5000 AXa IU x 1		Placebo saline x 1		p
Patients	58		54		
Total DVT (FUT)	9	16%	19	35%	<0.02
DVT confirmed by venography	8*		16**		
Proximal DVT	0	0%	14	26%	<0.01
PE (non fatal)	0		1		
Total blood loss (ml)	1668		1825		NS
Transfusions (g erythrocytes)	905		940		NS

* 1 venography not possible.
** 3 venographies not possible.

COMMENTS

❑ Prophylaxis in hip surgery drastically reduced the incidence of DVT.

❑ As observed in a previous study (see Eriksson, 1988) no proximal DVT was observed with the dosage of 5000 AXa IU.

❑ A delay in the onset of DVT was observed in the dalteparin group (after D4); in the placebo group, DVT occurred within the first four days.

❑ The type of anesthesia was not related with the incidence of DVT.

❑ No increase in pre- and postoperative bleeding was observed with this dalteparin regimen (2500 AXa IU before and 12 hours after surgery then 5000 IU once daily).

Prevention of deep-vein thrombosis and pulmonary embolism after total hip replacement.
Comparison of low-molecular-weight heparin and unfractionated heparin

AUTHORS	ERIKSSON B.I., KÄLEBO P., ANTHMYR B.A. et al.
REF	J. Bone and Joint Surg. 1991; 73: 484-493

STUDY	Randomized, double-blind, comparative	
CENTERS (n)	1	
COUNTRY	Sweden	
PATIENTS (n)	included	136
	evaluated	122

TYPE OF SURGERY
Hip replacement:
cemented prosthesis ≈ 80%,
non cemented ≈ 20%

ANESTHESIA
Extradural ≈ 90%, general ≈ 10-15%

STUDY DRUG	**Dalteparin**	sc daily dose: 5000 AXa IU o.d. + 2 placebo injections
		first injection: evening before operation
		second injection: in the evening of operation
		treatment duration: 10 days
REFERENCE DRUG	**UFH**	sc daily dose: 5000 IU t.i.d.
		first injection: 2h preop + a placebo evening before operation
		treatment duration: 10 days

Mobilization and physiotherapy started on D1 after surgery for all patients

ASSESSMENTS
- Bilateral venography on D12 ± 2.
- Pulmonary scintigraphy before venography.
- Bleeding complications.
- Biological activity (AXa).

ERIKSSON B.I. et al. 1991

	Dalteparin 5000 AXa IU x 1		UFH 5000 IU x 3		p
Patients	67		69		
Venography performed	63		59		
Total DVT	19	30.2%	25	42.4%	NS
Proximal DVT (lateral to prosthesis)	6	9.5%	18	30.5%	0.01
PE (lung scan)	8/65	12.3%	19/62	30.6%	0.01
Major bleeding	1		5		
Transfusions (red cell units ± SD)	2.3 ± 1.7		3.2 ± 1.9		0.01
Major hematomas	2		7		
AXa activity mean value IU/ml (range) at D7 (10h after injection)	0.07 (0-0.25)		0.02 (0-0.11)		

COMMENTS

❑ Efficacy of dalteparin (5000 AXa IU o.d.) was superior to that of UFH 5000 IU t.i.d. in the prevention of femoral (proximal) thrombosis and PE.

❑ Optimization of the venographic technique may have influenced the total number and distribution of thrombi detected, especially in muscular veins (same observations as in Eriksson's study in 1988, where the incidence of total DVT was surprisingly high). Relevant rate of PE detected by lung scan.

❑ Safety was improved with dalteparin. No thrombocytopenia in both groups.

❑ Of 44 confirmed cases of DVT, 40 were asymptomatic and out of 20 PE, only 3 patients had clinical symptoms.

Prolonged thromboprophylaxis following hip replacement surgery. Results of a double-blind, prospective, randomised, placebo-controlled study with dalteparin (Fragmin®)

AUTHORS	DAHL O.E., ANDREASSEN G., ASPELIN T. et al.
REF	Thromb. Haemostasis 1997; 77: 26-31

STUDY	Multicenter, randomized, double-blind, placebo-controlled
CENTERS (n)	2
COUNTRY	Norway
PATIENTS (n)	*included* 308
	randomized 265
	evaluated 227 for intention-to-treat analysis

TYPE OF SURGERY
Elective hip arthroplasty: primary and secondary

ANESTHESIA
Spinal

OBJECTIVE
Evaluation of DVT rate on D7 and on D35 after surgery in patients treated with dalteparin during 7 or 35 days after surgery

INITIAL TREATMENT
In-hospital

Dalteparin   sc daily dose: 5000 AXa IU
from D0 (12h preop) up to D7±2
+ dextran IV infusion 500ml at D0 and D1
+ elastic stockings
then randomization at D7±2 for:

PROLONGED TREATMENT
Home treatment

• **Dalteparin**   sc daily dose: 5000 AXa IU o.d.
treatment duration: 4 weeks
or
• **Placebo**   sc daily dose: 0.2ml o.d.
treatment duration: 4 weeks

ASSESSMENTS
❑ DVT: bilateral venography on D7 and D35 with blind assessment. Patients with proven clinical DVT on D7 were not randomized for prolonged prophylaxis.
❑ PE: lung scan and chest X-rays on D7 and D35.
❑ Bleeding complications.

DAHL O.E. et al. 1997

	Dalteparin 5000 AXa IU x 1		Placebo 0.2ml x 1		p
Initial treatment (D7)					
Clinical DVT	0	0%			
Evaluable venograms	258				
total DVT	41	15.9%	(no placebo,		
proximal DVT	14	5.4%	only dalteparin)		
PE - clinical	0				
- lung scan	33*	12.1%			
Prolonged treatment (D35)	**Dalteparin**		placebo		
Evaluable venograms	114		104		
Total DVT (prevalence) D7-D35	22	19.4%	33	31.7%	0.034
Proximal DVT	10	8.8%	14	13.4%	
Clinical DVT (confirmed)	8 (4)		4 (3)		
Patients without DVT at D7	93		89		
Total DVT (incidence) D7-D35	11	11.8%	23	25.8%	0.017
Proximal DVT	4	4.3%	9	10.1%	
PE - clinical	0		3 (1 fatal)	2.8%	
- lung scan	4/111	3.6%	6/105	5.7%	
Safety	No hemorrhagic or allergic event				

* All asymptomatic.

COMMENTS
- This study clearly showed that the DVT onset can be delayed.
- Extended prophylaxis significantly reduced the incidence of late DVT (and PE) and should be recommended for (at least) 5 weeks after hip replacement.

Prolonged prophylaxis with a low molecular weight heparin (dalteparin) after total hip arthroplasty — a placebo controlled study

AUTHORS	LASSEN M.R., BORRIS L.C. (on behalf of the Danish prolonged prophylaxis group)
REF	Thromb. Haemostasis 1995; 73: 1104 (Abst.)

STUDY	Multicenter, randomized double-blind, placebo-controlled
CENTERS *(n)*	8
COUNTRY	Denmark
PATIENTS *(n)*	*included* 281
	evaluated 215 (intention-to-treat)
	188 (per protocol)

TYPE OF SURGERY
Elective hip surgery for total hip arthroplasty (primary or revision)

ANESTHESIA
General ≈ 37%, regional ≈ 63%

OBJECTIVE
Evaluation of DVT rate 35 days after surgery in patients treated by dalteparin

INITIAL TREATMENT
In-hospital

Dalteparin To all patients:
sc daily dose: 5000 AXa IU from D0 (12h preop) up to D7±2
then randomization at D7±2 for:

PROLONGED TREATMENT
Home treatment

• **Dalteparin** sc daily dose: 5000 AXa IU o.d. from D7±2 up to D35±2

or

• **Placebo** sc daily dose: 0.2ml o.d. from D7 up D35±2

ASSESSMENTS
❑ DVT: bilateral venography at D35±2, clinical signs of DVT examined by color Doppler ultrasound.
❑ PE: lung scan if clinical suspicion.
❑ Bleeding complications, adverse events.

The Danish Group. 1995

	Dalteparin 5000 AXa IU x 1		Placebo 0.2ml x 1		p
Patients (included)	140		141		
Prolonged treatment	**(D0-D37)**		**(D8-D37)**		
Total DVT (from D8-D35 ± 2)					
per protocol (n=189)	4/101	4.0%	8/88	9.1%	NS
intention-to-treat (n=215)	5/113	4.4%	12/102	11.8%	0.04
Proximal DVT (from D8-D35 ± 2)					
per protocol (n=187)	0/99	0.0%	4/88	4.5%	0.03
intention-to-treat (n=212)	1/111	0.9%	5/101	5.0%	NS

COMMENTS
- In this study, the overall rate of total and proximal DVT was lower than expected.
- Prolonged prophylaxis reduced the number of thromboembolic complications
  (4 patients developed clinical symptoms of PE, none of them was confirmed by lung scan).
- One major bleeding has been recorded after discharge from hospital in the dalteparin group
  and 4 in the placebo-treated patients.

**Enoxaparine low molecular weight heparin:
its use in the prevention of deep venous thrombosis following
total hip replacement**

AUTHORS	PLANES A., VOCHELLE N., FERRU J. et al.
REF	Haemostasis. 1986; 16: 152-158

STUDY	Open-label, dose-ranging with blind phlebographic assessment
CENTERS (n)	1
COUNTRY	France
PATIENTS (n)	*included* 228

TYPE OF SURGERY	Total hip replacement (THR), iterative THR
ANESTHESIA	General

STUDY DRUG   **Enoxaparin**   sc daily doses: 4 dose regimens:
60mg o.d./ 30mg b.i.d./ 40mg o.d./ 20mg b.i.d.
first injection: 12h preop
treatment duration: at least 12 days

REFERENCE DRUG   **None**

Elastic bandaging, early ambulation for all patients

ASSESSMENTS
- ❏ DVT: bilateral venography at D12, blind assessment.
- ❏ Clinical symptoms for DVT and PE.
- ❏ Bleeding complications.
- ❏ Biological investigation: AXa activity.

PLANES A. et al. 1986

	Enox. 60mg x 1	Enox. 30mg x 2	Enox. 40mg x 1	Enox. 20mg x 2
Patients	50	28	50	100
Total DVT	6%	8%	8%	8%
Proximal DVT	6%	0%	4%	6%
PE	0	0	1 (fatal)	0
Local hematomas	12%	22% (severe)	0	0
Prophylaxis discontinued	no	yes	no	no
Maximal AXa activity (U/ml) 4h after injection	0.60	0.31	0.55	0.26

COMMENTS

❑ This dose-ranging study did not clearly determine which is the best regimen but 40mg o.d. offered good protection without major hemorrhagic risk.

❑ Increasing the dose did not increase the degree of protection but did increase the bleeding risk.

❑ Severe hematomas only occurred in patients treated with 30mg b.i.d.

❑ The AXa activity was not correlated either with the antithrombotic activity or with the hemorrhagic effects.

A randomized controlled trial of a low-molecular-weight heparin (enoxaparin) to prevent deep-vein thrombosis in patients undergoing elective hip surgery

AUTHORS	TURPIE A.G.G., LEVINE M.N., HIRSH J. et al.
REF	N. Engl. J. Med. 1986; 315: 925-929

STUDY	Multicenter, double-blind, randomized, placebo-controlled
CENTERS *(n)*	3
COUNTRY	Canada
PATIENTS *(n)*	*included* 142
	evaluated 100

TYPE OF SURGERY
Elective hip surgery

ANESTHESIA
General 2/3, spinal 1/3

STUDY DRUG	**Enoxaparin**	sc daily doses: 30mg b.i.d.
		first injection: 12-24h postop
		treatment duration: 14 days
REFERENCE DRUG	**Placebo**	sc daily doses: 0.3ml b.i.d. (saline)
		first injection: 12, 24h postop
		treatment duration: 14 days

ASSESSMENTS
- ❑ DVT: venography only if positive FUT or impedance phlethysmography in the initial group: group I (24 patients); venography mandatory at D14 in the second group: group II (76 patients)
- ❑ Major/minor hemorrhage.
- ❑ Biological investigation: AXa activity.
- ❑ Death.

TURPIE A.G.G. et al. 1986

	Enoxaparin 30mg x 2		Placebo		p
Group II	37		39		
Successful venography	30		33		
Total DVT	4	10.8%	20	51.3%	<0.001
Proximal DVT	2	5.4%	9	23.1%	<0.01
Entire study (gr I + gr II)	50		50		
Total DVT	6	12.0%	21	42.0%	<0.001
Proximal DVT	2	4.0%	10	20.0%	<0.01
Major bleeding	1		2		
Minor bleeding	1		0		
AXa level in IU/ml (+6h) D1/ D14	0.10 / 0.20		—		
Death	0		1 (adrenal hemorrhage)		

COMMENTS

❏ Study conducted in two phases: unfortunately for the first 24 patients, venography was not mandatory.

❏ This fixed regimen, 30mg b.i.d., started postoperatively, was effective and safe.

Prevention of postoperative venous thrombosis: a randomized trial comparing unfractionated heparin with low molecular weight heparin in patients undergoing total hip replacement

AUTHORS	PLANES A., VOCHELLE N., MAZAS F., et al.
REF	Thromb. Haemostasis 1988; 60: 407-410

STUDY	Multicenter, randomized, double-blind, comparative
CENTERS *(n)*	7
COUNTRY	France
PATIENTS *(n)*	*included* 237
	evaluated 228

TYPE OF SURGERY	Elective hip replacement (cemented and non cemented arthroplasty)
ANESTHESIA	General

STUDY DRUG	**Enoxaparin**	sc daily dose: 40mg o.d. + 2 placebo injections
		first injection: 12h preop (evening before surgery)
		and one placebo injection morning before surgery
		treatment duration: 14 days
REFERENCE DRUG	**UFH**	sc daily doses: 5000 IU t.i.d.
		first injections preop: evening and morning before surgery
		treatment duration: 14 days

Adjunctive therapy: elastic bandaging, early ambulation for all patients

ASSESSMENTS
- ❑ DVT: bilateral venography at D12-D15.
- ❑ PE: clinical symptoms; if suspicion, lung scan or angiography.
- ❑ Major/minor hemorrhage.
- ❑ Laboratory assays; AXa activity.
- ❑ Death.

PLANES A. et al. 1988

	Enoxaparin 40mg x 1		UFH 5000 IU x 3		p
Patients	124		124		
Venography performed	120		108		
Total DVT	15	12.5%	27	25.0%	0.03
Distal DVT	6	5.0%	7	6.0%	NS
Proximal DVT	9	7.5%	20	18.5%	0.01
PE clinical symptoms	2		3		
PE after angiogram	0		1		
Major bleeding	2		0		NS
Transfusions units (mean)	3.4		3.8		NS
Minor bleeding	1		2		NS
AXa activity (mcg/ml) 4h after last injection	1.5		0.5-0.8		
Death	0		0		

COMMENTS

❑ At this dosage (40mg o.d., and first dose administered before surgery) enoxaparin was more effective than, and as safe as, UFH 5000 IU t.i.d.

❑ These results confirmed those obtained in the dose-ranging study (Planes 1986) with the 40mg o.d. dose.

Efficacy and safety of perioperative enoxaparin regimen in a total hip replacement under various anesthesias

AUTHORS	PLANES A., VOCHELLE N., FAGOLA M., et al.
REF	Am. J. Surg. 1991; 161: 525-531

PUBLICATION	Retrospective analysis of 4 different trials
STUDY	Second trial: prospective, double-blind, randomized, comparing two dosing regimens
CENTERS (n)	2
COUNTRY	France
PATIENTS (n)	*included* 120
	evaluated 118

TYPE OF SURGERY
Total hip replacement

ANESTHESIA
General

STUDY DRUG	**Enoxaparin**	sc daily doses:	• 20mg b.i.d.
		versus	• 40mg o.d.
		first injection: 12h preop	
		treatment duration: 12 days	

REFERENCE DRUG	**None**

ASSESSMENTS
- ❏ DVT: bilateral venography at D12 to D15.
- ❏ PE: clinical observations.
- ❏ Wound hematomas.

PLANES A. et al. 1991: second trial

	Enoxaparin 20mg x 2		Enoxaparin 40mg x 1		p
Patients (for efficacy)	59		59		
Total DVT	1	1.7%	6	10.5%	NS
Proximal DVT	1	1.7%	3	5.2%	NS
PE	0		0		
Wound hematomas	3	5.0%	3	5.0%	NS
Major/minor bleeding complications	0		0		

COMMENTS
- In this publication, the study presented as "second trial" has been presented here for the comparison of the two dosing regimens.
- According to the authors, the regimen of enoxaparin (40mg 12h preoperatively and 40mg o.d. thereafter) was appropriate even though the same daily dosage divided in two injections   appeared at least as effective but without gain in safety.

Efficacy and safety of perioperative enoxaparin regimen in a total hip replacement under various anesthesias

AUTHORS	PLANES A., VOCHELLE N., FAGOLA M., et al.
REF	Am. J. Surg. 1991; 161: 525-531

PUBLICATION	Retrospective analysis of 4 different trials
STUDY	*Fourth part:* prospective, randomized, comparing 3 preop dosing regimens and 2 types of anesthesia
CENTERS (n)	2
COUNTRY	France

PATIENTS (n)	*included* 188
	evaluated 187

TYPE OF SURGERY
Total hip replacement

ANESTHESIA
General in 1/3, spinal in 2/3 of patients

STUDY DRUG **Enoxaparin**

sc daily dose: three groups
group I: spinal anesthesia
enox 40mg o.d. 12h after surgery
group II: spinal anesthesia
enox 20mg one hour after anesthesia
and just before operation
then 40mg o.d. 12h postop
group III: general anesthesia
enox 40mg o.d., first injection 2h preop
second injection: 12h postop
treatment duration: 12 days for all groups

ASSESSMENTS
- ❑ DVT: bilateral venography at D12 to D15.
- ❑ Bleeding, wound hematomas.
- ❑ PE: clinical observation.

PLANES A. et al. 1991; fourth trial

	Enoxaparin 40mg x 1 postop			p
Group	I	II	III	
Anesthesia	spinal	spinal	general	
First injection	40 mg 12h postop	20mg just before operation	40 mg 2h preop	
Venography performed	65	60	62	
Total DVT	11 17.0%	7 11.7%	4 6.5%	NS
Proximal DVT	4 6.0%	4 6.7%	4 6.5%	NS
Major bleeding	1	1	2	

COMMENTS

❑ This fourth part of Planes' publication showed that the standard fixed dosage of enoxaparin (40mg/day) is effective and safe regardless of the first dosing time and type of anesthesia. Even though the dose administered just before operation has been reduced to 20mg with spinal anesthesia.

Low molecular weight heparin (enoxaparin) versus Dextran 70.

The prevention of postoperative deep vein thrombosis after total hip replacement

AUTHORS	The Danish Enoxaparin Study Group
REF	Arch. Intern. Med. 1991; 151: 1621-1624

STUDY	Open-label, multicenter, randomized, comparative
CENTERS *(n)*	4
COUNTRY	Denmark
PATIENTS *(n)*	*included* 246 *evaluated* 219

TYPE OF SURGERY	Elective hip replacement (cemented prosthesis ≈ 80%)
ANESTHESIA	General in ≈ 1/3, spinal in ≈ 2/3 of patients

STUDY DRUG	**Enoxaparin**	sc daily dose: 40mg o.d. first injection: 12h preop treatment duration: 7 days
REFERENCE DRUG	**Dextran 70**	1st dose 500ml: during operation 2nd dose: +4h 3rd and 4th doses: D1, D3

Early deambulation for all patients

ASSESSMENTS

❏ DVT: bilateral venography between D7 and D11 or earlier if suspicion.

❏ Postoperative blood loss.

❏ 30-day follow-up.

❏ Laboratory assays: AXa activity.

The Danish Enoxaparin Study Group. 1991

	Enoxaparin 40mg x 1		Dextran		p
Venography performed	108		111		
Total DVT	7	6.5%	24	21.6%	0.01
Distal DVT	5	4.6%	18	16.2%	
Proximal DVT	2	1.8%	6	5.4%	
Postop blood loss (mean and range in ml)	550	(130-1175)	625	(75-2340)	<0.01
Total blood transfusion (mean units and range)	2	(0-8)	2	(0-7)	NS
Maximal AXa activity (IU/ml) 4h after last injection	0.14- 0.18				
Thirty-day follow-up					
DVT (confirmed)	0		3		
PE/Death	0/1 (AMI?)		0		

COMMENTS

❏ Surprisingly low incidence of total and proximal DVT after enoxaparin 40mg o.d.

❏ The type of anesthesia did not interfere with the results.

❏ AXa activity was not correlated with occurrence of DVT.

**Prevention of deep vein thrombosis after elective hip surgery.
A randomized trial comparing low molecular weight heparin
with standard unfractionated heparin**

AUTHORS	LEVINE M.N., HIRSH J., GENT M., et al.
REF	Ann. Intern. Med. 1991; 114: 545-551

STUDY	Multicenter, double-blind, randomized, comparative
CENTERS (n)	5
COUNTRY	Canada
PATIENTS (n)	randomized 665
	evaluated 521

TYPE OF SURGERY
Total hip replacement
(cemented: circa 50%)

ANESTHESIA
Not stated

STUDY DRUG	**Enoxaparin**	sc daily doses: 30mg b.i.d.
		first injection: 12-24h postop
		treatment duration: max. 14 days
REFERENCE DRUG	**UFH**	doses: 7500 IU b.i.d.
		first injection: 12-24h postop
		treatment duration: max. 14 days

Adjunctive therapy: anti-inflammatory drugs in 24 enoxaparin patients and in 17 UFH patients

ASSESSMENTS
- ❏ DVT: FUT daily, impedance plethysmography (IPG): 5, 7, 9, 11, 13 days after surgery, venography if FUT and/or IPG positive.
- ❏ Major/minor bleeding.
- ❏ PE clinically; if suspicion, lung scan

LEVINE M.N. et al. 1991

	Enoxaparin 30mg x 2		UFH 7500 IU x 2		p
Patients	333		332		
Total DVT*	57	17.1%	63	19.0%	NS
Proximal DVT	16	4.8%	18	5.4%	NS
Evaluable venograms	258	77.5%	263	79.2%	NS
Total DVT (venographic evidence)	50	19.4%	61	23.2%	NS
Proximal DVT	14	5.4%	17	6.5%	NS
PE	0		2 (non fatal)		
Hemorrhagic complications	17	5.1%	31	9.2%	0.04
Major bleeding	11	3.3%	19	5.7%	NS
Minor bleeding	6	1.8%	12	3.6%	NS
Transfusions	No difference				
Thrombocytopenia	0		2 (D8-D11)		

* Diagnosed by venography or non-invasive tests.

COMMENTS

❑ LMWH 30mg twice daily appeared to be less hemorrhagic than UFH 7500 IU twice daily.

❑ The difference in the rate of DVT although not statistically significant indicated a trend in favor of LMWH.

❑ No difference between cemented and not cemented prosthesis regarding the incidence of DVT.

**Prevention of deep vein thrombosis after major knee surgery.
A randomized, double-blind trial comparing a low molecular weight heparin
fragment (enoxaparin) to placebo**

AUTHORS	LECLERC J.R., GEERTS W.H., DESJARDINS L. et al.
REF	Thromb. Haemostasis 1992; 67: 417-423

STUDY	Multicenter, randomized, double-blind, placebo-controlled
CENTERS (n)	4
COUNTRY	Canada
PATIENTS (n)	*randomized* 131
	evaluated 129 (for efficacy)
	131 (for safety)

TYPE OF SURGERY
Knee arthroplasty, tibial osteotomy

ANESTHESIA
General in about 60% and epidural
in 40% of patients

STUDY DRUG	Enoxaparin	sc daily doses: 30mg b.i.d.
		first injection: 24h postop (up to 48h)
		treatment duration: 14 days or until discharge

REFERENCE DRUG	Placebo (saline)	sc doses: 0.3ml b.i.d.
		first injection: 24h postop
		treatment duration: 14 days or until discharge

ASSESSMENTS
- ❏ DVT: FUT, preop and postop. Bilateral venography at D14, impedance plethysmography (IPG) if venography not possible.
- ❏ Clinical PE confirmed by lung scan.
- ❏ Major/minor hemorrhage.
- ❏ 6-week follow-up.

LECLERC J.R. et al. 1992

	Enoxaparin 30mg x 2		Placebo		p
Patients	65		64		
Total DVT (FUT/IPG)	11	17%	37	58%	<0.001
Proximal DVT	0	0%	12	19%	<0.001
DVT after arthroplasty	5/50	10%	31/54	57%	<0.001
DVT after osteotomy	6/15	40%	6/10	60%	NS
Venography performed	41		54		
Total DVT	8	19%	35	65%	<0.001
Proximal DVT	0	0%	11	20%	<0.001
PE	0		1 (non fatal)		
Major hemorrhage	0	0%	1	2%	NS
Minor hemorrhage	4	6%	4	6%	NS
Six-week follow-up PE	1		no event		
Death	1 (MI)				

COMMENTS
- ❑ Small number of patients mainly for those who underwent tibial osteotomy.
- ❑ This prophylactic treatment started after surgery, mainly after 24h (up to 48h) was well-tolerated and significantly reduced the incidence of DVT (mainly proximal); efficacy was more evident for knee arthroplasty than for tibial osteotomy.

Prophylaxis for the prevention of venous thromboembolism after total knee arthroplasty

AUTHORS	FAUNØ P., SUOMALAINEN O., REHNBERG V. et al.
REF	J. Bone and Joint Surg. 1994; 76: 1814-1818

STUDY	Multicenter, double-blind, randomized, comparative
CENTERS (n)	3
COUNTRIES	Denmark, Finland
PATIENTS (n)	randomized 185
	evaluated 185

TYPE OF SURGERY
Total knee arthroplasty
(about 2/3 cemented prosthesis)

ANESTHESIA
General in 20%,
epidural/spinal in 80% of patients

STUDY DRUG	Enoxaparin	sc daily dose: 40mg o.d. + 2 placebo injections
		first injection: 12h preop
		treatment duration: 6-9 days

REFERENCE DRUG	UFH	sc doses: 5000 IU t.i.d.
		first injection: 12h preop
		treatment duration: 6-9 days

+ Elastic compression stockings in both groups

ASSESSMENTS
- DVT: bilateral venography at D6/ D9.
- PE: if clinically suspected, lung scan.
- Perioperative blood loss, wound hematomas.
- Two-month follow-up.

FAUNØ P. et al. 1994

	Enoxaparin 40mg x 1	UFH 5000 IU x 3	p
Patients	92	93	
Total DVT	23%	27%	NS
Proximal DVT	3%	5%	NS
Distal DVT	20%	22%	
PE	0	0	
Wound hematomas (benign)	8	12	NS
Perioperative blood loss	No difference		
Two-month follow-up (DVT)	0	1	

COMMENTS

❏ In knee surgery, it seems that incidence of total DVT is higher than in hip surgery despite prophylactic regimen (mainly distal DVT).

❏ However, the rate of proximal DVT was low with these two regimens started before surgery.

❏ Excellent tolerance of both treatments: no discontinuation of treatment, no reoperation.

Use of enoxaparin, a low-molecular weight-heparin and unfractionated heparin for the prevention of deep vein thrombosis after elective hip replacement

AUTHORS	COLWELL C.W., SPIRO T.E., TROWBRIDGE A.A. et al.
REF	J. Bone and Joint Surg. 1994; 76: 3-14

STUDY	Open-label, multicenter, randomized, parallel groups, controlled
CENTERS (n)	32
COUNTRY	United States
PATIENTS (n)	*randomized* 610
	evaluated 604 (for intent-to-treat analysis)

TYPE OF SURGERY
Elective hip replacement
(cemented ≈ 25%, not cemented 75%)

ANESTHESIA
General in ≈ 2/3
and regional in ≈ 1/3 of patients

STUDY DRUG	**Enoxaparin**	sc daily doses: 2 groups:
		• 30mg b.i.d.
		• 40mg o.d.
		first injection: within 24h postop
		treatment duration: ≤ 7 days
REFERENCE DRUG	**UFH**	sc daily doses: 5000 IU t.i.d.
		first injection: within 24h postop
		treatment duration: ≤ 7 days

ASSESSMENTS
- ❑ DVT incidence in patients who have received at least 75% of the study medication and who underwent bilateral venography (414 patients) at D7 (exclusion of patients with previous DVT or with DVT confirmed by non-invasive method within 14D before operation).
- ❑ PE (assessment not stated).
- ❑ Major/minor hemorrhage.
- ❑ Death.
- ❑ 6-week follow-up.

COLWELL C.W. et al. 1994

| | Enoxaparin | | UFH |
	30mg x 2	40mg x 1	5000 IU x 3
Patients	194	203	207
Evaluable venograms	136	136	142
Total DVT (venographic evidence)	8 6%	28 21%	21 15%
Total DVT (intention-to-treat)	9 5% *	30 15%	24 12%
Proximal DVT	4 2%	8 4%	10 7%
PE	0	0	1 (fatal)
Major hemorrhage	8 4%	3 1%	13 6%
Minor hemorrhage	16 8%	18 9%	12 6%
In-hospital death	1 (AMI)	0	2 (1 PE)
Readmission for DVT/PE (within 6 weeks after discharge)	3 DVT	1 DVT	1DVT/3 PE

* p= 0.03 vs UFH and 0.0002 vs Enoxaparin 40mg x 1.

COMMENTS

- Very good results with enoxaparin 30mg b.i.d., first injection postop.
- Surprising good efficacy with UFH 5000 IU b.i.d. in this study.
- The results obtained with enoxaparin 40mg o.d. were consistent with those observed in Planes' studies (1988,1991).

Efficacy and safety of enoxaparin to prevent deep venous thrombosis after hip replacement surgery

AUTHORS	SPIRO T.E., JOHNSON G.J., CHRISTIE M.J. et al.
REF	Ann. of Intern. Med. 1994; 121: 81-89

STUDY	Multicenter, double-blind, randomized, dose-ranging
CENTERS *(n)*	32
COUNTRY	United States
PATIENTS *(n)*	*randomized* 572
	evaluated 568 (intent-to-treat analysis)

TYPE OF SURGERY

Elective hip surgery
(cemented ≈ 40%)

ANESTHESIA

General in 2/3,
regional in 1/3 of patients

STUDY DRUG   **Enoxaparin**   sc daily dose:
- enoxaparin 10mg o.d.
- enoxaparin 40mg o.d.
- enoxaparin 30mg b.i.d.

first injection: within 24h postop

REFERENCE DRUG   **None**.

ASSESSMENTS

- ❏ DVT: daily clinical evaluation, bilateral venography at D7.
- ❏ PE: clinical evaluation.
- ❏ Major/minor hemorrhage.
- ❏ Follow-up.

SPIRO T.E. et al. 1994

| | Enoxaparin | | |
	10mg x 1	40mg x 1	30mg x 2
Patients	161	199	208
Evident DVT*	40 25%	27 14%	22 11%
Evaluable venography	116	149	143
Total DVT	36 31%	21 14%	16 11%
Proximal DVT	16 14%	9 6%	8 6%
Distal DVT	20 17%	12 8%	8 6%
PE	1	1	0
Major hemorrhage	3 2%	7 4%	11 5%
Minor hemorrhage	5 3%	14 7%	15 7%
In-hospital death	0	2 (AMI)	0
Readmission for DVT/PE	2 (1 PE)	2 (1 PE)	2

* Evidence: included venography, non-invasive methods, clinical evidence.

COMMENTS
- ❏ The number of inadequate or no venography was ranging between 24-31%.
- ❏ The number of patients treated who did not complete the study (discontinued) was about 30% in each of the three groups.
- ❏ 40mg o.d. and 30mg b.i.d. were more effective in preventing DVT than 10mg o.d.
- ❏ Once again, the difference in efficacy and safety between the two effective doses (giving an incidence of proximal DVT of 6%) is not clear.
- ❏ No mention of hemorrhagic risk with spinal anesthesia. The overall incidence of major hemorrhage was low in all three treatments.

Low molecular weight heparin (enoxaparin) compared with unfractionated heparin in prophylaxis of deep venous thrombosis and pulmonary embolism in patients undergoing hip replacement

AUTHORS	AVIKAINEN V., von BONSDORFF H., PARTIO E. et al.
REF	Ann. Chir. Gynaecol. 1995; 84: 85-90

STUDY	Open-label, randomized, comparative	**TYPE OF SURGERY**	Total hip replacement
CENTERS *(n)*	1	**ANESTHESIA**	
COUNTRY	Finland	Regional in 2/3, general in 1/3 of patients	
PATIENTS *(n)*	*included* 167 *evaluated* 167		

STUDY DRUG	**Enoxaparin**	sc daily dose: 40mg o.d. first injection: 12h preop treatment duration: 10 days
REFERENCE DRUG	**UFH**	sc daily doses: 5000 IU b.i.d. first injection: 12h preop treatment duration: 10 days

Early ambulation in both groups
Elevation of lower extremities on a special pillow until D3

ASSESSMENTS

❑ DVT: bilateral ultrasonography confirmed by venography.
❑ PE: clinical symptoms confirmed by lung scan, angiography.
❑ Bleeding complications.

AVIKAINEN V. et al. 1995

	Enoxaparin 40mg x 1		UFH 5000 IU x 2		p
Patients	83		84		
Proximal DVT	1	1.2%	4	4.8%	< 0.05
PE	0	0%	1	1.2%	NS
Large local hematomas (D4)	15		17		
Number of patients with transfusion requirements (peri-postop) ≥ 3 units	29		27		

COMMENTS

❑ The patients who developed DVT were evenly distributed with respect to the type of anesthesia.

❑ The patient who developed PE had spinal anesthesia.

❑ The low incidence of DVT observed in this study could be partly due to the type of anesthesia, more frequently epidural or spinal than general, the elevation of the lower extremities and the early ambulation of the patients.

❑ No spinal hematoma has been reported despite the preop injection of LMWH (–12h).

Prevention of venous thromboembolism after knee arthroplasty;
a randomized, double-blind trial comparing enoxaparin with warfarin

AUTHORS	LECLERC J.R., GEERTS W.H., DESJARDINS L. et al.
REF	Ann. Intern. Med. 1996; 124: 619-626

STUDY	Multicenter, randomized, double-blind, comparative
CENTERS *(n)*	8
COUNTRY	Canada
PATIENTS *(n)*	*randomized* 670
	evaluated 417

TYPE OF SURGERY	Knee arthroplasty
ANESTHESIA	General in about 89%, regional in about 14% of patients

STUDY DRUG	**Enoxaparin**	sc daily doses: 30mg b.i.d. + oral placebo
		first injection: 12h postop
		treatment duration: 14 days or up to hospital discharge
REFERENCE DRUG	**Warfarin**	first dose (not stated) administered the evening of surgery + 1 placebo injection
		oral daily dose adjusted to get an INR 2-3 and 2 placebo injections
		treatment duration: 14 days or up to hospital discharge

ASSESSMENTS

- ❏ DVT: bilateral venography at D14 or earlier if necessary (before venography, bilateral compression ultrasonography "CUS").
- ❏ If suspected clinical DVT, CUS or impedence plethysmography; if abnormal, venography.
- ❏ PE: clinical symptoms confirmed by lung scan or angiography.
- ❏ Major/minor hemorrhage.
- ❏ Adverse events.
- ❏ Death.

LECLERC J.R. et al. 1996

	Enoxaparin 30mg x 2		Warfarin		p
Patients	336		334		
Evaluable venography	206	61.3%	211	63.2%	
Total DVT	76	36.9%	109	51.7%	0.003
Proximal DVT	24	11.7%	22	10.4%	NS
PE	1	0.3%	3	0.9%	NS
Major hemorrhage	7	2.1%	6	1.8%	NS
Minor hemorrhage	94	28.0%	83	24.9%	NS
Thrombocytopenia	0		2 (on D3)		
In-hospital death	0		0		

COMMENTS

❏ As observed in the other studies, there was a high incidence of total DVT after knee surgery despite prophylaxis, but it must be pointed out that one center had a higher incidence of DVT in both groups, 58.8% for enoxaparin and 88.2% for warfarin.

❏ Lower incidence of proximal DVT, equally reduced by enoxaparin 30mg b.i.d. (postop) and by warfarin.

Risk of deep venous thrombosis after hospital discharge in patients having undergone total hip replacement: double-blind randomized comparison of enoxaparin versus placebo

AUTHORS	PLANES A., VOCHELLE N., DARMON J.Y. et al.
REF	Lancet. 1996; 348: 224-228

STUDY	Randomized, double-blind, placebo-controlled	**OBJECTIVE** To evaluate the risk of DVT in patients with total hip replacement after hospital discharge and to assess the efficacy of a prolonged prophylactic treatment
CENTERS (n)	1	
COUNTRY	France	
PATIENTS (n)	*included* 179 at hospital discharge (13-15 days after surgery) without DVT	**TYPE OF SURGERY** Total hip replacement 12-14 days before randomization

INITIAL TREATMENT
In-hospital

Enoxaparin 40mg sc o.d. from D1 until hospital discharge for all patients
then, randomization after venography at hospital discharge to:

PROLONGED TREATMENT
Home treatment

• **Enoxaparin** sc daily dose: 40mg o.d.
treatment duration: from hospital discharge up to D35 after surgery (about 21 days of treatment)
or

• **Placebo** dose: 0.4ml saline o.d.
treatment duration: from hospital discharge up to D35 after surgery

ASSESSMENTS

❏ DVT: bilateral venography (with non ionic contrast media) at D14 (at hospital discharge) and D35 after surgery.
❏ PE: lung scan if clinically suspected (DVT and/or PE: primary outcomes).
❏ Hemorrhage.
❏ Adverse events.
❏ Death.

PLANES A. et al. 1996

Events D14-D35	Enoxaparin 40mg x 1		Placebo		p
Intent-to-treat analysis					
Patients with venography (at D35)	85		88		
total DVT	6	7.1%	17	19.3%	0.08
proximal DVT	5	5.9%	7	7.9%	NS
distal DVT	1	1.2%	10	11.4%	0.006
Per-protocol analysis					
Patients with venography (at D35)	75		80		
total DVT	2	2.7%	16	20,0%	0.001
proximal DVT	1	1.3%	7	8.8%	NS
distal DVT	1	1.3%	9	11.3%	0.02
Clinical symptoms of DVT	14		16		
Confirmed DVT	3	3.5%	7	8.7%	
Hemorrhage (minor)	17	18.9%	4	4.5%	
Death or PE	0		0		

COMMENTS

❏ Without long-term prophylaxis, the risk of late total or proximal DVT remained high for at least 35 days after surgery (despite initial therapy).

❏ Prolonged prophylaxis with LMWH drastically reduced this risk.

❏ The clinical symptoms of DVT did not significantly differ between the two (short and prolonged) regimens.

❏ The rate of delayed DVT was only related with history of neoplasia.

**Low-molecular weight heparin (enoxaparin)
as prophylaxis against venous thromboembolism after
total hip replacement**

AUTHORS	BERGQVIST D., BENONI G., BJÖRGELL O. et al.
REF	N. Engl. J. Med. 1996; 335: 696-700

STUDY	Double-blind, randomized, placebo-controlled
CENTERS *(n)*	1
COUNTRY	Sweden
PATIENTS *(n)*	*included* 288
	at hospital discharge, without venography
	randomized 262
	evaluated 233 for efficacy

OBJECTIVE
To verify the efficacy of a prolonged vs short-term prophylaxis after hip surgery

TYPE OF SURGERY
Total hip replacement (cemented or non cemented) 10 days before randomization

INITIAL TREATMENT	**Enoxaparin**	40mg sc o.d. from D1 to D10 after surgery for all
In-hospital		patients, *then randomization (without venography) to:*
LONG-TERM PROPHYLAXIS	**• Enoxaparin**	sc daily dose: 40mg o.d.
Home treatment		1st day of hospital discharge
		treatment duration: 21 days
		(total duration: 10 + 21 = 31 days)
		or
	• Placebo	dose: 0.4ml saline o.d.
		1st day of hospital discharge
		treatment duration: 21 days

ASSESSMENTS

❑ DVT: bilateral venography 18-23 days after hospital discharge (no venography at hospital discharge; difference with Planes' study).

❑ PE: clinical symptoms confirmed by lung scan or angiography.

❑ Hemorrhagic complications.

❑ DVT clinical symptoms.

❑ 3-month follow-up.

BERGQVIST D. et al. 1996

After hospital discharge ≈ D30	**Enoxaparin** 40mg x 1		**Placebo**		**p**
Patients (randomized)	131		131		
Evaluable venography	117		116		
Total thromboembolism (D0-D30)	21	18%	45	39%	<0.001
Proximal DVT	8	7%	28	24%	<0.001
Clinical symptoms of DVT*	2	1.7%	8	6.7%	
PE	0		2 (confirmed)		
Rehospitalization (n)	11		32		
Rehospitalization (total days)	99		269		
Major complications	0		0		
Death during 3-month follow-up	0		0		

* all confirmed.

COMMENTS

❑ Curiously enough, the rate of DVT (total and/or proximal) was similar after 30 days of prophylaxis or after 10 days of prophylaxis (in line with the results observed in other studies).

❑ The location of DVT was mainly in the leg operated.

❑ At D30, a dramatic higher incidence of DVT was observed in the placebo group (short-term prophylaxis) with more rehospitalizations

❑ It seems clear that a "long-term" prophylaxis after orthopedic surgery should be recommended.

❑ It can be interesting to note that regional anesthesia was used in 95% of the patients.

Low molecular weight heparin associated with spinal anaesthesia and gradual compression stockings in total hip replacement surgery

AUTHORS	SAMAMA C.M., CLERGUE F., BARRE J., et al (ARAR Study Group)
REF	Br.J. Anaesth. 1997; 78 : 660-665

STUDY	Multicenter, randomized, double-blind, placebo-controlled
CENTERS (n)	11
COUNTRY	France
PATIENTS (n)	included 170
	evaluated 153

TYPE OF SURGERY
total hip replacement
(cemented or not)

ANESTHESIA
Spinal

STUDY DRUG **Enoxaparin** sc daily dose: 40mg o.d.
first injection: 6±1h postop (after spinal puncture)
treatment duration: during hospital stay (10±2 days)

REFERENCE DRUG **Placebo** sc daily dose: 0.4ml saline o.d.
treatment duration: during hospital stay (10±2 days)

+ Elastic compression stockings from D0-D10 for both groups
Then Enoxaparin 40mg o.d. for 28 days in open-label regimen in both groups after hospital discharge

ASSESSMENTS

- ❑ DVT: daily clinical evaluation, bilateral Doppler on D3 and D6 and bilateral venography on D10±2.
- ❑ PE: in case of suspicion, lung scan or angiography.
- ❑ Hemorrhagic complications.
- ❑ 3-month follow-up for DVT, PE, mortality.

SAMAMA C.M. et al. 1997

	Enoxaparin 40mg x 1 + elastic stocking		Placebo 0.4ml x 1 + elastic stocking		p
Total patients	85		85		
Evaluable patients (intention-to-treat)	78		75		
Total DVT	11	14.1%	28	37.3%	<0.01
Proximal DVT	2	2.6%	12	16.0%	
Patients with clinical symptoms	1*		1*		
PE	0		0		
Major hemorrhage (without discontinuation of therapy)	1		1		
Spinal hematomas	0		0		
Wound hematomas	33		20		
Transfusions	16		7		<0.01
3-month follow-up (D12-D90)					
DVT/PE	0		0		
death	0		0		

* Confirmed by venography.

COMMENTS

❑ In the placebo group, the association of spinal anesthesia with compression stockings alone was not sufficient to protect against the risk of postoperative DVT after hip surgery.

❑ No neurological sequelae in either group.

❑ In both groups, it is interesting to note that no clinical thromboembolic event was observed during the 3-month follow-up. Was this result related to prolonged prophylaxis (enoxaparin 40mg o.d. for 28D) after hospital discharge?

Prevention of deep vein thrombosis after hip replacement: randomized comparison between unfractionated heparin and low molecular weight heparin

AUTHORS	LEYVRAZ P.F., BACHMANN F., HOEK J. et al.
REF	B.M.J. 1991; 303: 543-548

STUDY	Open-label, multicenter, randomized, comparative
CENTERS (n)	28
COUNTRIES	Belgium, France, Italy, Switzerland, The Netherlands
PATIENTS (n)	randomized 409
	evaluated 349

TYPE OF SURGERY
Elective total hip replacement
(2/3 cemented)

ANESTHESIA
General

STUDY DRUG **Nadroparin** one sc daily body weight adjusted dose:
- 100 AXa ICU/kg from D1 to D3 corresponding to ≈ 40 IU/kg, then,
- 150 AXa ICU/kg from D4 to D10 corresponding to ≈ 60 IU/kg
first injection: 12h preop, second injection 12h postop
treatment duration: 10 days

REFERENCE DRUG **UFH** three sc daily doses daily adjusted to APTT values
(+2 to +5 sec. above control values)
(mean dose, less than 4000 IU x 3)
first injections: 4000 IU 16h preop then, 2h preop (APTT-adjust.)
third injection: 12h postop

+ Elastic compression stockings in both groups

ASSESSMENTS

- ❑ DVT: bilateral venography (D9-D11).
- ❑ PE, confirmed by lung scan or angiography.
- ❑ Major, minor hemorrhage, wound hematomas.
- ❑ Thrombocytopenia.
- ❑ Follow-up: 30-50 days.
- ❑ Death.

LEYVRAZ P.F. et al. 1991

	Nadroparin x 1 (Time and BW-adjusted)		**UFH** x 3 (APTT-adjusted dose)		**p**
Evaluated patients	174		175		
Total DVT	22	12.6%	28	16.0%	NS
Proximal DVT	5	2.9%	23	13.1%	<0.001
Confirmed PE	1	0.6%	4*	2.3%	
Major hemorrhage	1/198		3/199		
Hematomas (site of injection)	26	13.3%	62	31.1%	0.001
Thrombocytopenia	0		2		
Death	1 (AMI)		2		
30/50-day follow-up	1 death (D34)		4 DVT/1 PE		

* 1 fatal.

COMMENTS
- With this scheduled regimen, nadroparin o.d. was more effective than sc monitored UFH in preventing proximal DVT after elective hip replacement. This activity was significantly more evident on proximal DVT than on distal DVT.
- Tolerance regarding transfusion requirements, major hemorrhage, wound hematomas was good and similar in the two groups (data not shown).
- Good correlation between the two dosages and AXa levels but not between AXa activity and DVT incidence (results not shown).

Prevention of deep vein thrombosis with low molecular-weight heparin in patients undergoing total hip replacement

AUTHORS	The German Hip Arthroplasty Trial (GHAT) Group
REF	Arch. Orthop. Trauma Surg. 1992; 111: 110-120

STUDY	Multicenter, double-blind, randomized, comparative	
CENTERS (n)	15	
COUNTRY	Germany	
PATIENTS (n)	*randomized*	341
	treated	335
	evaluated for efficacy	267

TYPE OF SURGERY
Total hip replacement:
cemented prosthesis 45%,
non cemented 55%

ANESTHESIA
General in 90%, regional and combined
in about 10% of patients

STUDY DRUG	**Nadroparin**	sc daily dose: 10 000 AXa ICU (3800 AXa IU)= 0.4ml o.d. + 2 placebo injections per day first injection: evening before operation treatment duration: 16 ± 1 days

REFERENCE DRUG	**UFH**	sc daily doses: 5000 IU t.i.d. one injection (placebo) evening before operation first injection: 2h preop treatment duration: 16 ± 1 days

+ Elastic compression stockings and early ambulation in both groups

ASSESSMENTS
❑ DVT: bilateral venography at D14 ± 1.
❑ Clinical PE: lung scan, angiography.
❑ Major/minor hemorrhage, wound hematomas.

The GHAT Group. 1992

	Nadroparin 0.4ml x 1		UFH 5000 IU x 3		p
Treated patients	167		168		
Evaluable patients	136		137		
DVT Total	45	33.1%	47	34.3%	NS
Proximal	14	10.3%	27	19.7%	0.05
Distal	21	15.4%	14	10.2%	NS
Muscle	10	7.4%	4	2.9%	NS
DVT < 60 years	9/44	20.5%	8/44	18.2%	NS
> 60 years	36/92	39.1%	39/93	41.9%	NS
Clinical DVT	1		6		
PE	2	1.2%	6 (2 fatal)	3.6%	
Major hemorrhage	2		2		
Severe wound hematomas	1		4		
Six-week follow-up:					
Thromboembolic events	0		0		

COMMENTS

❑ Surprisingly high DVT incidence in both groups, probably attributable to the specific method which takes into account calf muscle vein thromboses. Mention of intra-operative autotransfusion by "cell saver" system (only simple blood filtration?) see Palareti's study for similar problem.

❑ DVT incidence was not influenced by prosthesis type (cemented or not); but strongly influenced by age (> 60 years) and in the LMWH group, by BW (25% <70kg, 38% >70kg).

❑ The UFH dosage (5000 IU t.i.d.) was higher than in Leyvraz's study and despite this, a higher incidence of DVT was observed. Is APTT-adjustment better than fixed dose for UFH?

Subcutaneous low molecular weight heparin or oral anticoagulants for the prevention of deep-vein thrombosis in elective hip and knee replacement

AUTHORS	HAMULYAK K., LENSING A.W.A., van der MEER J. et al.
REF	Thromb. Haemostasis 1994; 74: 1428-1434

STUDY	Multicenter, single-blind, randomized, comparative
CENTERS (n)	12
COUNTRY	The Netherlands
PATIENTS (n)	*included* 672
	evaluated 517 (for efficacy)

TYPE OF SURGERY
Hip or knee replacement

ANESTHESIA
General in about 50%,
regional in 50% of patients

STUDY DRUG	**Nadroparin**	sc daily dose: ≈ 60 AXa IU/kg
		i.e. 0.3ml for BW ≤ 60kg
		0.4ml for BW 60-80kg
		0.6ml for BW > 80kg
		first injection: 0.3ml 12h preop
		treatment duration: 10 days

REFERENCE DRUG	**Acenocoumarol**	oral daily dose: INR-adjusted (2-3)
		first dose: 4mg preop; 2mg day of surgery
		treatment duration: 10 days

+ *Elastic compression stockings in both groups*

ASSESSMENTS
- DVT: bilateral venography at D10 ± 2.
- PE if clinical symptoms confirmed by lung scan or angiography.
- Bleeding complications.
- Side effects (thrombocytopenia).

HAMULYAK K. et al. 1994

	Nadroparin ≈ 60 AXa IU/kg x 1		Acenocoumarol		p
Evaluated patients for:					
efficacy	260		257		
tolerance	330		342		
Hip arthroplasty	195		195		
Total DVT	27	13.8%	27	13.8%	NS
Proximal DVT	12	6.2%	9	4.6%	NS
Severe bleeding	3	1.2%	7 (1 fatal)	2.6%	NS
Knee arthroplasty	65		61		
Total DVT	16	24.6%	23	37.7%	NS
Proximal DVT	5	7.7%	5	9.8%	NS
Severe bleeding	2	2.6%	1	1.3%	NS
Symptomatic DVT	0		0		
Thrombocytopenia	0		0		
PE	suspected in 3 patients but not confirmed (group not mentioned)				

COMMENTS
- ❏ With fixed body-weight adapted dose, nadroparin appeared to have an efficacy similar to oral anticoagulant in hip surgery and to be slightly better in knee surgery even though the results are not significantly different.
- ❏ Tolerance was similar in the two groups although one patient treated with oral anticoagulant died from hemorrhage.
- ❏ As observed in other studies, the incidence of total DVT remained high after 10 days of prophylaxis in knee arthroplasty.

**Postoperative versus preoperative initiation
of deep vein thrombosis prophylaxis with a low-molecular-weight heparin
(nadroparin) in elective hip replacement**

AUTHORS	PALARETI G., BORGHI B., COCCHERI S. et al.
REF	Clin. Appl. Thrombosis Haemostasis. 1996; 2: 18-24

STUDY	Multicenter, double-blind, randomized, comparison of two timing regimens: preop vs postop injection	
CENTERS *(n)*	7	
COUNTRY	Italy	
PATIENTS *(n)*	*included*	180
	evaluated	131 (for efficacy)
		179 (for tolerance)

TYPE OF SURGERY
Elective hip replacement

ANESTHESIA
General

STUDY DRUG   **Nadroparin**   sc daily dose:
- 0.3ml up to D3 then,
- 0.4ml from D4 up to D14
first injection: 12h **preop**
second injection evening of operation

versus

- same dosage regimen
first injection: 12h **postop**
treatment duration: ≥ 14 days

ASSESSMENTS
- ❑ DVT: bilateral venography at D10/D15 after surgery.
- ❑ Major/minor hemorrhage.
- ❑ PE: clinical observation; if suspicion, lung scan.

PALARETI G. et al. 1996

	Nadroparin 0.3ml up to D3, then 0.4ml from D4 until hospital discharge		
	1st inj. preop	**1st inj. postop**	p
Evaluable patients for:			
Efficacy	65	66	
Safety	90	89	
Total DVT	27 41.5%	24 36.4%	NS
Proximal DVT	7 10.8%	4 6.1%	NS
Clinical DVT	4 6.1%	4 6.1%	NS
PE	0	0	
Major hemorrhage	2 2.2%	3 3.4%	NS

COMMENTS

❏ Inadequate venography in ≈ 30% of patients.

❏ Surprisingly high incidence of confirmed total DVT exactly as in the GHAT study. Mention is made of "intraoperative blood salvage" either with reinfusion of blood — after simple filtration — or with washed erythrocytes. Did these transfusional practices affect postoperative hypercoagulability (high incidence of total DVT in both groups and in the two studies)?

❏ No difference between pre- and post-surgery prophylaxis either in terms of efficacy or in terms of bleeding complications.

The use of low molecular weight heparins for post-surgical DVT prevention in orthopaedic patients

AUTHORS	CHIAPUZZO E., ORENGO G.B., OTTRIA G. et al.
REF	J. Internat. Med. Research. 1988; 16: 359-366

STUDY	Open-label, controlled
CENTERS (n)	1
COUNTRY	Italy
PATIENTS (n)	*evaluated* 140

TYPE OF SURGERY

Major orthopedic surgery
(hip prosthesis ≈ 30%, osteosynthesis
of fractured inferior limbs ≈ 30%,
osteotomy ≈ 10%)

ANESTHESIA

Not stated

STUDY DRUG	**Parnaparin**	sc daily doses: 7500 AXa U b.i.d. (corresponding to about 3200 AXa IU) first injection: 2h before surgery treatment duration: 7 days
REFERENCE DRUG	**UFH**	sc daily doses: 5000 IU t.i.d. first injection: 2h before surgery treatment duration: 7 days

ASSESSMENTS

❑ DVT: Doppler ultrasonography (FUT in 20 patients).

❑ PE: clinical or radiological findings.

❑ Laboratory tests.

CHIAPUZZO E. et al. 1988

	Parnaparin 7500 AXa U x 2		UFH 5000 IU x 3	
Patients	70		70	
Total DVT PE	5	7.1% 0	7	10.0% 0
Hematomas	3		5	
Treatment stopped	0		0	
AXa level U/ml (at peak) mean value D1 to D7	0.23		0.06	

COMMENTS

❑   In this first Italian orthopedic trial using a LMWH, the daily regimen of parnaparin about 6400 AXa IU has been subdivided in two administrations with the first dose administered 2h before surgery.

❑   The efficacy of this regimen appeared as effective and safe as UFH 5000 IU t.i.d.

Comparison of antithrombotic efficacy and hemorrhagic side effects of reviparin sodium versus enoxaparin in patients undergoing total hip replacement surgery

AUTHORS	PLANES A., CHASTANG Cl., VOCHELLE N. et al.
REF	Blood Coag. and Fibrinolysis. 1993; 4: S 33-S 35

STUDY	Randomized, double-blind, 2 parallel groups
CENTERS (n)	1
COUNTRY	France
PATIENTS (n)	included 440
	evaluated 416

OBJECTIVE
To compare the efficacy of reviparin vs enoxaparin

TYPE OF SURGERY
Total hip replacement

ANESTHESIA
Not stated

STUDY DRUG	Reviparin	sc daily doses: 4200 AXa IU (0.6ml) + 1 placebo injection (0.4ml) o.d. first injection: 12h preop treatment duration: at least 10 days
REFERENCE DRUG	Enoxaparin	sc daily doses: 40mg (0.4ml) + 1 placebo injection (0.6ml) o.d. first injection: 12h preop treatment duration: at least 10 days

ASSESSMENTS

- ❏ Incidence of DVT: bilateral venography at D10-D13.
- ❏ PE: assessment not stated.
- ❏ Bleeding complications, wound hematomas.
- ❏ AXa activity.

PLANES A. et al. 1993

	Reviparin 4200 AXa IU x 1		Enoxaparin 40mg x 1	
Patients	219		221	
Venography performed	207		209	
Total DVT	21	10%	18	9%
Proximal DVT	12	6%	13	6%
PE	2		0	
Major bleeding	1		1	
Wound hematomas	7	3%	12	5%
AXa levels at D8 (IU ± SD)				
4h after injection	0.36±0.17		0.46±0.10	
after injection 12h	0.06±0.07		0.11±0.07	
Death	0		0	

COMMENTS

❑ First direct comparison between two LMWHs.

❑ The clinical efficacy in preventing DVT after hip surgery was equivalent with reviparin at the dose of 4200 IU and enoxaparin 40mg (corresponding to 4000-4200 IU). It appeared that equivalent doses of LMWHs gave equivalent efficacy.

❑ Surprisingly, the plasma AXa activities were different in the two groups, with a constant lower AXa level in reviparin-treated patients.

Prevention of thromboembolism in 190 hip arthroplasties,
comparison of low molecular weight heparin and placebo

AUTHORS	LASSEN M.R., BORRIS L.C., CHRISTIANSEN H. et al.
REF	Acta. Orthop. Scand. 1991; 62: 33-38

STUDY	Multicenter, randomized, double-blind, placebo-controlled
CENTERS (n)	2
COUNTRY	Denmark
PATIENTS (n)	*included* 210
	evaluated 190

TYPE OF SURGERY

Hip arthroplasty
(cement or cementless prosthesis)

ANESTHESIA

General in about 70%,
regional in about 30% of patients

STUDY DRUG	**Tinzaparin**	sc daily dose: 50 AXa IU/kg o.d.
		first injection: 2h preop
		treatment duration: 7 days
REFERENCE DRUG	**Placebo**	sc daily dose: saline injection
		first injection: 2h preop
		treatment duration: 7 days

+ Elastic compression stockings in both groups; early mobilization on the 4th postoperative day

ASSESSMENTS

❑ DVT: bilateral venography at D8 or D10 or earlier if clinical suspicion.

❑ PE: if clinical suspicion, lung scan.

❑ Bleeding complications.

❑ Distribution of thromboembolism in relation to mobilization policy.

LASSEN M.R. et al. 1991

	Tinzaparin 50 AXa IU/kg x 1		Placebo		p
Patients	93		97		
Total DVT	29	31%	44	45%	0.02
Proximal DVT	24	26%	35	36%	
Clinical symptoms	0		0		
PE	1 (fatal)	1%	1	1%	
Thromboembolism					
Early mobilization	18/77	23%	38/85	45%	0.002
Late mobilization	12/16	75%	7/12	58%	NS
Mean transfusions — in units — (range)	2.7	(0-8)	2.2	(0-6)	0.02
Wound hematomas	13		7		NS
Death	1	(D11)	1	(D6)	

COMMENTS

❑ Surprising high incidence of proximal DVT in this study for tinzaparin-treated patients, especially for those with late mobilization (results totally different from those obtained in Matzch's study, see following study).

❑ None of the patients with DVT developed any clinical symptoms.

❑ Postoperative blood loss and total number of blood transfusions higher in the LMWH group. However, these differences were of no clinical importance.

Comparison of the thromboprophylactic effect of a low molecular weight heparin versus dextran in total hip replacement

AUTHORS	MÄTZSCH T., BERGQVIST D., FREDIN H. et al.
REF	Thromb. Haemor. Disord. 1991; 3: 25-29

STUDY	Open-label, multicenter, randomized, comparative
CENTERS (n)	2
COUNTRIES	Sweden, Denmark
PATIENTS (n)	randomized 243
	evaluated 219

TYPE OF SURGERY

Hip arthroplasty

ANESTHESIA

Epidural or spinal: 95% of patients

STUDY DRUG	Tinzaparin	sc daily dose: 50 AXa IU/kg o.d.
		first injection: 2h preop
		treatment duration: 7 days

REFERENCE DRUG	Dextran 70	route iv: 500ml during surgery
		500ml at D0, D1, D3, D5

ASSESSMENTS

❏ Isotopic DVT: FUT every day until D10; if positive, venography.

❏ PE: lung scan if clinical suspicion.

❏ Bleeding complications.

MÄTZSCH T. et al. 1991

	Tinzaparin 50 AXa IU/kg x 1	Dextran	p
Patients	111	108	
In-hospital DVT* total	19 17.1%	31 28.7%	0.04
proximal	4 3.6%	3 2.8%	NS
Post-hospital DVT**	2 (D15-D17) 1.8%	1 (D18) 0.9%	
PE (time not stated)	2	0	
Total transfusion requirements (units ± SD)	4.3±2.4	3.8±2.4	NS
Wound hematomas	4	10	
	No bleeding complications needing discontinuation of therapy in either group.		
Death	1	1	

*   Venographically verified in patients receiving correct prophylaxis.
** Clinical symptoms confirmed by venography.

COMMENTS

❑ Tinzaparin 50 AXa IU/kg was at least as effective as dextran 70 and was safer with regard to bleeding in total hip replacement.

❑ The results obtained in this study were very different from those of Lassen with the same product, same indication, same dosage, but with different anesthesia: in this study almost all patients had regional anesthesia.

A comparison of subcutaneous low molecular weight heparin with warfarin sodium for prophylaxis against deep-vein thrombosis after hip or knee implantation

AUTHORS	HULL R.D., RASKOB G.E., PINEO G.F. et al.
REF	N. Engl. J. Med. 1993; 329: 1370-1376

STUDY	Multicenter, randomized, double-blind, comparative
CENTERS (n)	4
COUNTRIES	United States, Canada
PATIENTS (n)	*included* 1436
	evaluated 1207

TYPE OF SURGERY
Hip surgery (795 patients)
Knee surgery (641 patients)
Primary or revised procedures

ANESTHESIA
General in about 50%, regional or combined in about 50% of patients

STUDY DRUG	**Tinzaparin**	sc daily dose: 75 AXa IU/kg o.d.
		first injection: 18- 24h postop
		treatment duration: 14 days or up to hospital discharge
REFERENCE DRUG	**Warfarin**	first dose: 10mg postop (evening D0)
		then adjusted to INR 2-3
		treatment duration: 14 days or up to hospital discharge

ASSESSMENTS

❏ DVT: bilateral venography on D14 (blind lecture).
❏ Clinical assessments for DVT, PE.
❏ Major/minor bleeding.
❏ 3-month follow-up.
❏ Adverse events.

HULL R.D. et al. 1993

	Tinzaparin 75 AXa IU/kg x 1				**Warfarin**			
	hip		knee		hip		knee	
Patients	398		317		397		324	
Successful venography	332		258		340		277	
Total DVT	69	20.8%	116	45.0%	79	23.2%	152	54.9%
Proximal DVT	16	4.8%	20	7.8%	13	3.8%	34	12.3%
Major bleeding	11	2.8%	9	2.8%	6	1.5%	3	0.9%
Wound hematomas	23	5.8%	28	8.8%	10	2.5%	19	5.9%
	Tinzaparin (pooled data)				**Warfarin** (pooled data)			
Thrombocytopenia (non severe)	12	1.7%			3	0.4%		
Death (not thrombosis/ or bleeding related)	5	0.7%			5	0.7%		
3-month follow-up								
DVT	7	1.0%			3	0.4%		
PE	1	(D28)			1	(D69)		

COMMENTS

❏ In orthopedic surgery, tinzaparin 75 AXa IU/kg was slightly more effective than warfarin, especially in knee surgery, but this benefit was offset by an increase in the number of bleeding complications and wound hematomas.

❏ Regarding the incidence of total or proximal DVT, the greater variability was related to centers (for example from 11% up to 34% with LMWH in hip surgery).

Expert comments

DAVID BERGQVIST. *LMWHs and the prophylaxis against postoperative venous thromboembolism*

Prophylaxis against postoperative venous thromboembolism has actually been discussed and studied since the turn of this century although the era of modern investigations with randomization and objective diagnostic principles started with the by now classical study by Sevitt and Gallagher in 1959 (1). With 40 years perspective it is interesting to see how the diagnostic pendulum is swinging. When it was realized that clinical diagnosis of deep vein thrombosis was inaccurate with both false positives and false negatives, venographic diagnosis became mandatory but cumbersome. Moreover, it is not readily feasible for repeated investigations to follow a course such as postoperative surveillance. For some 20 to 25 years, venography was replaced by the fibrinogen uptake test when it became clear that at least in orthopedic surgery this was suboptimal and venography was considered necessary again. Now the fibrinogen uptake test is forbidden in most countries because of the risk for viral transmission. In addition, the discussion is again focused on the clinical consequences of venous thromboembolism, that is, symptomatic deep vein thrombosis and pulmonary embolism. The frequency of symptomatic venous thromboembolism is much lower than the total frequency as diagnosed with some objective test. This obviously has significant importance for the sample size calculation, when new studies are planned.

Parallel to the philosophy of diagnostic requirements in venous thromboembolism can be discussed the development of prophylactic measures. From the first biochemical reports on the relation between the molecular weight of heparin fragments and heparin effects in 1976 there has been tremendous and fascinating research activity regarding the several commercial substances which have been approved as pharmacological agents. Without doubt it can be stated that low molecular weight heparin is the thromboprophylactic principle with the best documentation throughout prophylactic history. The documentation now is so great that it is difficult to keep all publications actual. Therefore the present volume, *LMWH Therapy: an Evaluation of Clinical Trials Evidence,* is extremely welcome, summarizing as it does the important data in the individual studies with short pertinent comments.

It seems without doubt that low molecular weight heparins are effective and safe, the evidence in fact indicating that they are somewhat better than unfractionated heparin. In addition, being more practical with once daily injection, the current use of low molecular weight heparins creates a logistic problem in future thromboprophylactic research. Any new substances must be compared with low molecular weight heparins and to show better and/or safer prophylaxis necessitate very large trials, and the question must be asked if they are at all worthwhile doing. In orthopedic and trauma surgery, and probably also cancer surgery, there is, however, still room for improvements.

Nonetheless, there are still questions which can be asked concerning the use of low molecular weight heparins in prophylaxis against venous thromboembolism. One important question, which is briefly hinted at in the chapter on orthopedic surgery, deals with prolonged prophylaxis. In four studies on hip arthroplasty the frequency of venographically proven deep vein thrombosis at around one month postoperatively is significantly lower if the prophylaxis is continued until the venographic investigation than if it is given for around one week (2,3,4,5). Another obvious group of patients where this concept of prolonged prophylaxis must be evaluated is those operated on for various types of malignant disorders, where there is a reason to believe that the thrombotic challenge continues for more than the duration of conventional prophylaxis. There are several questions concerning prolonged prophylaxis, some of them listed below:

- For how long is there an increased risk of venous thromboembolism postoperatively?
- Does prolonged prophylaxis only delay the development of thromboembolism?
- For how long should prolonged prophylaxis continue?
- Are late postoperative thrombi as dangerous as early ones, with respect to pulmonary embolism?
- Does prolonged prophylaxis prevent the development of late venous insufficiency?
- Which are the risk groups where prolonged prophylaxis really is of benefit?
- Are low molecular weight heparins the optimal regimen for prolonged prophylaxis or should oral anticoagulation be used?
- Which are the health economic implications of prolonged prophylaxis?
- Is there motivation to perform a study on prolonged prophylaxis with clinical endpoints (fatal pulmonary embolism, mortality, clinical thromboembolism)?

It is important not to accept routine prolonged prophylaxis without answering the above questions on a scientific basis.

Another group where our knowledge on prophylaxis is insufficient is various types of laparoscopic procedures. After laparoscopic cholecystectomy at least, fatal pulmonary embolism seems to be extremely rare (6). As laparoscopic surgery is made for more advanced disorders the risk for thromboembolism will probably increase. Although minimally invasive, there are problems which may potentially increase the thrombogenicity: prolonged procedures with increased abdominal pressure with impaired venous emptying and vena caval compression. Again there is an urgent need to evaluate when low molecular weight heparins are indicated before routine use is recommended.

REFERENCES

1 - Sevitt S, Gallagher NG. Prevention of venous thrombosis and pulmonary embolism in injured patients. Lancet 1959;i:981-984

2 - Bergqvist D, Benoni G, Björgell O, Fredin H, Hedlundh U, Nicolas S, Nilsson P, Nylander G. Low-molecular-weight heparin (enoxaparin) as prophylaxis against venous thromboembolism after total hip replacement. N Engl J Med 1996;335:696-700.

3 - Planes A, Vochelle N, Darmon J-Y, Fagula M, Belland M, Huet Y. Risk of deep-venous thrombosis after hospital discharge in patients having undergone total hip replacement : double-blind randomized comparison of enoxpararin versus placebo. Lancet 1996;348:224-228.

4 - Dahl O, Andreassen G, Aspelin T, Müller C, Mathiesen P, Nyhus S, Abdelnoor M, Solhaug J-H, Arnesen H. Prolonged thromboprophylaxis following hip replacement surgery-results of a double-blind, prospective, randomized placebo-controlled study with dalteparin (Fragmin). Thromb Haemost 1997;77:20-31.

5 - Lassen M, Borris L. Prolonged thromboprophylaxis with low molecular weight heparin(Fragmin) after elective total hip arthroplasty : a placebo-controlled trial. Drugs 1996;52 Suppl 7:47-54.

6 - Caprini J. A., Arcelus J. I. Prevention of postoperative venous thromboembolism following laparoscopic cholecystectomy. Surg Endosc 1994; 8:741-747

ANDRÉ PLANÈS. *LMWHs in orthopedic and traumatologic surgery*

After a decade of prophylactic use of low molecular weight heparins (LMWHs) in orthopedic and trauma surgery, it is important to summarize and report on the clinical experience acquired with these compounds. This comprehensive review gives us the opportunity to consider the contribution of these drugs to the prophylaxis of venous thromboembolism, subsequent progression of the concepts of prophylactic management and stimulation of further research. In this context, we welcome the initiative of this overview and find it more informative than the usual meta-analysis of studies with their known limitations.

At the time of their introduction into the international pharmacopoeia, LMWHs were considered as "distinct and separate compounds". We now recognize that the opinions of Barrowcliffe, Johnson and Thomas, expressed in 1992 (1) that LMWH are "siblings and not distant cousins" is entirely justified, since, as these authors pointed out, "their mean molecular weight is in the range of 4,000 to 6,000 daltons". Results reported in comparative trials of the most widely studied LMWHs have confirmed this point of view. With the advent of an appropriate and accepted International Standard for LMWHs, we are now convinced that a dosage range of between 4000 and 5000 anti-factor Xa (AXa) IU, once daily, is appropriate for prevention of venous thromboembolism. Nevertheless, for each compound, the correct dosage must be demonstrated and such dosages are not interchangeable.

The main advantage provided involves efficacy, in particular, regarding the reduction in occurrence of deep vein thrombosis (DVT). This advantage is associated with simplified prophylactic use, with once-daily subcutaneous injection without the need for laboratory monitoring. This advance promoted improved compliance, and resulted in generalized use of this type of heparin compound. Based on our own experience with 300 to 400 hip and knee replacements performed every year, complete disappearance of symptomatic cases of thrombo-embolism has occurred. One injection daily is the regimen commonly used except in the US and Canada, where surgeons are reluctant to use heparin in the preoperative and immediate peri-operative period. Accordingly, a postoperative, twice-daily dosing regimen is used.

The case for pre- or postoperative administration is still unresolved. The solution can only be obtained by comparing these two concepts "head to head" in a prospective, randomized, double-blind trial on two parallel groups of patients. In the future, this question could possibly lose its importance if the concept of "extended prophylaxis", as described below, demonstrates its validity and becomes generally accepted.

Fixed-dosage adjusted to variable time of first administration (i.e. 2 or 12 hour before, 6,12 or 24 hour after surgery), or by body weight of the patient, are also sources of debate among experts and pharmaceutical manufacturers. In light of a recent, still unpublished trial, adjustment of dosage to body weight for prophylactic therapy does not seem necessary. Nevertheless, we must recognize that the correct scientific explanation for a standard dosage remains to be elucidated.

In comparison with unfractionated heparin (UFH), an increased margin of safety between bleeding tendency induced by an unnecessarily high dosage and an effective and safe, prophylactic, antithrombotic dosage is possible with LMWHs, when considering the wide variations in recommended dosages expressed in AXa IU made by manufacturers. Between 4000 and 6000 anti-factor Xa IU provide approximately equivalent efficacy and safety. Such a wide margin, associated with a stable and effective dose-response, represents an undisputed advance in the prophylaxis of venous thromboembolism with LMWHs, compared to conventional UFH.

Whatever the increased margin of safety may be, LMWHs may induce an increased bleeding tendency if the proper dosage is not chosen. This bleeding tendency is proportional to the amount of AXa activity administered (an unexpected observation at the beginning of research on LMWHs). Whether or not they induce a lesser bleeding tendency than UFH in patients when the correct dosage is administered is still an unsolved question. Confusion in this matter arises from the differences in dosages used in clinical trials, in the definition of bleeding, methods of assessment of bleeding and also possibly in operative methods. In this context, meta-analysis, in our opinion, is unreliable, since there are substantial differences between studies. Only placebo-controlled trials could help to solve this problem. But, the latter are unacceptable for ethical reasons. In our experience, the risk of bleeding, with proper dosage of LMWH, is low and major bleeding generally is associated with a latent hemorrhagic lesion (i.e. cancer, gastro-duodenal ulcer).

Methods of research and diagnostic tools have improved considerably over the past decade. Initially, research on UFH was conducted based on clinical diagnosis of venous thrombo-embolic disease. Given the technological methods of clinical diagnosis that existed at the time, results between trials were inconsistent and unreliable. Autopsy findings improved this research, but postmortem examination has become increasingly difficult to carry out over the last ten years and results, based on a procedure performed on at best 30% of patients, are of little value.

The radioactive fibrinogen uptake test has been abandoned for reasons related to sterility as well as intrinsic reliability, in particular, overestimation of distal DVT, especially in orthopedics.

Nevertheless, results observed with this technique were not very different from those observed with venography. Ascending lower extremity contrast venography remains the "gold standard" test for documentation of the presence or absence of lower limb thrombosis in well-designed, prospective randomized trials. Its technique has been improved by recent improvements in contrast media and refinements in methodology. Interpretation of venograms must be performed by a central committee of experts. However, results observed with the same dosage of compound have varied considerably across clinical trials. Such variations have been attributed to differences in samples of patients, but also in the manner in which committees of experts "interpret" this objective investigation, and significant inter-observer variability is observed. Also criteria used for radiologic diagnosis of DVT are not always the same, nor is the use of unilateral or bilateral venographies. Finally, a center-related and country-related effect have been described. As previously stated for varible safety outcomes, only placebo-controlled trials can determine the absolute risk reduction afforded by a compound. These wide variations, in our opinion, can lead to flaws in simple meta-analysis.

Objective diagnosis of pulmonary embolism (PE) has changed considerably, since the publication of the PIOPED study (1). With regard to ventilation and perfusion scintigraphic lung scans, only normal results which can exclude a PE, or a high probability scan which can confirm it, must be considered in clinical trials. Pulmonary angiography, an invasive method, remains the "gold standard" for the diagnosis of PE, but in the future, could be supplanted by generalization of spiral CT chest scan. Thus, objective confirmation of a PE is now perfectly reliable for all patients, regardless of their PIOPED classification.

Similarly, objective diagnosis of symptomatic DVT has also improved. Non-invasive duplex-ultrasound examination has demonstrated quite acceptable sensitivity and specificity, compared to venography. Thus, the general impression is that at last we now have at our disposal methods of investigation for venous thromboembolism which allow for the conduct of clinical research with strong scientific basis.

This indisputable scientific advance should not conceal the problems which remain to be solved. Diagnosis of venous thromboembolism based on coagulation tests in these patients at high risk has been disappointing. But increasing knowledge and understanding of thrombophilia has emerged. A number of new biological risk factors for thrombosis have been discovered. In our day-to-day practice, such disorders are relatively rare, but require thorough preoperative evaluation of the patient to rule them out.

Prophylaxis of venous thromboembolism in orthopedics continues to be imperfect and a number of patients are discharged from the hospital with a DVT. Though the vast majority of these DVTs will resolve spontaneously, some will extend and give rise to late, symptomatic venous thromboembolism, including fatal PE and post-thrombotic syndrome.

Moreover, well-conducted, placebo-controlled trials have provided venographic evidence of the extended risk for venous thromboembolic disease after hospital discharge. At least 20% of patients with negative venograms on discharge may develop late DVTs. This observation has led to the concept of extended prophylaxis. But this concept must be defined more precisely and no consensus is possible at the present time. Current recommendations for duration of prophylaxis after orthopedic surgery vary from 12 to 15 up to 90 postoperative days.

Finally, the main bone of contention is that venographically-detected DVTs are only a marker of disease, a "surrogate endpoint". The important clinical outcome continues to be sudden death from fatal PE or symptomatic DVT or PE with the risk of recurrence and late complications. Thus, new trials based on these clinical endpoints are necessary to define mortality and morbidity associated with the use of these compounds, and their possible reduction with extended prophylaxis.

New prospects for the next decade include research on new drugs, possibly including more effective ultra- LMWHs. Currently, a pentasaccharide, a pure anti-factor Xa inhibitor, obtained by chemical synthesis, has demonstrated promising results. Recombinant hirudin, desirudin, has demonstrated better efficacy than LMWH in one clinical trial using the "gold standard" test, venography, as its primary efficacy outcome measure. New anti-factor IIa oral inhibitors are under development and could provide an elegant solution to this complex, multi-factorial disease. The task we are faced with is daunting and so research in this field must continue.

REFERENCE

(1) The PIOPED Investigators. Value of the Ventilation/perfusion scan in acute pulmonary embolism : results of the Prospective Investigation of Pulmonary Embolism Diagnosis (PIOPED).JAMA 1990 ; 263 : 2753-2759.

JACQUES R. LECLERC. *LMWHs and duration of prophylaxis in arthroplastic surgery*

The optimal duration of prophylaxis after arthroplastic surgery of the lower extremity, and possibly other high risk surgical sub-groups, is unknown. This controversy revolves around the clinical significance of residual venous thrombi after in-hospital prophylaxis and those who arise de novo over the ensuing weeks.

Most thromboprophylaxis studies in arthroplastic surgery have relied on pre-discharge venography for the assessment of efficacy, thus allowing residual thrombi to be detected and treated (1). The most efficacious regimens are associated with rates of residual thrombosis of approximately 20% and 30% in hip and knee arthroplasty patients, respectively (2-9). Approximately one-quarter of residual thrombi in hip and one-third of those in knee patients involve the proximal veins. Pre-discharge venography is not commonly performed in routine practice and screening compression ultrasonography is insensitive to the usually asymptomatic post-operative thrombi (10,11). The issue is further compounded by the fact that patients have increasingly shorter hospital stays. Thus, it is likely that in routine practice, a significant number of patients are discharged with residual deep vein thrombi, some of them involving the proximal veins.

Recent studies have shown that de novo thrombi occur during the first few weeks following discharge and that their incidence can be reduced by continuing out prophylaxis after discharge (12-14). In these trials, patients who underwent hip replacement received initial low molecular weight heparin prophylaxis. Upon discharge, they were randomized to continue prophylaxis for three to four weeks or to discontinue it. Venography was performed at the end of the three to four weeks period. All three studies showed a significant reduction in the incidence of late deep vein thrombosis in patients who received extended prophylaxis. The majority of these thrombi, however, were asymptomatic. It is unknown whether these late thrombi will increase the risk of late complications, e.g., recurrence or postphlebitic syndrome.

Two recent prospective studies have focused on the clinical outcome of arthroplastic patients (11, 15). In the Canadian cohort study, 1,984 knee and hip arthroplasty patients who received in-hospital low molecular weight prophylaxis, only two percent of patients developed symptomatic venous thromboembolism post hospital discharge (15). In the Post-Arthroplasty Screening Study (PASS), totaling 1,024 patients, only one percent of patients who received in-hospital warfarin prophylaxis developed symptomatic venous thromboembolism over a three-month follow-up period (11). In both the Canadian and the PASS studies, however, in-hospital prophylaxis was given for an average of nine days. Thus, the very good clincial outcome results obtained in these studies may not be directly applicable to patients who receive shorter prophylaxis courses.

In conclusion:

1. Two prospective studies totaling approximately 3,000 patients suggest that patients who have received in-hospital prophylaxis for an average nine days have a very favorable clinical outcome at three months.

2. The clinical significance of the mostly asymptomatic residual venous thrombi or those which arise *de novo*, is unknown. Further studies with longer patient follow-up will be needed in this area.

REFERENCES

1. Mohr D, Silverstein M, Murtaugh P, Harrison J. Prophylactic agents for venous thrombosis in elective hip surgery. Meta-analysis of studies using venographic assessment. Arch. Intern Med. 1993 ;153 :2221-8.

2. Nurmohamed MT, Rosendaal FS, Buller HR, Dekker E, Hommes DW, Vandenbroucke JP et al. Low-molecular weight heparin versus standard heparin in general and orthopedic surgery : a meta-analysis.Lancet 1992 ;340 :152-6.

3. Leizorovicz A, Haugh MC, Chapuis FR, Samama MM, Boissel JP. Low molecular weight heparin in prevention of perioperative thrombosis. Br Med J. 1992; 305 :913-20.

4. Hull R, Raskob G, Pineo G, Rosenbloom D, Evans W, Mallory T, et al. A comparison of subcutaneous low-molecular weight heparin with warfarin sodium for prophylaxis against deep-vein thrombosis after hip or knee implantation. N Engl J Med 1993 ;329 :1370-6.

5. Jorgensen LN, Wille-Jorgensen P, Hauch O. Prophylaxis of postoperative thromboembolism with low molecular weigh heparins. Br J Surg. 1993 ;80 :689-704.

6. The RD Heparin Arthroplasty Group. RD heparin compared with warfarin for prevention of venous thromboembolic disease following total hip or knee arthroplasty. J Bone Joint Surg (Am) 1994;76:1174-85.

7. Leclerc JR, Geerts WH, Desjardins L, Laflamme GH, l'Espérance B, Demers C, et al. Prevention of Venous Thromboembolism after Knee Arthroplasty - A Randomised, Double-Blind Trial Comparing Enoxaparin to Warfarin. Ann Intern Med 1996;124:619-26.

8. Heit JA, Berkowitz SD, Bona R, Cabanas V, Corson JD, Elliott CG, et al. Efficacy and safety of low-molecular weight heparin (ardeparin sodium) compared to warfarin for the prevention of venous thromboembolism after total knee replacement surgery : a double-blind, dose-ranging study. Thromb Haemostas. 1997;77:32-8.

9. Erikson BI, Wille-Jorgensen P, Kalebo P, Mouret P, Rosencher N, Bosch P, et al. A comparison of recombinant hirudin with a low-molecular-weight-heparin to prevent thromboembolic complications after total hip replacement. New Engl J Med 1997;337:1329-35.

10. Ascani A, Radicchia S, Parise P, Nenci GG, Agnelli G. Distribution and occlusiveness of thrombi in patients with surveillance detected deep vein thrombosis after hip surgery. Thromb. Haemostas. 1996;75:239-41.

11. Robinson KS, Anderson DR, Gross M, Petrie D, Leighton R, Stanish W, et al. Ultrasonographic screening before hospital discharge for deep venous thrombosis after arthroplasty : the post-arthroplasty screening study. A randomized, controlled trial. Ann Intern Med. 1997;127:439-45.

12. Planes A, Vochelle N, Darmon JY, Fagola M, Bellaud M, Huet Y. Risk of deep-venous thrombosis after hospital discharge in patients having undergone total hip replacement : double-blind randomized comparison of enoxaparin versus placebo. Lancet 1996 ;348 :224-8.

13. Dahl OE, Andreassen G, Aspelin T, Muller C, Mathiesen P, Nyhus S, et al. Prolonged thromboprophylaxis following hip replacement surgery - Results of a double-blind, prospective, randomised, placebo-controlled study with dalteparin (Fragmin). Thromb Haemostas. 1997;77:26-31.

14. Bergqvist D, Benoni G, Bjorgell O, Fredin H, Hedlundh U, Nicolas S. et al. Low-molecular weight heparin (enoxaparin) as prophylaxis against venous thromboembolism after total hip replacement. New Engl J Med.1996;35:696-700.

15. Leclerc JR, Gent M, Hirsh J, Ginsberg JS, Geerts, WH. The incidence of symptomatic venous thromboembolism during and after prophylaxis with enoxaparin : A multi-institutional cohort study in patients who underwent hip or knee arthroplasty. Arch Intern Med 1998;158:873-878.

3.3
Prophylaxis
of venous thromboembolism
in traumatology

Prevention of deep vein thrombosis in patients with hip fractures: low molecular weight heparin versus dextran

AUTHORS	OERTLI D., HESS P., DÜRIG M. et al.
REF	World J. Surg. 1992; 16: 980-985

STUDY	Open-label, randomized
CENTERS (n)	1
COUNTRY	Switzerland
PATIENTS (n)	*randomized* 216
	evaluated 198

TYPE OF SURGERY
Fractures of the femoral neck treated by cemented bipolar endoprosthesis (53%), dynamic hip screw (42%)

ANESTHESIA
Regional 85%, general 15%

STUDY DRUG   **Certoparin**   sc daily dose: 3000 AXa IU o.d.
first injection: preop (time not stated)
treatment duration: 10 days

REFERENCE DRUG   **Dextran 70**   route iv:
• 500ml during surgery
• 500ml 8h and 24h postop
• 500ml on D5 (if incomplete mobilization)

ASSESSMENTS
❏ Isotopic DVT (FUT) every day for 7 days. If positive, duplex scanning or venography.
❏ Bleeding complications.
❏ PE.
❏ Death.

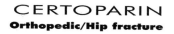

OERTLI D. et al. 1992

	Certoparin 3000 AXa IU x 1		Dextran		p
Patients	113		103		
FUT (complete screening)	103		95		
Total DVT	16	15.5%	31	32.6%	<0.005
Proximal DVT	2	1.9%	1	1.1%	NS
PE	2 (1 fatal)		2 (2 fatal)*		
Wound hematomas	2		5		NS
Mortality at D30	10	8.8%	6	5.8%	NS

* One at D14 and one fatal fat embolism several hours after surgery.

COMMENTS

❑ Certoparin 3000 IU daily was effective and well tolerated and showed a better thromboprophylactic effect than dextran 70.

❑ The very low rate of proximal DVT is probably related to failure to obtain routine venography.

❑ Mortality in these patients mainly due to cardiac failure or myocardial infarction.

Thromboprophylaxis
with low molecular weight heparin in outpatients
with plaster-cast immobilisation of the leg

AUTHORS	KOCK H-J., SCHMIT-NEUERBURG K.P., HANKE J. et al.
REF	Lancet. 1995; 346: 459-461

STUDY	Open-label, randomized, control group
CENTERS (n)	1 for outpatients
COUNTRY	Germany
PATIENTS (n)	*included* 429
	evaluated 339

PATIENTS
Outpatients with leg injuries (sprains, fractures) managed with plaster cast

STUDY DRUG **Certoparin** sc daily dose: 0.3ml (3000 AXa IU o.d.)

first injection: just after plaster cast was applied

treatment duration: until plaster cast removed

REFERENCE DRUG **Control group**: no prophylaxis

ASSESSMENTS
- ❏ DVT: after removal of the cast, assessment by IPG, B-mode compression ultrasonography; venography if positive findings.
- ❏ Bleeding complications.

KOCK H-J. et al. 1995

	Certoparin 3000 AXa IU x 1		Control		p
Patients	176		163		
Mean duration of immobilization (days)	15		19		
DVT all patients	0	0%	7	4.3%	0.006
DVT in patients with fractures	0/38	0%	2/34	5.9%	
DVT in patients with distorsion and contusion	0/68	0%	4/54	7.4%	
Bleeding complications	4*		0		

* Minor hematomas.

COMMENT

❑ The results of this study suggested that certoparin 3000 AXa IU was effective against thrombosis in outpatients with plaster casts even though the incidence of DVT was low in control subjects.

❑ Only 21% of patients had fractures.

❑ The number of patients who had venography was not reported.

A prospective double-blind trial of a low molecular weight heparin once daily compared with convential low-dose heparin three times daily to prevent pulmonary embolism and venous thrombosis in patients with hip fracture

AUTHORS	MONREAL M., LAFOZ E., NAVARRO A. et al.
REF	J. Trauma 1989; 29: 873-875

STUDY	Randomized, double-blind		TYPE OF SURGERY	Hip fracture operated on the day of fracture
CENTERS (n)	1			
COUNTRY	Spain			
			ANESTHESIA	Not stated
PATIENTS (n)	included	96		
	evaluated	90		

STUDY DRUG	Dalteparin	sc daily dose: 5000 AXa IU o.d.
		first injection: 2h preop 2500 AXa IU
		second injection: 5000 AXa IU postop morning D1
		+ 2 placebo injections
		treatment duration: 9 days
REFERENCE DRUG	UFH	sc daily dose: 5000 IU t.i.d.
		first injection: 2h preop
		treatment duration: 9 days

ASSESSMENTS
- Ventilation/perfusion lung scan on D8 after surgery.
- Bilateral venography if suspicion of clinical thrombosis for the first 57 patients.
- Bilateral venography routinely for the next 33 patients on D9.
- Bleeding complications.

MONREAL M. et al. 1989

	Dalteparin 5000 AXa IU x 1		UFH 5000 IU x 3		p
Patients	46		44		
PE lung scan					
high probability	6	1.3%	0	0%	0.02
indeterminate	8		6		NS
normal	30		36		
Venography performed	32		30		
Total DVT	14/32	43.7%	6/30	20.0%	0.04
Proximal DVT	12	37.5%	5	16.7%	NS
Wound hematomas	2		2		NS
Intestinal bleeding	2		1		NS
Death	2		3		NS

COMMENTS

❑ Low-dose heparin patients had significantly fewer DVT and PE than those given dalteparin.

❑ No lung scan at D0.

❑ Venography was performed in 69% of patients.

The thromboprophylactic effect
of a low-molecular-weight heparin (Fragmin)
in hip fracture surgery. A placebo-controlled study

AUTHORS	JORGENSEN P.S., KNUDSEN J.B., BROENG L. et al.
REF	Clin. Orthop. 1992; 278: 95-100

STUDY	Randomized, double-blind	
CENTERS (n)	1	
COUNTRY	Denmark	
PATIENTS (n)	*included*	82
	evaluated	68

TYPE OF SURGERY
Hip replacement

ANESTHESIA
general ≈ 60%
spinal ≈ 40%
combined ≈ 3%

STUDY DRUG	**Dalteparin**	sc daily dose: 5000 AXa IU o.d. (D1-D7)
		first injection: 2h preop 2500 AXa IU (DO)
		second injection: 12h postop 2500 AXa IU (DO)
		treatment duration: 7 days
REFERENCE DRUG	**Placebo**	saline sc: 0.2ml o.d.
		treatment duration: 7 days

ASSESSMENTS
❑   DVT: FUT on D1, 3, 5, 7, 9; if positive, venography.
❑   Bleeding complications.
❑   PE (assessment not stated).
❑   Clinical follow-up: 6 to 12 weeks postop.

JORGENSEN P.S. et al. 1992

	Dalteparin 5000 AXa IU x 1		Placebo		p
Patients	30		38		
DVT	9	30%	22	≈ 58%	<0.03
PE	0		1		
Bleeding in drainage (ml)	58		100		NS
Transfusion (g erythrocytes)	915		605		< 0.05
Hb difference (D7-D1)	−0.45		−0.90		NS
Death	3		4 (1 PE)		

COMMENTS

❑ The prophylactic dalteparin regimen (5000 IU) has significantly reduced the rate of postsurgical DVT, even though the incidence remained high.

❑ 46% of patients had venography and only 34% of patients had adequate venography.

❑ False positive FUT tests not addressed.

❑ This trial did not distinguish between distal and proximal DVT.

❑ Compared to placebo group, the tolerance regarding bleeding was good.

A comparison of low-dose heparin with low-molecular-weight heparin as prophylaxis against venous thromboembolism after major trauma

AUTHORS	GEERTS W.H., JAY R.M., CODE K.I. et al.
REF	N. Eng. J. Med. 1996; 335: 701-707

STUDY	Randomized, double-blind
CENTERS *(n)*	1
COUNTRY	Canada
PATIENTS *(n)*	*randomized* 344
	evaluated 265

PATIENTS
- Patients with injury severity score ≥ 9 (mean 23)
- Spinal cord injury 5%, lower extremity fracture 54%
- Surgery in 85% of patients
- Patients with intracranial bleeding excluded

STUDY DRUG	Enoxaparin	sc daily dose: 30mg b.i.d.
		first injection: within 36h of the injury
		treatment duration: up to 14 days

REFERENCE DRUG	UFH	sc daily doses: 5000 IU b.i.d.
		first injection: within 36h of the injury
		treatment duration: up to 14 days

ASSESSMENTS
- ❑ DVT: bilateral venography at D10-D14.
- ❑ Clinical PE confirmed by lung scan.
- ❑ Major hemorrhage.

GEERTS W.H. et al. 1996

	Enoxaparin 30mg x 2		UFH 5000 IU x 2		p
Patients (with evaluable venograms)	129		136		
Total DVT	40	31.0%	60	44.1%	0.014
Proximal DVT	8	6.2%	20	14.7%	0.012
Patients with leg fractures:	80		88		
Total DVT	31	38.8%	43	48.9%	NS
Proximal DVT	4	5.0%	16	18.2%	0.01
Patients without leg fractures:	49		48		
Total DVT	9	18.4%	17	35.4%	NS
Proximal DVT	4	8.2%	4	8.3%	NS
Major hemorrhage	5	2.9%	1	0.6%	NS
PE	1 (non fatal)		0		

COMMENTS

❑ Enoxaparin 30mg b.i.d. was significantly more effective than UFH 5000 IU b.i.d. in patients with leg fractures for proximal DVT; even though the results were not statistically significant, there was a trend in favor of LMWH in the reduction of total DVT.

❑ Two patients treated with UFH developed heparin-induced thrombocytopenia and symptomatic DVT.

❑ LMWH seems to be an effective prophylaxis method for most trauma patients without intracranial bleeding.

Incidence and prophylaxis
of deep veinous thrombosis in outpatients with injury
of the lower limb

AUTHORS	KUJATH P., SPANNAGEL V., HABSCHEID W.
REF	Haemostasis 1993; 23 (suppl. 1): 20-26

STUDY	Open-label, randomized		
CENTERS (n)	1		
COUNTRY	Germany		
PATIENTS (n)	*included*	306	
	evaluated	253	

PATIENTS

Young outpatients (mean age 33± 14 years) with leg injuries (soft tissue 70%; fracture 30%) managed nonoperatively with plaster casts

STUDY DRUG	**Nadroparin**	sc daily dose: 0.3ml (≈ 3000 AXa IU) o.d.
		first injection: D1
		treatment duration: until removal of plaster cast (mean 16D)
REFERENCE DRUG	**No prophylaxis**	

ASSESSMENTS

❑ DVT: compression ultrasound (CUS) of thigh and calf veins when plaster cast was removed, or if DVT clinically suspected

❑ If CUS positive or non diagnostic, venography.

❑ Relationship between DVT and individual risk factors.

KUJATH P. et al. 1993

	Nadroparin 0.3ml x 1		No prophylaxis		p
	DVT/patients		DVT/patients		
Total DVT	6/126	4.8%	21/127	16.5%	<0.05
DVT with soft tissue injuries	2/87	2.4%	10/89	11.3%	<0.05
DVT with fractures	4/39	10.3%	11/38	29.0%	<0.05
Treatment duration* (days ± SD)	15.6± 6.8		15.8± 9.8		
PE	0		1**		

* Or removal of plaster cast.
** Clinical symptoms not confirmed.

COMMENTS

❏ 70% had casts for soft tissue injuries only.

❏ Once daily LMWH regimen was associated with a reduced risk of DVT without any complications in these patients.

❏ Risk factors for thrombosis included: presence of fracture, age > 40 y, obesity and varicose veins.

Thromboembolic prophylaxis in orthopaedic trauma patients: a comparison between a fixed dose and an individually adjusted dose of a low molecular weight heparin (nadroparin calcium)

AUTHORS	HAENTJENS P. and the Belgian Fraxiparine study group
REF	Injury. 1996; 27: 385-390

STUDY	Open-label, multicenter, randomized, comparison of two dosage regimens
CENTERS (n)	29
COUNTRY	Belgium
PATIENTS (n)	*randomized* 283
	evaluated 215 at D10
	150 at week 6

PATIENTS

Spinal, pelvic or lower extremity fractures (51% with hip fracture)
Surgery for ≈ 87% of randomized patients with general anesthesia (≈ 73%) or loco-regional anesthesia (≈ 27%)

STUDY DRUG **Nadroparin** sc daily dose comparing

1) fixed dose 3075 AXa IU (0.3ml) versus
2) BW-adjusted dose (Leyvraz's schema):
   ≈ 40 AXa IU/kg from D0 to D3 after surgery
   ≈ 60 AXa IU/kg from D4 after surgery

first injection: within 8h of injury

treatment duration: up to 6 weeks

ASSESSMENTS

❑ DVT: duplex ultrasound or impedance plethysmography at D10 and week 6. If positive, bilateral venography.

❑ Clinical PE confirmed by lung scan or angiography.

❑ Major hemorrhage and other complications.

HAENTJENS P. et al. 1996

	Nadroparin x 1	
	Fixed dose	B.W.-adjusted dose
Patients	142	141
Evaluable patients for efficacy		
At D10	106	109
At week 6	76	74
DVT at D10	0 0%	3 2.8%
DVT at week 6	1 1.3%	4 5.4%
PE	1	2 (1 fatal)
DVT + PE	2 2.6%	6 8.1%
Major hemorrhage	5	5
Thrombocytopenia	1 (D10)	1 (D3)
Death	8	4

COMMENTS

- ❑ Recruitment only 5 patients/center/year.
- ❑ 24% post-randomization drop-outs.
- ❑ Only 53% of patients had 6-week screening for DVT.
- ❑ The remarkably low incidence of DVT was probably the combined result of inaccurate screening tests and large proportion of not screened patients. DVT occurred in patients with hip surgery and increased with age.
- ❑ This study suggests that there may be no advantage to individual dosing.

Low molecular weight heparin (Alfa LMWH) compared with unfractionated heparin in prevention of deep vein thrombosis after hip fractures

AUTHORS	PINI M., TAGLIAFERRI A., MANOTTI C. et al.
REF	Int. Angiol. 1989; 8: 134-139

STUDY	Open-label, randomized		TYPE OF SURGERY
			Fracture of femoral neck
CENTERS (n)	1		
COUNTRY	Italy		ANESTHESIA
			Not stated
PATIENTS (n)	included	70	
	randomized	49	
	evaluated	49	

STUDY DRUG	Parnaparin	sc daily doses: 7500 AXa U b.i.d.
		(corresponding to ≈ 3200 AXa IU b.i.d.)
		first injection: as soon as possible and before surgery
		treatment duration: up to 14 days

REFERENCE DRUG	UFH	sc daily doses: 5000 IU t.i.d.
		first injection: as soon as possible and before surgery
		treatment duration: up to 14 days

ASSESSMENTS

- ❏ FUT x 7D and strain-gange plethysmography on D14; if positive, venography.
- ❏ PE: clinical symptoms.
- ❏ Bleeding complications.
- ❏ Laboratory tests (not reported).

PINI M. et al. 1989

	LMWH 7500 AXa U x 2		UFH 5000 IU x 3		p
Patients	25		24		
Total DVT	5	20.0%	7	29.2%	NS
Proximal DVT	2	8.0%	1	4.2%	NS
PE	0		1		NS
Death	0		2		
Bleeding complications	No difference				

COMMENTS

❏ Similar results for parnaparin and UFH, but unblinded study with a sample size too small to conclude that the interventions are equivalent.

❏ No routine venography.

Prevention of thromboembolism
in spinal cord injury:
role of low molecular weight heparin

AUTHORS	GREEN D., CHEN D., CHMIEL J. et al.
REF	Arch. Phys. Med. Rehabil. 1994; 75: 290-292

STUDY	Open-label and retrospective	
CENTERS (n)	1	
COUNTRY	United States	
PATIENTS (n)	*included*	60
	evaluated	48

PATIENTS

Acute spinal cord injury with complete motor paralysis

STUDY DRUG **Tinzaparin** sc daily dose: 3500 AXa IU o.d.

first injection ≤ 72h post injury; if surgery, after operation

treatment duration: 8 weeks

REFERENCE DRUG **Retrospective historical studies**

ASSESSMENTS

❏ Daily clinical symptoms for DVT, PE, bleeding.

❏ Color Doppler ultrasonography at week 8 and then weekly x 4 if negative.

❏ If suspicion of thromboembolism, venography and/or lung scan/angiography.

❏ Comparison with previous UFH experiences.

GREEN D. et al. 1994

	Tinzaparin 3500 AXa IU x 1		UFH Historical retrospective*	
Eight-week follow-up *(with prophylaxis)*				
Patients who completed full period or had an event	48		79	
Total DVT	6	13%	16	20%
Proximal DVT	4	8%		
Major bleeding	1		9	
PE	2 (1 fatal)	4%	2 (fatal)	2.5%
Post 8-week follow-up *(prophylaxis discontinued)*				
Patients	33			
Total DVT	1			
PE	1 (fatal)			

* 29 patients received UFH 5000 IU x 2; 21 patients received 5000 IU x 3; 29 patients with adjusted doses.

COMMENTS

❑ 20% of patients dropped out of the study before week 8.

❑ In this retrospective analysis, tinzaparin compared favorably with UFH and appeared to be safer, but no direct comparison to control.

Expert comments

WILLIAM H. GEERTS. *Prophylaxis of DVT in hip fracture/trauma*

Hip fracture patients and trauma patients have a number of features in common. Both groups have experienced a traumatic insult, both are at increased risk of venous thromboembolism and, in both situations, there are very few methodologically-sound clinical trials to guide prophylaxis decisions. However, major differences exist between these two groups:

1. While the vast majority of hip fracture patients are older than age 65, the mean age of trauma patients is in the 30s.

2. Most hip fracture patients are female while the majority of trauma patients are male.

3. Hip fracture is generally an isolated injury while many trauma patients have had multiple injuries affecting more than one body system.

4. Many hip fracture patients have pre-existing medical conditions while the overwhelming majority of trauma patients are healthy prior to the injury.

5. Without prophylaxis, the thrombosis risk is relatively uniform across hip fracture patient groups (50-60 %). The spectrum of thrombosis risk in trauma is much more variable with rates from < 10 % to > 80 % depending on which trauma subgroup is studied.

6. The risk of bleeding in hip fracture patients is largely confined to the operative site while trauma patients with head or pelvic injuries or injuries involving the liver or spleen have the additional potential for bleeding at these and other sites.

For all of these reasons, hip fracture patients and those with major or minor trauma should be considered as distinct risk groups.

Hip Fracture

Hip fracture patients are clearly at high risk for venous thromboembolism [Clagett,1995]. In prospective studies with objective outcome measures and in which prophylaxis was not used, the pooled rates of DVT, proximal DVT, and fatal pulmonary embolism are 54% (377/697), 30% (91/305), and 2.4% (10/417), respectively. Among hip fracture patients who have not received prophylaxis, PE is the most common cause of death within the first month after surgery.

In addition to the injury itself and its subsequent surgical repair, the factors that increase the thromboembolic risk in hip fracture patients include age, delayed admission following fracture, and use of a general anesthetic. There is less certainty about the role of other factors, including the site of the fracture, the specific surgical procedure, and patient mobility, in modifying the DVT rates. DVT is most commonly ipsilateral to the fracture although up to 30% of patients have bilateral or contralateral thrombosis [Monreal, 1989; Oertli, 1992]. In 8-19% of hip fracture patients, DVT has been demonstrated preoperatively [Freeark, 1967; Roberts, 1990].

The first important observation about thromboprophylaxis studies in hip fracture is the poor accuracy of noninvasive testing [Moskovitz, 1978; Pini, 1989; Fauno, 1990; Oertli, 1992; Bergqvist, 1993]. For example, in the study by Oertli (1992), 33 of the 80 patients with positive fibrinogen leg scans (41%) did not have DVT by venography and none of the 57 patients with abnormal scans in the proximal thigh had DVT. Other studies have confirmed the poor accuracy of noninvasive diagnostic tests, including fibrinogen leg scanning, impedance plethysmography, and Doppler-ultrasound, for asymptomatic DVT in orthopedic surgery patients [Cruickshank, 1989;Wells; l995; Magnusson, 1996; Lensing, 1997]. Routine bilateral contrast venography remains the screening modality of choice for high risk (orthopedic and trauma) patients undergoing thromboprophylaxis trials [Bergqvist, 1993; Agnelli, l995]. Unfortunately, none of the hip fracture studies reviewed in this chapter utilized this outcome measure.

The available prophylaxis trials in patients with hip fracture suggest that LMWH is significantly more efficacious than placebo in preventing DVT [Jorgensen, 1992] and more effective than dextran [Oertli, 1992] or aspirin [Gent, 1996]. The only two studies that directly compared LMWH to LDH did not resolve the relative protection of these agents [Monreal, 1989; Pini, 1989]. The trial by Monreal found that heparin 5000 U TID was significantly more efficacious than dalteparin 5000 U once daily [Monreal, 1989] while the small study by Pini failed to show a difference between heparin 5000 U TID and parnaparin 3200 AXa IU BID [Pini, 1989].

Prophylaxis trials in elective hip and knee arthroplasty patients demonstrate that LMWH is superior to LDH. Future studies may also confirm this observation in hip fracture patients although LDH may be more effective in hip fracture than after elective orthopedic surgery since the usual prophylactic heparin dose (10,000 or 15,000 U per day) is not "low dose" in many of these elderly, low body-weight patients [Pini, 1989].

Thromboprophylaxis is clearly warranted in hip fracture patients to reduce fatal PE, symptomatic DVT and PE, and also to avoid the significant resource expenditures associated with a failure to prevent these complications [Clagett, 1995; Todd, 1995].

Although there are few level 1 clinical trials of prophylaxis in hip fracture, the options for which there is reasonable evidence for efficacy include LMWH, warfarin and LDH. There is currently insufficient evidence to definitively recommend one option over the others in this patient population. If there will be a significant delay between admission and surgery, prophylaxis should be initiated preoperatively [Jorgensen, 1996]. The optimal duration of prophylaxis has not been resolved.

REFERENCES

Agnelli G, Radicchia S, Nenci GG: Diagnosis of deep vein thrombosis in asymptomatic high-risk patients. Haemostasis 1995;25:40-8.

Berggvist D: Endpoints for diagnosis of postoperative thromboembolism in hip fracture surgery. Semin Thromb Hemostas 1993;19(suppl 1):175-7.

Clagett GP, Anderson FA, Heit J, et al: Prevention of venous thromboembolism. Chest 1995;108(suppl):312S-334S.

Cruickshank MK, Levine MN, Hirsh J, et al: An evaluation of impedance plethysmography and l25I-fibrinogen leg scanning in patients following hip surgery. Thromb Hemostas 1989;62:830-4.

Faunø P, Suomalainen O, Bergqvist D, et al: The use of fibrinogen uptake test in screening for deep vein thrombosis in patients with hip fracture. Thromb Res 1990;60: 185-90.

Freeark RJ, Boswick J, Fardin R: Posttraumatic venous thrombosis. Arch Surg 1967;95:567-75.

Gent M, Hirsh J, Ginsberg JS, et al: Low-molecular-weight heparinoid Orgaran is more effective than aspirin in the prevention of venous thromboembolism after surgery for hip fracture. Circulation 1996;93:80-4.

Jorgensen PS, Knudsen JB, Broeng L, et al: The thromboprophylactic effect of a low molecular-weight heparin (Fragmin) in hip fracture surgery. A placebo-controlled study. Clin Orthop 1992;278:95-100.

Jorgensen PS, Strandberg C, Wille-Jorgensen P, et al: Early preoperative thromboprophylaxis with Klexane® in hip fracture surgery. A placebo controlled study. [abstract] Haemostasis 1996;26(Suppl 3):003.

Lensing AW, Doris CI, McGrath FP, et al: A comparison of compression ultrasound with color doppler ultrasound for the diagnosis of symptomless postoperative deep vein thrombosis. Arch Intern Med 1997;157:765-8.

Magnusson M, Eriksson Bl, Kalebo P, Sivertsson R: Is colour doppler ultrasound a sensitive screening method in diagnosing deep vein thrombosis after hip surgery? Thromb Haemostas 1996;75:242-5.

Monreal M, Lafoz E, Navarro A, et al: A prospective double-blind trial of a low molecular weight heparin once daily compared with conventional low-dose heparin three times daily to prevent pulmonary embolism and venous thrombosis in patients with hip fracture. J Trauma 1989;29:873-5.

Moskovitz PA, Ellenberg SS, Feffer HL, et al: Low-dose heparin for prevention of venous thromboembolism in total hip arthroplasty and surgical repair of hip fractures. J Bone Joint Surg 1978;60-A: 1065-70.

Oertli D, Hess P, Durig M, et al: Prevention of deep vein thrombosis in patients with hip fractures: low molecular weight heparin versus dextran. World J Surg 1992;16:980-5.

Pini M, Tagliaferri A, Manotti C, et al: Low molecular weight heparin (Alfa LMWH) compared with unfractionated heparin in prevention of deep-vein thrombosis after hip fractures. International Angiology 1989;8: 134-9.

Roberts TS, Nelson CL, Barnes CL, et al: The preoperative prevalence and postoperative incidence of thromboembolism in patients with hip fractures treated with dextran prophylaxis. Clin Orthop 1990;255: 198-203.

Todd CJ, Freeman CJ, Camilleri-Ferrante C, et al: Differences in mortality after fracture of hip: the East Anglia audit. BMJ 1995;310:904-8.

Wells PS, Lensing AW, Davidson BL, et al: Accuracy of ultrasound for the diagnosis of deep venous thrombosis in asymptomatic patients after orthopedic surgery. Ann Intern Med 1995,122:47-53.

Trauma

Venous thromboembolism also occurs very commonly in trauma patients. The epidemiology of thromboembolism in these patients was evaluated by means of a prospective study in which routine contrast venography was performed in 443 major trauma patients who did not receive thromboprophylaxis [Geerts, 1994]. The incidence of DVT was 58% while proximal DVT was present in 18% of patients. Although the majority of thrombi that develop in trauma (as in other risk groups) are asymptomatic, PE is the third most common cause of death occurring more than 24 hours after injury. The incidence of fatal PE following trauma is in the range of 0.5% to 3.0% [Geerts, 1994; Sevitt, 1961].

The factors which independently interact to increase the risk of DVT in major trauma include the age of the patient, the presence of a spinal cord injury, lower extremity fracture, or femoral venous line, the need for a surgical procedure, and the duration of immobility [Geerts, 1994] .

Among patients with isolated lower extremity injuries, the incidence of DVT by contrast venography has been found to range from 30% to 45% [Hjelmstedt 1968; Abelseth, 1996] while lower extremity fractures in major trauma patients are associated with a venographic incidence of DVT of 60-80 % [Geerts,1994] .

Routine use of thromboprophylaxis in trauma was first recommended more than 50 years ago although prospective studies in this patient group have only been conducted within the past decade [Bauer, 1944]. While mechanical methods of DVT prophylaxis are commonly used in trauma, there is little evidence supporting the protection of these modalities. In fact, the bulk of the data suggests that intermittent pneumatic compression devices are no better than no prophylaxis in these patients (except possibly in those with isolated major intracranial trauma).

A double-blind randomized trial of 344 major trauma patients recently compared heparin 5000 U SC BID with the low molecular weight heparin, enoxaparin 30 mg SC BID, using contrast venography on or before day 14 as the primary outcome measure [Geerts, 1996]. All study patients commenced the study drug within 36 hours of their injury and none received concomitant mechanical prophylaxis. Enoxaparin was found to be significantly more efficacious than LDH for all DVT (risk reduction 30%) and for proximal DVT (risk reduction 58%). In both groups, major bleeding was seen in less than 3% of patients and was not significantly different between groups. There is considerable additional data demonstrating the lack of protection afforded by LDH in trauma [Upchurch, 1995].

Further support for the use of LMWH comes from two randomized trials in outpatients with isolated lower extremity injuries [Kujath, 1993; Kock, 1995]. In both studies, prophylactic LMWH resulted in significant reductions in DVT, detected by duplex ultrasound, compared with the control groups. The study by Haentjens et al, which compared prophylaxis with nadroparin, given either as a fixed-dose or as a body-weight adjusted dose in orthopedic trauma patients, suggests that there may be no advantage for individualized dosing of LMWH in trauma [Haentjens, 1996].

Thromboprophylaxis should be a mandatory component of the care of major trauma patients including those with spinal cord injuries. Currently, the prophylaxis method of choice for the majority of trauma patients is subcutaneous low molecular weight heparin, started when primary hemostasis has occurred. Patients with frank intracranial bleeding or uncontrolled bleeding elsewhere should have the LMWH prophylaxis delayed until there is no further evidence of bleeding. Although the optimal duration of prophylaxis is not known for these patients, it should probably continue at least until hospital discharge. If trauma patients require rehabilitation, prophylaxis should continue in this phase as well.

Conclusion

The studies of LMWH in hip fracture and trauma reviewed in this chapter illustrate the poor quality of evidence for prophylaxis in these two important patient groups. Clearly, more methodologically-rigorous trials are urgently needed to guide our decisions about thromboprophylaxis in these patients. In the meantime, however, LMWH should be considered the prophylaxis method of choice for these high risk populations based on the available evidence from studies in these two patient groups and from data derived from other, related patient groups.

REFERENCES:

Abelseth G, Buckley RE, Pineo GE, et al: Incidence of deep-vein thrombosis in patients with fractures of the lower extremity distal to the hip. J Orthop Trauma 1996;10: 230-5.

Bauer G: Thrombosis following leg injuries. Acta Chir Scand 1944;90:229-48.

Geerts WH, Code KI, Jay RM, et al: A prospective study of venous thromboembolism after major trauma. N Engl J Med 1994;331: 1601-6.

Geerts WH, Jay RM, Code KI, et al; A comparison of low-dose heparin with low molecular-weight heparin as prophylaxis against venous thromboembolism after major trauma. N Engl J Med 1996;335:701-7.

Haentjens P and The Belgian Fraxiparine Study Group: Thromboembolic prophylaxis in orthopaedic trauma patients: a comparison between a fixed dose and an individually adjusted dose of a low molecular weight heparin (nadroparin calcium). Injury 1996;27:385-90.

Hjelmstedt U, Bergvall U: Phlebographic study of the incidence of thrombosis in the injured and uninjured limb in 55 cases of tibial fracture. Acta Chir Scand 1968; 134:229-34.

Kock H-J, Schmit-Neuerberg KP, Hanke J, et al: Thromboprophylaxis with low molecular-weight heparin in outpatients with plaster-cast immobilisation of the leg. Lancet 1995;346:459-61.

Kujath P, Spannagel U, Habscheid W: Incidence and prophylaxis of deep venous thrombosis in outpatients with injury of the lower limb. Haemostasis 1993;23 (Suppl 1):20-6.

Sevitt S, Gallagher N: Venous thrombosis and pulmonary embolism. A clinico pathological study in injured and burned patients. Br J Surg 1961;48:475-89.

Upchurch GR, Demling RH, Davies J, et al: Efficacy of subcutaneous heparin in prevention of venous thromboembolic events in trauma patients. Am Surg 1995; 61 :749-55.

MANUEL MONREAL. *Prophylaxis of thromboembolic events in traumatology*

Venous thromboembolism (VTE) is a common, life-threatening complication of major trauma. Autopsy studies have found deep vein thrombosis in the majority of fatally injured patients while pulmonary embolism is the third most common cause of death in patients who survive the first 24 hours (1). A consensus panel of the American College of Chest Physicians cited trauma patients as being at high risk for VTE, implying that prophylaxis with either oral anticoagulants or low molecular weight heparin (LMWH) is warranted (2).

However, there is a paucity of information documenting the safety and efficacy of VTE prophylaxis in patients with major trauma. Such data would be invaluable, since trauma patients with central nervous system injury or abdominal injury may have an absolute contraindication to the use of anticoagulant prophylaxis. Therefore, a knowledge of the factors that might increase the "relative" risk of VTE would be beneficial in allowing the clinician to make judgements regarding the need for prophylaxis. Geerts et al recently reported the results of a prospective study of VTE in 349 patients with trauma (3). Deep venous thrombosis was found by contrast venography in 58% of the patients. The factors associated with an increased risk of thrombosis included increasing age, surgery, blood transfusion, fracture of the femur or tibia, and spinal cord injury. In another study, we found preoperative platelet count levels to be associated to an increased risk of postoperative pulmonary embolism in a series of 459 consecutive patients operated on because of either hip fracture or elective hip replacement (4).

Of the possible prophylaxis options, graduated-compression stockings and intermittent pneumatic compression have limited efficacy and cannot be used in many patients with leg fractures (because of the presence of lower extremity plaster immobilizers, traction, or external fixators). Oral anticoagulants have several disadvantages: they have a delayed onset of action, require regular laboratory monitoring, have effects difficult to reverse in the event of a surgical procedure, and create concern about the risk of bleeding. The alternatives are either unfractionated heparin or LMWH.

Several studies have compared the effectiveness and safety of LMWH with that of either unfractionated heparin or no prophylaxis in patients with trauma. All studies comparing LMWH with no prophylaxis found a significantly higher VTE rate in patients without the drug. As to the studies comparing LMWH with unfractionated heparin, the results have been contradictory. The variability in the reported findings may be due to the methods used to make the diagnosis of VTE and to differences in LMWH dosage. In our opinion, further studies are needed to clearly demonstrate if LMWHs may be considered superior to unfractionated heparin in trauma patients.

REFERENCES

(1) SEVITT S., GALLAGHER N. Venous thrombosis and pulmonary embolism: a clinico-pathological study in injured and burned patients. Br. J. Surg. 1961; 48 : 475-489.

(2) CLAGET G.P., ANDERSON F.A., HEIT J., LEVINE M.N., WHEELER H.B. Prevention of venous thromboembolism. Chest 1995; 108 : 312S-334S.

(3) GEERTS W.H., CODE K.I., JAY R.M., CHEN E., SZALAI J.P. A prospective study of venous thromboembolism after major trauma. N. Engl. J ;Med. 1994; 331 : 1601-1606.

(4) MONREAL M., LAFOZ E., ROCA J., GRANERA X., SOLER J., SALAZAR X., OLAZABAL A., BERGQVIST D. Platelet count, antiplatelet therapy and pulmonary embolism. A prospective study in patients with hip surgery. Thromb. Haemostasis 1995; 73 : 380-385.

3.4
Low molecular weight heparins and regional anesthesia

Anticoagulation and safety guidelines for regional anesthesia

ANDRÉ KHER, FRANCIS TOULEMONDE

Spinal and epidural anesthesia are being increasingly used not only in obstetric practice but also in orthopedic, abdominal or vascular surgery. The regional anesthetic management has a number of potential advantages over general anesthesia, avoiding central nervous and cardiopulmonary system depression, and has been associated with a lower risk of deep vein thrombosis (see review by Prins H. and Hirsh J.).

Such anesthetic approaches are generally safe; however, they carry the risk (even though very rare, less than 1/100,000) of spinal hematoma with progressive cord compression and consequent permanent paraplegia if the hematoma is not promptly evacuated. This risk can be probably higher if patients have concurrent coagulation disorders, full dose anticoagulation -including anti-platelet therapy or recent thrombolysis.

Reports of spinal hematoma occurring spontaneously with concurrent anticoagulation have generated concern regarding the safety of LMWHs in patients undergoing regional anesthesia.

A definitive answer cannot be assumed since according to G. Lowe "This concern is a theoretical one". Therefore, this author suggests the use of national registers of spinal or epidural hematoma in order "to evaluate future risk assessment and to redress the unfounded, but widespread fears of anesthetists".

Nevertheless, this risk is judged very serious since at the end of 1997 the US FDA has issued an alert to physicians warning of a serious safety problem with low molecular weight heparins, following reports of epidural or spinal hematomas, some of which have resulted in long-term or permanent paralysis in patients receiving such products in combination with spinal or epidural anesthesia.

Of the cases so far reported, about 75% of the patients were elderly women undergoing orthopedic surgery. Doctors are being told to monitor patients frequently for signs and symptoms of neurological impairment, with urgent treatment to be started if neurologic compromise is noted. The risk/benefit potential must be considered fully before epidural/spinal anesthesia is given to patients anticoagulated for thromboprophylaxis.

The FDA has asked the manufacturers of these products to incorporate a boxed warning about the risk of spinal hematoma in their package inserts.

Recently, T.T. Horlocker and J.A. Heit published pertinent guidelines for regional anesthetic management in patients receiving perioperative LMWHs, which can be summarized as follow:

• for preoperative LMWH, needle placement should occur at least 10-12h after the last dose. Subsequent dosing should be delayed for at least 2h after needle insertion.

• for postoperative LMWH, patients may safely undergo single-dose and continuous catheter technique but the timing of catheter removal should be delayed for at least 10-12h after a dose of LMWH.

Some recent publications related to this concern are reported hereafter in the references below.

REFERENCES

BERGQVIST D. et al. Risk of combining low molecular weight heparin for thromboprophylaxis and epidural or spinal anesthesia. Semin. Thromb. Haemost. 1993; 13 (Suppl) : 147-151.

HORLOCKER T.T. and HEIT J.A. Low molecular weight heparin: biochemistry, pharmacology perioperative prophylaxis regimens, and guidelines for regional anesthetic management. Anesth. Analg. 1997; 85: 874-885.

LOWE G.D.O. Low-dose anticoagulation before spinal anaesthesia: a theoretical concern. Vessel 1997; 3 : 32-34.

LUMPKIN M.M. - FDA Alert - FDA public health advisory Anesthesiology 1998; 88: 27A-28A.

PARNASS S. et al. Adverse effects of spinal and epidural anaesthesia. Drug Safety 1990; 5 : 179-194.

PRINS M.J., HIRSH J. A comparison of general anesthesia and regional anesthesia as a risk factor for deep vein thrombosis following hip surgery : a critical review. Thromb. Haemostasis 1990; 64 : 497-500.

RALLAY F. Pro: neuraxial anesthesia should not be used in patients undergoing heparinalation for surgery. J. Cardioth. Vasc. Anesth. 1996; 10 : 957-960.

TURNBULL K.W. Con: neuraxial anesthesia is useful in patients undergoing heparinization for surgery. J. Cardiothor. Vasc. Anesth. 1996; 10 : 961-962.

WILIIAMS-RUSSO P. et al. Randomized trial of epidural versus general anesthesia. Clin. Orthop. Rel. Res. 1996; 33 : 199-208.

Low molecular weight heparins and locoregional anesthesia

CHARLES MARC SAMAMA

The risk of use of locoregional anesthesia in combination with low molecular weight heparins (LMWHs) has been underestimated by North American authors and some Scandinavian investigators (1,2) even though a French consensus conference had clearly established the existence of such a risk in 1991 (3,4). A recent warning from the FDA has again called attention to this subject. A certain number of adverse events are reported to have occurred. Thus, the occurrence of an epidural or subarachnoid hematoma, the adverse events involved, cannot be ruled out.

A comprehensive review (5) of events reported (since 1906) associated with combination use of anticoagulants or platelet antiaggregants and spinal anesthesia provides an objective overview of this topic. Vandermeulen et al searched the medical literature as far back as 1906 and identified 61 such published adverse events, 42 of which were related to use of anticoagulants in a broad sense (68%). Several cases have been published or reported, before or after an injection of LMWH (6,7) and a certain number of other cases probably have not been reported. The conclusion of the European Consensus Conference of Windsor (8) ruled out such a risk with heparin but did make any pronouncement regarding the use of LMWH. It is recommended that a prospective registry for recording such complications be established. Unfortunately, an analysis of the bibliographical references for this report has not found the articles describing adverse events published since 1950 (5,9). Similarly, an editorial (2), limits the scope of risk by reporting the many series of patients published in which anesthesia in combination with thromboprophylactic heparin was well-tolerated. As stated by the Windsor conference, the author is optimistic, and does not take into account (or only very little) the adverse events previously reported. In his opinion, there does not appear to be a risk. Nevertheless, this article is counterbalanced in the same issue by another editorial by Modig (10) who reminds us, and rightly so, that careful monitoring of a patient's neurological status is essential to avoid a catastrophe caused by an epidural or subarachnoid hematoma. Indeed, a therapeutic procedure to relieve pressure on the spinal cord performed within 12 hours after the onset of the first clinical signs of such an adverse event is only effective in achieving recovery from neurological damage in half of the cases. Furthermore, Modig repeats that use of anticoagulants increases the risk and that it is solely the anesthesiologist's responsibility based on his own experience to determine a favorable benefit-to-risk ratio.

The total absence of data from the literature confirming the usefulness of a preoperative injection continues to be a topic of surprise. Could this regimen have been in use since the early 1970s without any evidence of its value? Reality is even more sobering: dozens of studies have been conducted without having confirmed the hypothesis of perioperative formation of a thrombosis. Only one historical study, in France, showed a major reduction in the incidence of DVT when calcium heparin is given by injection prior to surgery (11). Summaries of product characteristics all mention the necessity of initiating heparin therapy (standard heparin of LMWH) before surgery, but this approach needs to be reevaluated.

Very recently, a randomized, prospective, double-blind study demonstrated the lack of usefulness of the preoperative dose of heparin (12). However, even though this study showed a trend, too few patients were studied to draw a conclusion. In addition, preventive anticoagulant therapy started after spinal anesthesia appeared effective and the rate of venographic thrombosis was similar (13) to those observed when heparin is started before general anesthesia. But, in this regard, the difference between dosage regimens used in North America and those in Europe takes on major significance because with a higher dose (50% higher in Europe) in two divided injections starting 12h after surgery, the incidence of neurological adverse events appears to be higher in North America. Thus, in the final analysis, is the schedule of administration of LMWH of less importance than an increase of dosage?

REFERENCES

(1) SHARROCK N.E., BRIEN W.W., SALVATI E.A., MINEO R., GARVIN K, SCULO T.P. The effect of intravenous fixed-dose heparin during total hip arthroplasty on the incidence of deep vein thrombosis. J. Bone Joint Surg. (Am) 1990; 72 A : 1457-1461.

(2) BERGQVIST D., LINDBLAD B., MATZSCH T. Low molecular weight heparin for thromboprophylaxis and epidural/spinal anaesthesia; is there a risk? Acta. Anaesth. Scand. 1992; 36 : 605-609.

(3) Conférence de Consensus : "Prophylaxie des thromboses veineuses profondes et des embolies pulmonaires postopératoires". Assistance Publique, Paris, 8 mars 1991. AP-HP éditeur.

(4) SAMAMA C.M., BARRE J., CLERGUE F., SAMII K. Bénéfices de l'anesthésie locorégionale. Traitement anticoagulant et anesthésie locorégionale. Ann. Fr. Anesth. Réanim. 1992; 11 : 282-287.

(5) VENDERMEULEN E.P., VAN AKEN H. VERMYLEN J. Anticoagulants and spinal-epidural anesthesia. Anesth. Analg. 1994 : 79 : 1165-1177.

(6) CHOQUET O., KRIVOSIE-HORBER R., DELECROIX M., HURIAU M., PRUVO J.P. Hématome sous arachnoïdien après rachianesthésie et héparine de bas poids moléculaire. Ann. Fr. Anesth. Réanim. 1993; 12 : 428-430.

(7) HYNSON J.M., KATZ J.A., BUEFF H.U. Epidural hematoma associated with enoxaparin. Anesth. Analg. 1996; 82 : 1072-1075.

(8) NICOLAIDES A.N. Prevention of venous thromboembolism. European consensus statement. Int. Angiol. 1992; 11 : 151-159.

(9) MODIG J. Spinal or epidural anaesthesia with low molecular weight heparin for thromboprophylaxis requires careful postoperative neurological observation. Acta. Anesth. Scand. 1992; 36 : 603-604.

(10) OWENS E.L., KASTEN G.W., HESSEL E.A. Spinal subarachnoid haematoma after lumbar puncture and heparinization: a case report, review of the literature, and discussion of anesthetic implications. Anesh. Analg. 1986; 65 : 1201-1207.

(11) DE MOURGES G., PAGNIER F., CLERMONT N., VILLE D., MOYEN B. Etude de l'efficacité de l'héparine sous cutanée utilisée selon deux protocoles dans la prévention de la thrombose veineuse post-opératoire après prothèse totale de hanche. Rev. Chir. Orthop. 1979; 65 : 74-76.

(12) PALARETI G., BORGHI B., COCCHERI S., LEALI N., GOLFIERI R., MONTEBUGNOLI M., INGHILLERI G., RONZIO A., BARBUI R., POGLIANI E.M., DI NINO G., SPOTORNO L. for the CITO study group. Postoperative versus preoperative initiation of deep vein thrombosis prophylaxis with a low molecular weight heparin (nadroparin) in elective hip replacement. Clin. Appl. Thrombosis Hemostasis 1996; 200 : 18-24.

(13) SAMAMA C.M., CLERGUE F., BARRE J., SAMII K., MONTEFIORE A., III P, the ARAR and the enoxaparin study group. Low molecular weight heparin (enoxaparin) versus placebo associated with elastic stockings and spinal anaesthesia in total hip replacement surgery: a double blind randomized study. Br. J. Anaesth. 1997; 78 : 3

3.5

Prophylaxis
of venous thromboembolism
in medicine

**Randomized controlled study
of heparin and low molecular weight heparin for prevention
of deep vein thrombosis in medical patients**

AUTHORS	HARENBERG J., KALLENBACH B., MARTIN V. et al.
REF	Thromb. Research 1990; 59: 639-650

STUDY	Multicenter, randomized, double-blind, controlled
CENTERS (n)	2
COUNTRY	Germany
PATIENTS (n)	*randomized* 166
	evaluated 166

INCLUSION CRITERIA
Patients confined to bed rest
for malignancy, heart disease, cerebral
infarction, infections, other

STUDY DRUG	**Certoparin**	sc daily dose: 1500 APTT units (corresponding to about 37mg or 3100 AXa IU) o.d. + 2 placebo injections treatment duration: 7-12 days
REFERENCE DRUG	**UFH**	sc daily doses: 5000 IU t.i.d. treatment duration: 7-12 days

ASSESSMENTS

❏ DVT: impedance plethysmography (IPG) or Doppler ultrasound; if clinical suspicion, venography.

❏ Bleeding complications, hematomas.

❏ Biological tolerance.

HARENBERG J. et al. 1990

	Certoparin 3000 AXa IU		UFH 5000 IU x 3	
Patients	84		82	
DVT	3	3.5%	4	4.8%
Death (not thrombosis-related)	3		1	
Cerebral embolism	0		1	
Large local hematomas >10cm	0		12	

COMMENTS

❑ The prophylactic regimen with o.d. sc LMWH was at least as effective and safe as UFH t.i.d.

❑ The dose of UFH used in this study may be too high given the risk category of these medical in-patients.

❑ Good local tolerance of certoparin.

Efficacy of low molecular weight heparin (Fragmin) for thromboprophylaxis in medical patients: a randomized double-blind trial
(German)

AUTHORS	PONIEWIERSKI M., BARTHELS M., KUHN M. et al.
REF	Med. Klin. 1988; 83: 241-245

STUDY	Randomized, double-blind, comparative	
CENTERS *(n)*	1	
COUNTRY	Germany	
PATIENTS *(n)*	*included*	200
	evaluated	192

INCLUSION CRITERIA

Medical patients stratified according to the risk of DVT;
- high risk: malignant diseases, previous thromboembolism
- low risk: myocardial infarction and/or coronary heart disease

STUDY DRUG	**Dalteparin**	sc daily dose: 2500 AXa IU o.d. treatment duration: 7-10 days
REFERENCE DRUG	**UFH**	sc daily doses: 5000 IU b.i.d. treatment duration: 7-10 days

ASSESSMENTS
- ❏ DVT: clinical symptoms, daily thermography; in case of positive findings, venography.
- ❏ PE: clinical symptoms.

PONIEWIERSKI M. et al. 1988

	Dalteparin 2500 AXa IU x 1		UFH 5000 IU x 2	
	low risk	high risk	low risk	high risk
Patients	49	47	49	47
DVT (thermography)	0	0	0	0
PE	0	0	0	0
Patients with hematomas (at injection site)	31		38	

COMMENTS

❏ In this trial, neither DVT (detected by thermography screening) nor clinically PE were observed.

❏ No relevant bleeding complications even in patients undergoing interventions such as spinal puncture, gastroscopy.

❏ This study suggested that dalteparin 2500 AXa IU was as effective and safe as UFH 5000 IU twice daily in high and low risk medical patients.

Prevention of deep vein thrombosis
in elderly medical in-patients by a low molecular weight heparin:
a randomized double-blind trial

AUTHORS	DAHAN R., HOULBERT D., CAULIN C. et al.
REF	Haemost. 1986; 16: 159-164

STUDY	Randomized, double-blind, placebo-controlled
CENTERS (n)	1
COUNTRY	France
PATIENTS (n)	*randomized* 270
	evaluated 253

INCLUSION CRITERIA

Hospitalized non surgical patients over 65-year old essentially for: heart failure/respiratory disease/ischemic stroke/malignant disease

STUDY DRUG	**Enoxaparin**	sc daily dose: 60mg o.d. (0.3ml)
		treatment duration: ≈ 10 days
REFERENCE DRUG	**Placebo**	sc daily dose: saline 0.3ml
		treatment duration: ≈ 10 days

ASSESSMENTS

❑ DVT (FUT): D0 and repeated every day until D10.
❑ Tolerance: systemic or local hemorrhage.
❑ Mortality.

DAHAN R. et al. 1986

	Enoxaparin 60mg x 1		Placebo 0.3ml x 1		p
Patients (evaluable)	132		131		
DVT	4	3.0%	12	9.1%	0.03
Major hemorrhage	1		3		
Death	6		6		
Fatal PE	1		3		
Mean number of hematomas (±SD) at injection site)	0.8±1.6		0.4±1.2		<0.05

COMMENTS
- ❑ Despite this high dosage of LMWH, no significant hemorrhagic events.
- ❑ Less DVT in treated patients without any reduction in mortality.

A multicenter randomized double-blind study of enoxaparin compared with unfractionated heparin in the prevention of venous thromboembolic disease in elderly in-patients bedridden for an acute medical illness

AUTHORS	BERGMANN J.F., NEUHART E.
REF	Thromb. Haemostasis 1996; 76: 529-534

STUDY	Multicenter, randomized, double-blind, comparative
CENTERS (n)	12
COUNTRY	France
PATIENTS (n)	*randomized* 442
	evaluated 439 (for safety)
	evaluated 423 (for efficacy)

INCLUSION CRITERIA
Patients 65 years old or more with recent acute illness and reduced mobility

STUDY DRUG	**Enoxaparin**	sc daily doses: 20mg o.d. + 0.2ml placebo treatment duration: 10 days
REFERENCE DRUG	**UFH**	sc doses: 5000 IU b.i.d. treatment duration: 10 days

ASSESSMENTS
- ❏ DVT: daily FUT up to D10; if positive, a bilateral venography could be performed.
- ❏ PE: clinical symptoms confirmed by lung scan or at autopsy.
- ❏ Death.

BERGMANN J.F. et al. 1996

	Enoxaparin 20mg x 1		UFH 5000 IU x 2	
Patients (efficacy/safety)	207/216		216/223	
Isotopic DVT	9	4.2%	10	4.6%
Confirmed DVT by venography	5 ⌉		7 ⌉	
Confirmed DVT by Doppler	2 ⌋	3.3%	1 ⌋	3.6%
PE	1 (non fatal)		0	
Total thromboembolic events	10	4.8%	10	4.4%
Major bleeding	1		2	
Death	7 (no PE)	3.2%	8 (no PE)	3.6%

COMMENTS

❑ Low incidence of thromboembolic events in elderly bedridden patients treated either with UFH or with enoxaparin (low dose).

❑ No difference between the two treatments in terms of efficacy and safety.

❑ Good tolerance in both groups.

The venous thrombotic risk in non surgical patients: epidemiological data and efficacy/safety profile of a low molecular weight heparin (enoxaparin)

AUTHORS	LECHLER E., SCHRAMM W., FLOSBACH C.W., the Prime Study Group
REF	Haemostasis 1996; 26 (Supp 2): 49-56

STUDY	Multicenter, randomized, double-blind, controlled
CENTERS (n)	26
COUNTRIES	Germany, Austria
PATIENTS (n)	*included* 959

INCLUSION CRITERIA

Bedridden patients at high risk of thromboembolism with at least one risk factor: age > 60y/malignancy/obesity/ previous thromboembolism/cardiac insufficiency/hemiplegia/severe infection

STUDY DRUG	**Enoxaparin**	sc daily doses: 40mg o.d. + 2 placebo injections (0.2ml) treatment duration: 7 days
REFERENCE DRUG	**UFH**	sc daily doses: 5000 IU t.i.d. treatment duration: 7 days

ASSESSMENTS

❏ DVT: at entry and at the end of study with B-mode scan or duplex sonography. Positive results confirmed by venography.

❏ PE: clinical symptoms confirmed by lung scan or angiography.

❏ Bleeding complications.

LECHLER E. et al. 1996

	Enoxaparin 40mg x 1		UFH 5000 IU x 3		p
Patients (per-protocol-analysis)	477	(393)	482	(377)	
Thromboembolic events (PPA)*	1	0.3%	5	1.3%	NS**
DVT	1		2		
PE	0		2		
DVT + PE	0		2		
Major hemorrhage	2		9		
Death (not thrombosis-related)	7		11		

* Per-protocol-analysis.
** Test for superiority: NS. Test for equivalence: p <0.0001.

COMMENTS

❑ Very low incidence of thromboembolic events in both groups; prophylactic dosages higher than in Bergmann's study (20 mg o.d.).

❑ Enoxaparin 40mg x 1 was better tolerated than UFH 5000 IU x 3.

**Tolerance to calcium nadroparin
for the prevention of thromboembolism in the elderly**
(French)

AUTHORS	FORETTE B., WOLMARK Y.
REF	Presse Med. 1995; 24,12: 567-571

STUDY	Multicenter, open-label, randomized
CENTERS *(n)*	35
COUNTRY	France
PATIENTS *(n)*	*included* 295
	evaluated 295

INCLUSION CRITERIA
Hospitalized bedridden patients (mean 82.5 years) with temporary locomotor disability

STUDY DRUG	**Nadroparin**	sc daily dose: 0.3ml once daily (= 2850 AXa IU) treatment duration: 28 days
REFERENCE DRUG	**UFH**	sc daily doses: • 5000 IU b.i.d. for patients < 70kg • 7500 IU b.i.d. for patients ≥ 70kg treatment duration: 28 days

ASSESSMENTS
❑ Premature discontinuation of treatment.
❑ DVT: echo Doppler; if abnormal findings, venography.
❑ Bleeding complications.
❑ Mortality.

FORETTE B. et al. 1995

	Nadroparin 0.3ml x 1		UFH 5000 IU/ 7500 IU x 2		p
Patients	146		149		
Premature discontinuation for death or other causes (total number)	16	11.0%	24	16.0%	NS
Premature discontinuation due to treatment	1	0.7%	10	6.7%	0.01
DVT	3		4		
PE	0		1		
Major hemorrhage	0		4		
Minor hemorrhage	2		5		
Hematomas at injection site	16	11.0%	41	27.5%	0.01
Thrombocytopenia	0		1		
Death (0-28 days)	6		7		

COMMENTS

❑   Excellent tolerance to nadroparin in elderly patients.

Heparin prophylaxis in bedridden patients

AUTHORS	BERGMANN J.F., CAULIN Ch.
REF	Lancet. 1996; 348: 205-206 (letter to Editor)

STUDY	Randomized, double-blind, placebo-controlled
CENTERS (n)	39
COUNTRIES	France, Italy, Spain
PATIENTS (n)	*included* 2474
	evaluated 2474

INCLUSION CRITERIA

High risk bedridden patients (mean age 76 years) admitted for acute condition:

cardiac disease:	25%
pulmonary disease:	22%
cancer:	14%
non pulmonary sepsis:	23%

OBJECTIVE

To test if a prophylactic antithrombotic drug may reduce overall mortality

STUDY DRUG	**Nadroparin**	sc daily dose: 7500 AXa ICU o.d. (2850 AXa IU) = 0.3ml treatment duration: up to 21 days
REFERENCE DRUG	**Placebo**	sc daily dose: saline 0.3ml treatment duration: up to 21 days

ASSESSMENTS

❑ Overall mortality during treatment.

❑ Fatal PE at autopsy.

BERGMANN J.F. et al. 1996

	Nadroparin 0.3ml x 1		Placebo 0.3ml x 1		p
Patients	1230		1244		
Overall mortality	63	10.1%	60	10.3%	NS
Fatal PE	10	0.8%	17	1.3%	NS

COMMENTS

❑ The use of a low molecular weight heparin (nadroparin) did not reduce overall mortality among population of bedridden medical patients.

❑ There was a trend toward less fatal PE in nadroparin-treated group than in placebo group.

Subcutaneous low-molecular weight heparin versus standard heparin and the prevention of thromboembolism in medical inpatients

AUTHORS	HARENBERG J., ROEBRUCK P., HEENE D. et al.
REF	Haemostasis. 1996; 26: 127-139

STUDY	Multicenter, double-blind, randomized, comparative
CENTERS (n)	10
COUNTRY	Germany
PATIENTS (n)	*randomized* 1968
	evaluated 1590 for safety
	1436 for efficacy

INCLUSION CRITERIA

Hospitalized bedridden patients 50 to 80 years old with increased risk of thromboembolism, cardiac insufficiency, coronary and cerebrovascular diseases

STUDY DRUG	**Nadroparin**	sc daily dose: 0.3ml o.d. + 2 placebo injections treatment duration: 10 days
REFERENCE DRUG	**UFH**	sc dose: 5000 IU t.i.d. treatment duration: 10 days

ASSESSMENTS

❑ DVT and PE: daily observation of clinical symptoms, compression ultrasonography at D1, 2, 8, 11; venography when abnormal findings.

❑ Bleeding complications.

❑ Adverse events.

HARENBERG J. et al. 1996

	Nadroparin 0.3ml x 1		UFH 5000 IU x 3	
Patients	726		710	
Total thromboembolic events:	6	0.8%	4	0.6%
PE	4 (1 fatal)		3	
DVT	2		1	
Major hemorrhage*	5		4	
Minor hemorrhage (injection site)	3		7	
Severe thrombocytopenia	0		0	

* No blood transfusions were required.

COMMENTS

❏ Low and equivalent incidence of thromboembolic events in both groups.

❏ The analysis of risk factors showed a correlation only with previous history of DVT and PE.

❏ No relationship with other risk factors such as adiposity, varicose veins, previous MI or stroke, cardiac failure.

❏ Better local tolerance with nadroparin than with UFH.

Efficacy and safety of the low molecular weight heparin, nadroparin calcium, in the prevention of deep vein thrombosis in acute, decompensated chronic obstructive pulmonary disease

AUTHORS	FRAISSE F., HOLZAPFEL L., COULAUD J.M. et al.
REF	*Submitted for publication*

STUDY	Multicenter, randomized, double-blind, placebo-controlled
CENTERS (n)	34
COUNTRY	France
PATIENTS (n)	*analyzed* 253
	169 (with venography)

INCLUSION CRITERIA

Patients with acute decompensated chronic obstructive pulmonary disease (COPD) hospitalized for mechanical ventilation without DVT at enrollment.

Patients with: chronic bronchitis ≈ 90%

emphysema ≈ 43%

asthma ≈ 20%

STUDY DRUGS **Nadroparin** sc daily dose, BW-adjusted:
- 0.4ml (3800 AXa IU) o.d. for BW 45-70kg (in 56% of patients) or
- 0.6ml (5700 AXa IU) o.d. for BW > 70kg (in 44% of patients)

treatment duration: maximum 21 days, mean duration 12 days

Placebo sc injection of saline 0.4ml or 0.6ml o.d.

treatment duration: maximum 21 days, mean duration 12 days

ASSESSMENTS
- ❑ DVT: bilateral Doppler once weekly.
- ❑ Venography at the end of study or in case of doubtful or uninterpretable Doppler (blind lecture).
- ❑ Daily clinical evaluation for DVT, PE.
- ❑ Bleeding complications.

FRAISSE F. et al. 1998

	Nadroparin BW-adjusted 3800-5700 AXa IU x 1		Placebo		p
Patients	109		114		
Venography performed	84		85		
Total DVT	13	15.5%	24	28.2%	0.045
Proximal DVT	3	2.7%	7	6.1%	NS
PE	1*		0		
Total hemorrhage	25		18		
Major hemorrhage	6		3		
Discontinuation of therapy	2		3		
Death	8		8		

* Not confirmed at angiography.

COMMENTS

❑ Critically ill patients with acute decompensated chronic obstructive pulmonary disease who require mechanical ventilation are at increased risk for developing deep vein thrombosis. Prophylaxis with nadroparin body-weight-adjusted dose significantly reduces the incidence of DVT.

Expert comments

JOB HARENBERG. *Prophylaxis of DVT in medicine*

Prophylaxis of DVT in medical hospitalized patients using heparin, low molecular weight heparin or other antithrombotic drugs differ substantially from those clinical studies investigating the effect in postoperative medicine. This is mainly due to the fact that patients in general medicine arrive at the hospital with an ongoing disease with an unknown start of origin. Thus, these patients arrive at the hospital at different stages of thrombotic risk. In contrast, in postoperative medicine the start of surgery is generally the well defined beginning of the risk of thromboembolic complications. Exceptions in postoperative medicine are cancer patients or repeated operations.

Another difference between postoperative and general medical patients in clinical studies is the possibility to perform the radiolabeled radiofibrinogen uptake test. In medical patients this test has only rarely been used due to various medical and historical reasons. Non-invasive methods or clinical endpoints have a much lower incidence of DVT or PE compared to the radiofibrinogen uptake test. Thus, studies from postoperative medicine and from general medicine can hardly be compared with regard to the incidence of DVT or PE during prophylaxis with heparin or low-molecular-weight heparin.

The studies published so far are referred to certoparin, dalteparin, enoxaparin and nadroparin have been studied in this indication so far. A total of about 4,000 patients have been randomized in these studies. The overall conclusion of these studies is that once daily low-molecular-weight heparin is almost as effective and safe as 3 times daily 5,000 IU unfractionated heparin for a time period of 10 days. The various low-molecular-weight heparins have been tested in different dosages. However, a meta-analysis of the available studies has not been performed so far.

Based on these data and on the results from studies of postoperative medicine, low-molecular-weight heparins are already widely used for prophylaxis of venous thromboembolism in hospitalized medical patients using 1 daily subcutaneous administration. The advantage of low-molecular-weight heparin is the lower incidence of side effects, i.e. thrombocytopenia type I or II, increase of liver enzymes, local allergy. The low incidence of endpoints will lead to the difficulty to convince local authorities to give general approval for the use of these drugs in this indication. However, upon a decision of the physician these drugs are valuable tools for this indication.

GÉRARD POTRON. *Prophylaxis of thrombosis in medicine*

Happy are those who are practitioners of surgery, a domain where the prophylaxis of thromboembolic events now has nearly become common practice! On the contrary, the situation in medicine remains unsatisfactory. The problems are complex, with different risks for a given patient and within patients, which accounts for the limited number of trials, generally on a restricted number of patients and carried out according to debatable protocols. It is difficult, from an ethical point of view, to propose venography to patients in poor conditions with an uncertain thrombotic risk.

Although there is no basis to extrapolate from the results obtained in surgery, heparins are now increasingly used in medicine, mostly due to the simplification (and probably to the limited risks) linked to LMWH use. But do we actually know whether we are dealing with hypothetical risks, and whether we are reducing mortality and/or post-thrombotic morbidity?

The risk, however, exists since medical bed-ridden patients have a risk of fatal PE which is three times higher than in the general population. Anderson et al (1) have shown that out of 1231 patients with DVT, 80% present a medical risk factor; controlled-population studies show a DVT incidence of 28 to 75% during stroke with paralysis, 17% to 34% of myocardial infarction, and 29% for patients in intensive care units. The Thromboembolic Risk Factor Consensus Group (THRIFT) (14), defines three different levels of risks, of which the high risk group also includes patients with stroke and lower limb paralysis or paraplegia severe illness, in elderly patients, congestive heart failure.

In practice, some situations appear simple even though results of published trials are unsatisfactory, both quantitatively and qualitatively.

The prophylactic efficacy of heparins has been studied in high risk disorders such as acute myocardial infarction (AMI). Previous studies conducted with unfractionated heparin (UFH) versus placebo have shown a risk of DVT close to 25% and a risk reduction of 71 to 83%. In 70 patients with cardiomyopathy, atrial fibrillation, prosthetic heart valves and venous thromboembolism, Harenberg et al (6) have shown that LMWH was succesfully used in patients intolerant to oral anticoagulant. The average duration of LMWH treatment was 26 weeks. Unfortunately, there was no control group; this study is not reported in this review. Scala P.J. (13) compared LMWH (dalteparin) by sc route twice daily versus UFH in continuous IV infusion, APTT-adjusted, on a limited number of patients with AMI in both groups not treated with a fibrinolytic agent, no DVT was found. Recently, findings reported by Nesvold A. (10) also suggest the efficacy of 2 to 3 daily injections of dalteparin in patients with AMI. Even though the results may be debatable, the advantages of prophylaxis with LMWH appear likely in patients with AMI. The duration of prophylaxis remains to be determined (generally up to 15 days).

In acute stroke, although the risk of DVT remains very high after onset of acute stroke with paralysis (40 to 60%), the number of trials based on a rigorous methodology is still limited. The recent results obtained in the FISS bis study show a significant reduction of PE in patients with acute stroke treated with nadroparin -Hommel M. (8)- compared with placebo patients (even though the first end point was not reduction of thromboembolism). Two studies with dalteparin versus placebo -Prins M.H. (11), Sandset P.M. (12)- are less conclusive even though in one study a significant reduction of total DVT was observed. Based on these results and an observation in clinical practice, prophylactic efficacy cannot be questioned and the risk of the ischemic injury progressing to hemorrhage appears to be low. Again the question of the length of treatment in a situation with extended risk remains valid.

Trials in various other fields of medicine prompt us to conclude that LMWHs and UFH are also efficacious when administered over a 7 to 10-day period with, however, a variable number of residual DVT which are undoubtely due to the heterogeneity of the studied population.

Few studies comparing LMWHs with UFH or placebo seem to favor LMWHS (unfortunately not always statistically significant difference). Enoxaparin in a large number of medical patients (Lechner E.) showed a trend for better efficacy in reducing the incidence of thromboembolic events compared with UFH. Nadroparin has been tested against placebo on the prevention of pulmonary embolism in elderly bed-ridden patients with no significant results -Bergman F .(2). Harenberg (7) in a large trial comparing nadroparin 0.3ml once daily with UFH 5000 IU x 3 in bed-ridden patients showed no difference between the two prophylactic regimens. Recently, a study carried out in bed-ridden patients with severe chronic pulmonary obstructive disease has demonstrated that administration of nadroparin significantly decreased the incidence of DVT detected by phlebography compared with placebo -Fraisse F. (4). One trial -Dahan R. (3)-compared enoxaparin with placebo and showed a significant reduction of DVT without any effect on mortality. Gardlung B et al. (5), out of 12,000 patients older than 55 years suffering from infection and being treated preventively by UFH versus placebo administered during three weeks, shows no difference in mortality (vascular included). Moreover, the authors observed a delay in mortality among the group treated with heparin, which could lead to conclude in a positive effect after three weeks of treatment, although this effect disappeared three weeks later.

The last study asks the questions of the necessity of such a prophylaxis and therefore of the selection of the patients who may benefit from such a prevention. Even if a large consensus, in a logical way, agrees on the fact that any patient showing at least one risk factor should receive preventive treatment, the benefits are not formally proven as yet. Early rising, physiotherapy and support stockings seen to be necessary have no iatrogenic consequences and are generally apparently sufficient, but their setting up is more difficult than a simple prescription. But this is only an extrapolation from surgical practice and may call for a demonstration.

It is necessary to pursue the trials with LMWHs in order to more clearly define not only the nature of the risk factors but also their real clinical weight which should lead to effective prophylaxis in medical contexts.

The length of preventive treatment should also be defined: orthopedics have recently shown that risk factors can persist over a long period in spite of walking.

In practice, what can we reasonably and logically suggest?

— Systematic prophylaxis for AMI is certainly needed (except in the case of a post-fibrinolytic heparinotherapy for example) and, with caution, in patients with stroke suffering from recent paralysis of one or two legs.

— Prophylaxis also for patients with several associated risk factors (cancer, infection, dehydration, etc.)

However, apart from the first case, there is no doubt that today systematic prophylaxis cannot be advocated but rather management adjusted to each patient according to clinical elements. Due to a lack of formal demonstration, each clinician, each department, each hospital should express their choices, their strategies, their scores and evaluate their efficacy in the long term. These procedures must take into account support and physiotherapy, even though the ease of use of LMWH makes them the first-line therapy, even more so now that their cost is decreasing. But will they continue be efficacious if we do not give ourselves the means to fight versus stasis, the main cause of DVT?

In conclusion, we can only hope that experience acquired in this field will convince pharmaceutical companies of the need to set up studies to guide therapeutic and preventive regimens, currently based in logical, strict methodology, but alas, still overly dependent on empirical choices.

REFERENCES

(1) ANDERSON F.A., WHEELER H.B. Venous thromboembolism. Risk factors and prophylaxis. Clin. Chest Med. 1995; 16 : 235-251.

(2) BERGMAN J.F., CAULIN Ch. Heparin prophylaxis in bed ridden patients. Lancet 1996; 318 : 205-206.

(3) DAHAN R., HOULBERET D., CAULIN C. et al. Prevention of deep vein thrombosis in elderly medical in-patients by a low molecular weight heparin : a randomized double-blind trial. Haemostasis 1986; 16 : 159-164.

(4) FRAISSE F., HOLZAPFEL L., COULAUD J.M. et al. Efficacy and safety of the low molecular weight heparin nadroparin calcium, in the prevention of deep vein thrombosis in acute decompensated chronic obstructive pulmonary disease. In press

(5) GARDLUNG B. Randomized, controlled trial of low dose heparin for prevention of fatal pulmonary embolism in patients with infectious diseases. Lancet 1996; 347 : 1357-1361.

(6) HARENBERG J. LEBER G., DEMPFLE C.E. et al. Long term anticoagulation with low molecular weight heparin in outpatients with side effets on oral anticoagulants. Nouv. Rev. Fr. Hematol. 1989; 31 : 363-369.

(7) HARENBERG J., ROEBRUCK P., HEENE P. et al. Subcutaneous low molecular weight heparin versus standard heparin in the prevention of thromboembolism in medical inpatients. Haemostasis 1996; 26 : 127-139.

(8) HOMMEL M. Fraxiparine in ischemic stroke. FISS bis study. Cerebrovascular Disease 1998; 8 (Abstract).

(9) LECHLER E., SCHRAMM W., FLOSBACH C.W. et al. The venous thrombotic risk in non surgical patients: epidemiological data and efficacy / safety profile of a low molecular weight heparin (enoxaparin). Haemostasis 1996; 26 supp 2 : 49-56.

(10) NESVOLD A. KONTNY F. ABILDGAARD U. DALE J. Safety of high doses of low molecular weight heparin (Fragmin) in acute myocardial infarction. A dose-finding study. Thromb. Res. 1991; 64 : 579-587.

(11) PRINS M.H., GELDSEMAR R., SING A.K. Prophylaxis of deep venous thrombosis with a low molecular weight heparin (Kabi 21/65 Fragmin) in stroke patients. Haemostasis 1989; 19 : 245-250.

(12) SANDSET P.M., DAHL T. STIRIS M. et al. A double-blind and randomized placebo-controlled trial of low molecular weight heparin once daily to prevent deep vein thrombosis in acute ischemic stroke. Sem. Thromb. Hemost. 1990; 16 (Suppl) : 25-33.

(13) SCALA P.J., THIOLLET M. MIDAVAINE M., KHER A., FUNCK-BRENTANO C., JAILLON P. ROBERTS A., VALTY J. Deep venous thrombosis and left ventricular thrombosis prophylaxis by low molecular weight heparin in acute myocardial infarction. Haemostasis 1990; 20 : 368-369.

(14) Thromboembolic Risk Factors (THRIFT) Consensus Group. Risk and prophylaxis for venous thromboembolism in hospital patients. BMJ 1992; 305 : 567-574.

3.6

Prophylaxis
of vascular thrombosis related
to venous catheter

Upper extremity deep venous thrombosis in cancer patients with venous access devices — prophylaxis with a low molecular weight heparin (Fragmin)

AUTHORS	MONREAL M., ALASTRUE A., RULL M. et al.
REF	Thromb. Haemostasis 1996; 75: 251-253

STUDY	Open-label, randomized
CENTERS (n)	1
COUNTRY	Spain
PATIENTS (n)	*included* 32
	evaluated 29

INCLUSION CRITERIA

Cancer patients undergoing placement of a long-term subclavian venous catheter (Port-a-Cath) with a projected survival >3 months, with a platelet count >100 x 109/l

OBJECTIVE

• To prevent catheter-related upper DVT
• To verify if thrombosis was related to high platelet count

STUDY DRUG	**dalteparin**	sc daily dose: 2500 AXa IU o.d.
		first injection: 2h before insertion of catheter
		treatment duration: 90 days
REFERENCE DRUG	**No prophylaxis**	

ASSESSMENTS

❏ Upper DVT: venography 90 days after placement of catheter or earlier if clinical symptoms (pain, swelling, dilation of the superficial veins of the arm or shoulder).
❏ Infection
❏ Major bleeding.

MONREAL M. et al. 1996

	Dalteparin 2500 AXa IU x 1	No prophylaxis	p
Patients	16	13	
DVT total	1	8	0.002
occlusive	1	4	
Infection	0	1	
Major bleeding	1*	0	
Thrombocytopenia (no discontinuation of treatment)	2	2	
Trend toward a higher platelet count (at catheter insertion) in patients who subsequently developed venous thrombosis but differences failed to reach statistical significance			

* sc hematoma around the procedural site (24h after placement) needing surgical repair.

COMMENTS
- The prophylactic regimen used in this trial (dalteparin 2500 AXa IU o.d.) proved to be effective and safe in preventing catheter-related upper venous thrombosis in cancer patients.

4

Low molecular weight heparins

International
Consensus Statement

Expert Comments

Andrew N. Nicolaides, Russell Hull   p. 250

Recommendations for use of LMWHs in the prevention of venous thromboembolism in the "International Consensus Statement"[1]

ANDREW N. NICOLAIDES, RUSSELL HULL

Only directly randomized comparisons were used to determine the risk reduction and the grades of recommendation and levels of evidence used were based on the criteria of Cook et al (2).

General surgery and urology

General considerations

In a multicenter study, low molecular weight heparin (LMWH) reduced not only the incidence of fatal pulmonary embolism (PE) but also the overall surgical mortality as compared to controls without prophylaxis (3). Three meta-analyses (4-6) of studies comparing LMWH with unfractionated heparin (UFH) indicated that LMWHs were at least as effective as UFH and possibly more (level II + evidence).

There is evidence from randomized controlled studies that combinations of LMWH and graduated elastic compression (5,7-9), are more effective than when used singly (10).

Recommendations

a) Moderate risk patients (eg major surgery, age over 40 years, without any additional risk factor).

The use of low dose heparin, LMWH, dextran or aspirin is recommended for all moderate risk patients. An alternative recommendation is intermittent pneumatic compression used continuously until the patient is ambulant, graduated elastic compression stockings, or a combination of both (11). These are grade A recommendations based on level 1 or level 2 (not all members of the faculty agree that meta-analyses can provide level 1 data). For the sake of uniformity the criteria of Cook et al. have been adhered to (2).

b) High risk patients (e.g. major surgery, age over 60 years or presence of additional risk factors).

All should receive prophylaxis as for moderate risk patients (grade A recommendation). In addition to single modalities such a low dose heparin, LMWH, combined modalities of pharmacological and mechanical methods should be considered as they may be more effective (table provided in consensus document) (grade B recommendations).

In moderate and high risk patients, dextran and aspirin are not the methods of choice because of their limited efficacy on DVT prevention, the anaphylactoid reactions and danger of cardiac overload associated with the former, the high dose of aspirin (1000-1500 mg per day) required and the fact that oral medications are not possible for several days in patients having abdominal surgery.

Additional considerations

In most randomized studies, prophylaxis with low dose heparin or LMWH was initiated before operation but prophylaxis starting after operation was also effective in a small number of studies (12-14). There are no studies comparing the two practices. There is an urgent need for a randomized study to compare the results of preoperative and postoperative commencement of pharmacological prophylaxis.

Orthopedic surgery and trauma

Recomendations

a) Elective hip replacement

LMWH may be superior to UFH in reducing both DVT and PE for hip replacement surgery (4-6, 13, 15, 16), but more studies are needed.

b) Elective knee replacement

There is evidence that LMWH is more effective than warfarin (17-21) and also more effective than UFH (22).

c) Emergency orthopedic surgery

The best results so far have been obtained from studies using LMWH (23) adjusted dose oral anticoagulants (24), dextran (25), one heparinoid (26, 27) and intermittent pneumatic compression (28-31), or foot impulse technology (32-36) (level 1 data). More studies are needed for all methods.

d) Duration of prophylaxis in elective orthopedic surgery

However, three recent randomized controlled studies in patients having hip arthroplasty indicate that prolonged thromboprophylaxis with LMWH decreases the frequency of venographically detected DVT (37-39).

Pregnancy

There are insufficient data on the use of LMWHs or mechanical methods in pregnancy. There is an urgent need for a multicenter trial comparing standard heparin with LMWH in high risk pregnant patients to assess efficacy, safety and possible side effects such as osteoporosis.

General medical patients

LMWH or one heparinoid appear to be as effective as standard heparin (40-42).

The evolution of consensus using evidence based medicine

A key challenge which is increasingly more successfully being met is the transfer of information from the research domain to the clinical front line. The increasing acceptance of evidence-based medicine as a scientific pathway to the clinical front line has resulted in the international Consensus Statement on the Prevention of Venous Thromboembolism.

In selecting the appropriate prophylaxis or treatment for venous thromboembolism the clinician must consider the levels of evidence. The levels of evidence and grades of recommendations for prophylaxis or therapy are shown below (2). Strong recommendations are possible if the evidence comes from level 1 data.

Level of evidence	Grade of recommendation
LEVEL I	**GRADE A**
Level 1	Results come from a single randomized clinical trial (RCT) in which the lower limit of the confidence interval (CI) for the treatment effect exceeds the minimal clinically important benefit.
Level 1+	Results come from a meta-analysis of RCTs in which the treatment effects from individual studies are consistent, and the lower limit of the CI for the treatment effect exceeds the minimal clinically important benefit.
Level 1−	Results come from a meta-analysis of RCTs in which the treatment effects from individual studies are widely disparate, but the lower limit of the CI for the treatment effect still exceeds the minimal clinically important benefit.

Level of evidence	Grade of recommendation
LEVEL II	**GRADE B**
Level II	Results come from a single RCT in which the CI for the treatment effect overlaps the minimal clinically important benefit.
Level II+	Results come from a meta-analysis of RCTs in which the treatment effects from individual studies are consistent and the CI for the treatment effect overlaps the minimal clinically important benefit.
Level II–	Results come from a meta-analysis of RCTs in which the treatment effects from individual studies are widely disparate and the CI for the treatment effect overlaps the minimal clinically important benefit.
LEVEL III	**GRADE C**
	Results come from non-randomized concurrent cohort studies
LEVEL IV	**GRADE C**
	Results come from non-randomized historic studies
LEVEL V	**GRADE C**
	Results come from cas series.

The acceptance of the need for prophylaxis is by no means uniform at the front line. Scepticism is still a major barrier to the transfer of information. There is reason to be optimistic, however, as the use of prophylaxis has steadily increased. Road blocks to clinical practice were identified during the consensus process. These included concern about the clinical relevance of data and the role of meta-analysis. The consensus process also allowed a clear identification of immediate clinical needs.

Future consensus updates will need to reexamine the role of meta-analysis. Findings based on meta-analysis may in the future be reported as a category separate from level 1 recommendations. It is possible that the belief that the results of a meta-analysis are equivalent to the findings by rigorous level 1 trials is an error (43). A recent editorial identifies that serious problems in the performance of meta-analyses are becoming widely recognized (44, 45). These are numerous and included egregious carelessness, insufficient understanding of the substantive issues, failure to consider relevant variables, gross heterogeneity in studies and even serious bias in the interpretation of pooled data. For these reasons it can be questioned as to whether the findings by meta-analysis should be used as level 1 evidence for recommendations.

Indeed, for most prophylactic measures against venous thromboembolism the availability of multiple individual randomized level 1 trials showing consistent findings make the use of meta-analysis redundant.

Key questions that need to be answered

The risk of venous thromboembolism may continue beyond hospitalization. This risk and methods to reduce it need to be assessed in prospective studies.

Cost-effectiveness studies of various preparations of LMWHs versus UFH are necessary.

The effectiveness and safety of LMWH in the treatment of PE should be determined by Level I randomized trials.

Further cost-effectiveness studies of LMWH prophylaxis versus strategies other than UFH such as foot impulse technology are required.

Further studies to assess the additive effects on the efficacy and safety of heparin or LMWH and mechanical technology in high and medium risk patients are needed.

A multicenter trial comparing standard heparin with LMWH in high risk pregnant patients assessing efficacy, safety and side effects such as osteoporosis and thrombocytopenia is needed.

The risk of DVT in the new minimally invasive abdominal surgical procedures needs to be established.

Note

The foundations for this International Consensus Statement were laid down in the European Consensus Statement on the Prevention of Venous Thromboembolism developed at Windsor (UK) in 1991 with support from the European Commission. This European statment was updated by an international faculty and was forged into its present form by extensive evaluation of the literature and debate during the International Union of Angiology World Congress in London in April 1995.

Subsequent work by the faculty and the editorial committee has ensured that recent major advances and the supporting evidence available in 1996 have been included.

The full consensus document was published in *International Angiology* 1997 (1) and is available as a paperback (ISBN 9963-592-57-0). It is also available on CD-Rom with the references (total 421) in both numerical and alphabetical order, together with commentaries (video presentations) by faculty members (70 minutes). The aim is educational and it is hoped that the multimedia presentation will help disseminate the messages throughout the medical world.

REFERENCES

(1) NICOLAIDES A.N., BERGQVIST D., HULL R. Prevention of Venous Thromboembolism. International Consensus Statement. Intern. Angiol. 1997; 16: 3-38

(2) COOK D.J., GUYATT G.H., LAUPACUS A. et al. Clinical recommendations using levels of evidence for antithrombotic agents. Chest 1995; 108 Suppl: 227-230s

(3) PEZZUOLI G., NERI SERNERI G.G., SETTEMBRINI G. et al. Prophylaxis of fatal pulmonary embolism in general surgery using LMWH CY 216; a multicentre, double blind, randomized, controlled clinical trial versus placebo (STEP). Int. Surg. 1989; 74 : 205-210

(4) LEIZOROVICZ A., HAUGH M.C., CHAPUIS F.R. et al. Low molecular weight heparin in prevention of perioperative thrombosis. Br. J. Med. 1992; 305 : 913-920

(5) NURMOHAMED M., ROSENDAAL F., BÜLLER H. et al. The efficacy and safety of low molecular weight heparin versus standard heparin in general and orthopedic surgery. Lancet 1992; 340 : 152-156

(6) JORGENSEN L.N., WILLE-JORGENSEN P., HAUCH O. Prophylaxis of postoperative thromboembolism with low molecular weight heparins. A review. Br. J. Surg. 1993; 80 : 689-704

(7) KALODIKI E., HOPPENSTEADT D.A., NICOLAIDES A.N. et al. Deep venous thrombosis prophylaxis with low molecular weight heparin and elastic compression in patients having total hip replacement; a randomized controlled trial. Int. Angio; 1996; 15 : 162-168

(8) LASSEN M.R., BORRIS L.C., CHRISTIANSEN H.M. et al. Prevention of thromboembolism in 190 hip arthroplasties. Acta Orthop. Scand. 1991; 62 (1) : 33-38

(9) LEYVRAZ P.F., BACHMANN F., HOEK J. Prevention of deep vein thrombosis after hip replacement; randomized comparison between unfractionated heparin and low molecular weight heparin. Br J. Med. 1991; 303 : 543-548

(10) MORRIS G.K. Prevention of venous thromboembolism: a survey of methods used by orthopedic and general surgeons. Lancet 1980; ii : 572-574

(11) WELLS PS., LENSING A.W.A., HIRSH J. Graduated compression stockings in the prevention of postoperative venous thromboembolism; a meta-analysis. Arch Intern. Med. 1994; 154 : 67-72

(12) LECLERC J.R., GEERTS W.H., DESJARDINS L., et al. Prevention of venous thromboembolism after knee arthroplasty; a randomized, double-blind trial comparing enoxaparin with warfarin. Ann. Intern Med. 1996; 124 : 619-626

(13) LEVINE M.N., HIRSH J., GENT M. et al. Prevention of deep vein thrombosis after elective hip surgery; a randomized trial comparing low molecular weight heparin with standard unfractionated heparin. Ann. Inter. Med. 1991; 114 : 545-551

(14) HULL R., RASKOB G., PINEO G. et al. A comparison of subcutaneous low molecular weight heparin with warfarin sodium for prophylaxis against deep vein thrombosis after hip or knee implantation. N. Eng. J. Med. 1993; 329 : 1370-1376

(15) COLWELL C.W.J., SPIRO T.E., TROWBRIDGE A.A. et al. Use of enoxaparin, a low molecular weight heparin, and unfractionated heparin for the prevention of deep venous thrombosis after elective hip replacement. J. Bone Joint Surg. 1994; 76-A : 3-14

(16) KALODIKI E., DOMJAN J., NICOLAIDES A.N. et al. V/Q defects and deep venous thrombosis following total hip replacement. Clin. Radio. 1995; 50 : 400-403

(17) HEIT J., BERKOWITZ S., BONA R. et al for the Ardeparin arthroplasty study group. Efficacy and safety of Normiflo (a LMWH) compared to warfarin for prevention of venous thromboembolism following total knee replacement: a double-blind, dose ranging study. Thromb. Haemostasis 1995; 73 : 978 (Abstr.)

(18) HULL R., RASKOB G., PINEO G. et al. A comparison of subcutaneous low molecular weight heparin with warfarin sodium for prophylaxis against deep vein thrombosis after hip or knee implantation. N. Eng. J. Med. 1993; 329 : 1370-1376

(19) LECLERC J.R., GEERTS W.H., DESJARDINS L. et al. Prevention of venous thromboembolism after knee arthroplasty; a randomized, double-blind trial comparing enoxaparin with warfarin. Ann. Inter; Med. 1996; 124 : 619-626

(20) RDHAG. RD heparin compared with warfarin for prevention of venous thromboembolic disease following total hip or knee arthroplasty. J. Bone Joint Surg. 1994; 76-A : 1174-1185

(21) SPIRO T.E., FITZGERALD R.H., TROWBRIDGE A.A. et al. Enoxaparin a low molecular weight heparin and warfarin for the prevention of venous thromboembolic disease after elective knee replacement surgery. Blood 1994; 84 Suppl 1 : 246 (Abstr.)

(22) COLWELL C.W.J., SPIRO T.E., TROWBRIDGE A.A. et al. for the enoxaparin clinical trial group. Efficacy and safety of enoxaparin versus unfractionated heparin for prevention of deep venous thrombosis after elective knee arthroplasty. Clin. Orth. Rel. Res. 1995; 321 : 19-27

(23) LASSEN M.R., BORRIS L.C. Thromboprophylaxis in hip fracture patients. Prevention of venous thromboembolism. BERGQVIST D., COMEROTA A. NICOLAIDES A.N., SCURR J. Eds. Med-Orion, London (1994) pp.281-95

(24) CLAGETT G.P., ANDERSON F.A., LEVINE M.N. et al. Prevention of venous thromboembolism. Chest 1992; 102 Suppl: 391-407s

(25) BERGQVIST D., KETTUNEN K., FREDIN H. et al. Thromboprophylaxis in patients with hip fractures; a prospective randomized comparative study between ORG 10172 and dextran 70. Surgery 1991, 109 : 617-622

(27) GERHART T.N., YETT H.S., ROBERTSON L.K. et al. Low molecular weight heparinoid compared with warfarin for prophylaxis of deep vein thrombosis in patients who are operated on for fracture of the hip. A prospective, randomized trial. J. Bone Joint Surg. (Am) 1991; 73-A : 494-501

(28) GALLUS A., ROMAN K., DARBY T. Venous thrombosis after elective hip replacement. The influence of preventive intermittent calf compression and of surgical technique. Br. J. Surg. 1983; 70 : 17-19

(29) HARTMAN J.T., PUGH J.L., SMITH R.D. et al. Cyclic sequential compression of the lower limb in prevention of deep venous thrombosis. J. Bone Joint Surg. 1982; 64-A : 1059-1062

(30) HULL R., DELMORE T.J., HIRSH J. et al. Effectiveness of intermittent pulsatile elastic stockings for the prevention of calf and thigh vein thrombosis in patients undergoing elective knee surgery. Thromb. Res. 1979; 16 : 37-45

(31) HULL R.D., RASKOB G.E., GENT M. et al. Effectiveness of intermittent pneumatic leg compression for preventing deep vein thrombosis after total hip replacement. JAMA 1990; 263 : 2313-2317

(32) BRADLEY J.G., KRUGENER G.H., JAGER H.J. The effectiveness of intermittent plantar venous compression in prevention of deep venous thrombosis after total hip arthroplasty. J. Arthropl. 1993; 8 : 57-61

(33) FORDYCE M.J.F., LING R.S.M. A venous foot pump reduces thrombosis after total hip replacement. J. Bone Joint Surg. 1992; 74-B : 45-49

(34) SANTORI F.S., VITULLO A., STOPPONI M. et al. Prophylaxis against deep vein thrombosis in total hip replacement; comparison of heparin and foot impulse pump. J. Bone Joint Surg. 1994; 76-B : 579-583

(35) WILSON N.V., DAS S.K., KAKKAR V.V. et al. Thromboembolic prophylaxis in total knee replacement; evaluation for the A-V impulse system. J. Bone Joint Surg. 1992; 74-B : 50-52

(36) STRANKS G.J., MACKENZIE N.A., GROVER M.L., FAIL T. The A-V impulse system reduces deep vein thrombosis and swelling after hemiarthroplasthy for hip fracture. J. Bone Joint Surg. 1992 : 74-B : 775-778

(37) DAHL O.E., ANDREASSEN G., MILLER C. et al. The effect of prolonged thromboprophylaxis with dalteparin on the frequency of deep vein thrombosis and pulmonary embolism 35 days after hip replacement surgery. Thromb. Haemostasis 1995; 73 : 1094

(38) LASSEN M.R., BORRIS L.C. on behalf of the Danish Prolonged Prophylaxis Study Group. Prolonged prophylaxis with low molecular weight heparin (Fragmin) after elective total hip arthroplasty, a placebo controlled study. Thromb. Haemostasis 1995; 73 : 1104

(39) PLANES A., VOCHELLE N., DARMON J.Y. et al. Risk of deep venous thrombosis after hospital discharge in patients having undergone total hip replacement: a double-blind randomized comparison of enoxaparin versus placebo. Lancet 1996; 348 : 224-228

(40) DAHAN R., HOULBERT D., CAULIN C. et al. Prevention of deep vein thrombosis in elderly medical in-patients by a low molecular weight heparin, a randomized double-blind trial. Haemostasis 1986; 16 : 159-164

(41) HARENBERG J. KALLENVBACH B., MARTIN U., ZIMMERMANN R. Randomized double-blind study of normal and a low molecular weight heparin in general medical patients. Thromb. Haemostasis 1987; 58-381 (Abstr)

(42) PONIEWIERSKI M., BARTHELS M., POLIWODA H. The safety and efficacy of a low molecular weight heparin (Fragmin) in the prevention of deep vein thrombosis in medical patients; a randomized double-blind trial. Thromb. Haemostasis 1987; 58-119 (Abstr)

(43) BORZAK S., RIDKER P.M. Discordance between meta-analyses and large-scale randomized, controlled trials. Ann. Intern. Med. 1995; 123 (11) : 873-877

(44) BAILAR J.C. III. Surgery for early breast cancer - can less be more. N. Engl. J. Med. 1995; 333 : 1496-1498

(45) BAILAR J.C. III. The practice of meta-analysis. J. Clin. Epidemiol. 1995; 48 : 149-157

5

Low molecular weight heparins
Treatment
of venous thromboembolism

Regression of deep vein thrombosis by iv administration of a low molecular weight heparin — results of a pilot study

AUTHORS	KIRCHMAIER C.M., LINDHOFF-LAST E., RÜBESAM D. et al.
REF	Thromb. Res. 1994; 73: 337-348

STUDY	Open-label, pilot
CENTERS (n)	1
COUNTRY	Germany
PATIENTS (n)	25 with confirmed DVT confined to bed rest for 6-8 days

OBJECTIVE
Efficacy of initial treatment on thrombus change (Marder's score) for thrombosis less than 4 weeks old

INITIAL DIAGNOSIS OF DVT
Venography

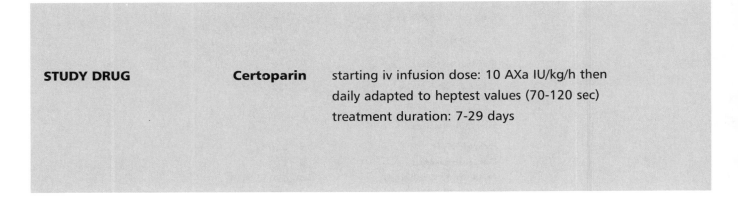

STUDY DRUG	**Certoparin**	starting iv infusion dose: 10 AXa IU/kg/h then daily adapted to heptest values (70-120 sec) treatment duration: 7-29 days

ASSESSMENTS
- ❏ Regression of the thrombus length according to Marder's score, venogram at inclusion and at the end of treatment.
- ❏ If PE suspected, angiography.
- ❏ Bleeding complications.
- ❏ Laboratory monitoring.

KIRCHMAIER C.M. et al. 1994

	Certoparin iv continuous infusion	
Patients	25	
Mean dose administered	15 ± 3 AXa IU/kg/h	
Venograms (Marder's score) with:		
complete recanalization	6	24%
improvement	11	44%
unchanged	8	32%
worsening	0	0%
Bleeding complications before cessation of treatment	3 (AXa IU/ml = 1.4-1.9) (AXa level expected range: 0.6-1.4 IU/ml)	

COMMENTS
- ❑ Therapeutic approach (iv infusion) specific for Germany since thrombolytics are often used for treatment of DVT. Despite the reduced number of patients, the results obtained by continuous infusion of a LMWH did not appear to be much better than after subcutaneous administration.
- ❑ The clinical values of complete recanalization compared to improvement regarding the thrombus size remains to be demonstrated with respect to long-term outcome.

Efficacy of a low molecular weight heparin administered intravenously or subcutaneously in comparison with intravenous unfractionated heparin in the treatment of deep venous thrombosis

AUTHORS	KIRCHMAIER C.M., WOLF H., BREDDIN H.K. for the certoparin study group
REF	Int. Angiol. 1998; 17:135–145

STUDY	multicenter, randomized, controlled
CENTERS (n)	23
COUNTRIES	Germany, Austria, Czech Republic
PATIENTS (n)	randomized 393
	evaluated 309

OBJECTIVE

To test thrombus regression (Marder's score) and prevention of PE in patients with recent DVT treated either by sc or iv LMWH (comparison with iv UFH)

STUDY DRUG	Certoparin	two groups:
		group I: iv bolus 3000 IU followed by infusion 14 IU/kg/h dose Heptest-adjusted
		group II: sc fixed-dose 4000 IU b.i.d.
		treatment duration: at least 14 days
REFERENCE DRUG	UFH	iv bolus 5000 IU followed by infusion 20 IU/kg/h for 14 days dose APTT-adjusted
		treatment duration: at least 14 days
LONG-TERM TREATMENT	Oral anticoagulant from D12-D14 up to 6 months	

ASSESSMENTS

- ❏ Venography at inclusion and at D12-D16 (central blind evaluation) (first end point: reduction of phlebographic Marder's score).
- ❏ Lung scan at inclusion and at D12-D16 (central PIOPED-criteria).
- ❏ Recurrent thrombosis — PE (6-month follow-up).
- ❏ Major, minor bleeding.

KIRCHMAIER C.M. et al. 1998

| | Certoparin | | UFH |
	iv infusion	sc 4000 IU x 2	iv infusion
Evaluated patients	103	101	105
Initial treatment Marder's score (median)			
at inclusion	23	22	25
at D12-D16	18	16	18.5
improvement > 30%	34.0%	42.6%	32.4%
Lung scan* (% of patients)			
at inclusion	33.0%	42.4%	38.7%
at D12-D16	15.3%	20.3%	19.1%
New PE during therapy	6.3%	7.1%	12.6% (1 fatal PE)
Total hemorrhage (major + minor)	9 (1 fatal at D17) + 6	1 + 3	4 + 4

* Intermediate, high probability according to PIOPED criteria.

COMMENTS

❏ First trial with direct comparison of LMWH administered by iv or by sc route during 2 weeks without OAC.

❏ It appeared that the sc route is at least as effective than iv route both for thrombus regression and PE prevention as the difference between LMWH sc and UFH iv (10.2%) is not significant.

❏ High incidence of asymptomatic PE in patients with recent DVT.

❏ Recurrent thromboembolic events were rare in all 3 treatment groups (results not shown).

❏ No difference in mortality (mainly cancer patients).

A comparison between low molecular weight heparin (Kabi 2165) and standard heparin in the intravenous treatment of deep vein thrombosis

AUTHORS	BRATT G., TÖRNEBOHM E., GRANQVIST S. et al.
REF	Thromb. Haemostasis 1985; 54: 813-817

STUDY	Two open, randomized, controlled studies	**OBJECTIVE** Comparison of the efficacy of dalteparin and UFH both administered by iv route in the initial treatment of proximal DVT based on venographic score outcome
CENTERS (n)	1	**DIAGNOSIS OF DVT** Venography within 12h after admission
COUNTRY	Sweden	
PATIENTS (n)	54	

INITIAL TREATMENT	*At entry, all symptomatic patients received UFH in iv bolus (5000 IU) followed by infusion 15,000 IU/12h before venography*		
STUDY DRUG	**Dalteparin**	iv route	• 1st study: 240 AXa IU/kg/12h • 2nd study: 120 AXa IU/kg/12h
REFERENCE DRUG	**UFH**	iv route	infusion initial dose 240 U/kg/12h
	Doses adjusted to APTT prolongation in both groups: *+ 10 to 30 sec in the 1st study, + 5 to 20 sec in the 2nd study*		
	treatment duration: about 5 days		
LONG-TERM TREATMENT	**Warfarin**	oral route from D2 up to 3 months at least thrombotest < 13% at cessation of infusion	

ASSESSMENTS
❑ Venographic Marder's score before and after treatment.
❑ Pulmonary perfusion scan.
❑ APTT and AXa values.

BRATT G. et al. 1985

	First study **Dalteparin iv** 240 AXa IU/kg/12h		Second study **Dalteparin iv** 120 AXa IU/kg/12h		UFH iv infusion	
Patients	12		13		29	
DVT Marder's score:						
improvement	6	50%	10	77%	14	48%
no change	6	50%	3	23%	12	41%
worsening	0	0%	0	0%	3	11%
Lung scan						
PE on 1st scan	4/12		4/13		11/29	
improvement on 2nd scan	2/4		2/4		8/11	
AXa level (range IU/ml)	1.5-2.0		0.7-1.3		0.5-0.7	
APTT values (sec)						
before treatment	25±3		27±4		25±3	
at D5	53±13		42±8		79±23	
Major bleeding complications	2 *		1		1**	

* First study discontinued (AXa: 2.9 IU/ml; APTT values x 2.5 for these 2 patients).
** Macroscopic hematuria in patient.

COMMENTS

❏ Pioneering study where a LMWH was tested in treatment of DVT and administered as conventional heparin therapy (by iv route).

❏ The lower dose (120 AXa IU/kg/12h) of dalteparin appeared effective and well tolerated.

❏ Neither APTT values nor AXa activity were informative regarding the efficacy of dalteparin; on the contrary, bleeding complications appeared to be correlated with high AXa activity and prolonged APTT values.

Subcutaneous heparin treatment of deep vein thrombosis: a comparison of unfractionated and low molecular weight heparin

AUTHORS	HOLM H.A., LY B., HANDELAND G.F., et al.
REF	Haemostasis. 1986; 16: 30-37

STUDY	Randomized, double-blind
CENTERS (n)	1
COUNTRY	Norway
PATIENTS (n)	56 with proven DVT (less than 14 days old) and without PE suspicion

OBJECTIVE

Comparison of administration of dalteparin vs UFH both subcutaneously in the initial treatment of DVT based on venographic score outcome

DIAGNOSIS OF DVT

Bilateral venography

INITIAL TREATMENT		*Before venography, all symptomatic patients were routinely treated with UFH in iv infusion for about 1 day then randomized*
STUDY DRUG	**Dalteparin**	sc doses b.i.d. 2 h after the end of UFH infusion
REFERENCE DRUG	**UFH**	sc doses b.i.d. 2 h after the end of UFH infusion
	initial dosage:	female ≥ 70 years = 0.40ml*
		female ≥ 60 years and male ≥ 70 years = 0.50ml*
		female < 60 years and male < 70 years = 0.75ml*

For both groups, dosage adjusted by AXa activity = 0.5-0.8 IU ml 2.5h after injection

treatment duration: 7 days

* 1ml = 10,000 IU for dalteparin, 20,000 IU for UFH

LONG-TERM TREATMENT	**Warfarin**	oral route started on D1 - thrombotest = 7-10% at cessation of initial heparin infusion. Duration: not stated

ASSESSMENTS

❏ Venographic Marder's score outcome before and after treatment (7 days) — evaluation by three independent radiologists.

❏ Bleeding complications.

HOLM H.A. et al. 1986

	Dalteparin 4000/7500 AXa IU x 2 (monitored)		UFH 8000/15,000 IU x 2 (monitored)		p
Venography performed	25		25		
Marder's score:					
before treatment	16.9±8.7		15.9±9.5		NS
after treatment	14.1±8.3		12.7±8.3		NS
improvement	10	40%	12	48%	NS
no change	14	56%	11	44%	
worsening	1	4%	2	8%	
PE	1		0		NS
Major bleeding	0		0		NS
AXa "peak" activity (IU/ml)					
mean ± SE at D2	0.60±0.09		0.58±0.07		
mean ± SE at D7	0.70±0.17		0.52±0.18		

COMMENTS
- ❏ This study experienced the sc route for LMWH. The results were not significantly different from sc UFH.
- ❏ Complex dosage based on age, sex and AXa values.
- ❏ More predictable AXa plasma activity with dalteparin (less adjustment in this group): 48% without no dose adjustment vs 24% in UFH group.
- ❏ Leg pain disappeared more rapidly in patients receiving dalteparin.

Treatment of acute venous thromboembolism with low molecular weight heparin (Fragmin). Results of a double-blind randomized study

AUTHORS	ALBADA J., NIEUWENHUIS H.K., SIXMA J.J.
REF	Circulation. 1989; 80: 935-940

STUDY	Randomized, double-blind
CENTERS (n)	1
COUNTRY	The Netherlands
PATIENTS (n)	219 stratified according to their bleeding risk category then randomized 194 treated

OBJECTIVE
Comparison of safety and efficacy of iv monitored dalteparin with monitored UFH in the initial treatment of DVT

INITIAL DIAGNOSIS OF DVT
Clinical symptoms confirmed in most of the cases with bilateral impedance plethysmography —IPG — (phlebography in exceptional cases)

STUDY DRUG	Dalteparin	iv bolus: 2500 AXa IU followed by iv infusion: 15,000 AXa IU/24h treatment duration: at least 5 days (6±1)
REFERENCE DRUG	UFH	iv bolus: 2500 IU followed by iv infusion: 30,000 IU/24h treatment duration: at least 5 days (5.9±1.3)

For both groups: dose adjusted according to AXa activity at 9AM and 4PM:
high bleeding risk group: *0.3-0.6 IU/ml*
low bleeding risk group: *0.4-0.9 IU/ml*

LONG-TERM TREATMENT	OAC	oral route (starting and duration at the physician's discretion)

ASSESSMENTS
- ❏ Daily physical examination.
- ❏ Major/ minor bleeding (primary end points)
- ❏ IPG before and just after stopping infusion therapy.
- ❏ PE: lung scan before and after treatment.
- ❏ Laboratory monitoring.

ALBADA. et al. 1989

	Dalteparin iv infusion		UFH iv infusion		p
Patients	96		98		
Major bleeding	10	10.4%	13	13.2%	NS
	(2 discontinuations)		(2 discontinuations)		
Minor bleeding	27	28.1%	35	35.7%	NS
DVT (IPG)					
improved	28/50	56.0%	22/43	51.2%	NS
worsened	2/96	2.0%	0/98	0%	NS
Disappearance of pain	54/59	88.1%	43/51	84.3%	
Decreasing of swelling					
upper leg	43/63	68.2%	38/49	77.6%	
lower leg	32/53	60.4%	33/47	70.2%	
PE, lung scan new defects	3/34	8.8%	6/46	13.0%	NS
Fatal PE	0		1		

COMMENTS

❑ This trial was conducted primarily to assess safety in the treatment of DVT with dalteparin. Both compounds were administered by iv infusion (in order to eliminate the questionable bioavailability related to sc route) and adjusted on equal AXa levels. There was no significant difference between the two studied treatments. Thrombocytopenia (<100,000/mcl) were observed in 3 Dalteparin and 2 UFH-group.

❑ Bleeding occurred more often in the high-risk group (17 major/26 minor) than in the low-risk group (6 major/29 minor) p=0.048.

❑ Despite different target in the protocol according to bleeding risk factors, AXa levels were not different: high risk group, 0.48 IU/ml, low risk group, 0.55 IU/ml. These results suggest the uselessness of laboratory monitoring.

**Deep vein thrombosis treatment. A comparative study: subcutaneous Fragmin®
versus unfractionated heparin administered by continuous infusion:
A French multicenter trial** *(French)*

AUTHORS	French Multicenter Study
REF	Rev. Med. Interne 1989; 4: 375-381

STUDY	Open-label, randomized	
CENTERS (n)	6	
COUNTRY	France	
PATIENTS (n)	*included*	66 with a (recent) confirmed DVT
	evaluated	60

OBJECTIVE

Efficacy and safety of sc AXa-adjusted doses of dalteparin in the initial treatment of symptomatic DVT

DIAGNOSIS OF DVT

Bilateral venography

INITIAL TREATMENT *Before venography, all patients were routinely treated with UFH infusion 240 IU/kg/12h, then randomized:*

STUDY DRUG | **Dalteparin** | sc initial doses: 100 AXa IU/kg b.i.d. the first day then adjusted to AXa activity (range 0.5-0.8 IU/ml) at D2, 5, 10 treatment duration: about 10 days

REFERENCE DRUG | **UFH** | iv infusion initial dose: 240 IU/kg/12h
APTT-adjusted (x 1.5-3) since D2
treatment duration: about 10 days

LONG-TERM TREATMENT   **Not stated**

ASSESSMENTS
❑ Quantitative venographic changes between D0-D10 (Marder's score). Blind assessment
❑ Bleeding complications.

French Multicenter Study. 1989

	Dalteparin 100 AXa IU/kg x 2	UFH infusion	p
Venography performed	31	29	
Marder's score (mean value ± SD): before treatment after treatment improvement worsening	20.5±11.9 16.2±10.5 71.0% 6.4%	20.0±12.3 15.9± 12.9 79.3% 3.4%	NS NS NS NS
PE (clinical observation)	0	0	
Bleeding complications	0	4	NS

COMMENTS
❏ With this dalteparin regimen sc administered twice daily and adjusted to AXa activity, 3h after injection:
  • no difference in thrombus extension or hemorrhagic complications in comparison with UFH.
  • no pulmonary embolism.
  • no decrease of ATIII levels at D10 in the dalteparin group, in UFH group, 7% decrease.
  • more predictable and stable AXa activity.
❏ Extending the target values: 0.5-0.8 U/ml to 0.5-1 U/ml was suggested.

Two daily subcutaneous injections of Fragmin as compared with intravenous standard heparin in the treatment of deep vein thrombosis (DVT)

AUTHORS	BRATT G., ABERG W., JOHANSSON M. et al.
REF	Thromb. Haemostasis 1990; 64: 506-510

STUDY	Open-label, randomized	
CENTERS (n)	1	
COUNTRY	Sweden	
PATIENTS (n)	*included*	110
	evaluated	94

OBJECTIVE

Efficacy of dalteparin in the initial treatment of symptomatic DVT based on venographic score modifications

DIAGNOSIS OF DVT

Bilateral venography

INITIAL TREATMENT		*Before venography, all symptomatic patients were routinely treated with UFH (iv bolus 5000 IU and 12h-infusion of 15,000 IU), then randomized*
STUDY DRUG	**Dalteparin**	sc doses: 120 AXa IU/kg b.i.d. then, adjusted to AXa activity (0.2-0.4 IU/ml) before injection and < 1.5 U/ml 4h after morning injection
REFERENCE DRUG	**UFH**	iv infusion daily adjusted to APTT (80-120 sec) (basal values 24-36 sec) treatment duration: at least 5 days
LONG-TERM TREATMENT	**Warfarin**	oral route from D1; dose not stated treatment duration: 3-6 months

ASSESSMENTS
- Venographic changes between D0-D5/6 (Marder's score); blind assessment.
- Laboratory data.
- Bleeding complications.
- Follow-up period.

BRATT G. et al. 1990

	Dalteparin AXa-adjusted		UFH infusion APTT adjusted		p
Patient	55 (45 evaluated)		55 (49 evaluated)		
Venographic changes in Marder's score:					
improvement	34	75.0%	30	61.2%	chi^2
no change	9	2.0%	16	32.0%	NS
worsening	2	4.4%	3	6.1%	
Major bleeding	0		2		
AXa levels IU/ml (at D3)*					
4h after injection	0.8				
1h before injection	0.3				
Twenty-two-month follow-up:					
death	11/55 (8)**		6/55 (4)**		
thromboembolic events	4 (DVT)		6 (DVT)		

* Evaluated from figure.
** (Patients with malignancy).

COMMENTS
❑ Dalteparin given subcutaneously b.i.d. was as effective and safe as UFH administered by intravenous route (infusion).
❑ No PE in either group.

Fragmin once or twice daily subcutaneously in the treatment of deep vein thrombosis of the leg

AUTHORS	HOLMSTRÖM M.C., BERGLUND S., GRANQVIST S. et al.
REF	Thromb. Res. 1992; 67: 49-55

STUDY	Open-label, randomized, comparison of two dose regimens
CENTERS (n)	1
COUNTRY	Sweden
PATIENTS (n)	*included* 101
	evaluated 87

OBJECTIVE

To determine whether dalteparin administered subcutaneously o.d. is as effective and safe as similar dosage administered as two daily injections in the initial treatment of DVT

DIAGNOSIS OF DVT

Bilateral venography

INITIAL TREATMENT *Before venography and randomization, all symptomatic patients were routinely treated with UFH in iv bolus 5000 IU followed by iv infusion not exceeding 24h*

STUDY DRUG **Dalteparin** sc daily starting doses either:
- 100 AXa IU/kg b.i.d. or
- 200 AXa IU/kg o.d. then
adjusted according to AXa activity = 0.1-0.3 IU/ml
2h before next injection
treatment duration: 5-7 days

LONG-TERM TREATMENT **Warfarin** oral route from D1-INR = 2-4
treatment duration: not stated

ASSESSMENTS
- ❑ Venographic score (Marder's score) before and after treatment (D5-D7). Blind assessment.
- ❑ Bleeding complications.
- ❑ Laboratory tests (AXa activity).

HOLMSTRÖM M.C. et al. 1992

Starting doses	Dalteparin 100 AXa IU/kg x 2	Dalteparin 200 AXa IU/kg x 1	p
Patients	51	50	
Evaluable venograms	45	42	
Marder's score (mean value ± SD):			
before treatment	15.1±10.2	11.5±9.5	NS
after treatment	13.4±10.2	9.8±9.2	NS
difference (Δ)	(−1.6±2.5)	(−1.8±3.1)	NS
Venogram improved	23 51%	23 55%	
Venogram worsened	2 (proximal DVT)	0	
PE	0	0	
Bleeding complications (minor/major)	3/1	0/1	
AXa level IU/ml			
mean value 2h before injection	0.4	0.2	
mean value 4h after injection	not stated	1.5	

*planned range 0.1-0.3.

COMMENTS
- This study was the first one published comparing once daily with twice daily sc administration of LMWH in the treatment of DVT.
- The total dose administered o.d. was as safe and effective as the daily dosage divided in two injections even though average of once daily dose was higher than the average dosage twice daily administered (188 vs 166 AXa U respectively).
- Failure of AXa activity monitoring, mainly in b.i.d. group, with AXa levels always higher than the highest planned dose (0.3 IU/ml).
- The authors concluded that an adequate fixed dose was more important than an AXa-adjusted dose.

Adjusted versus fixed doses
of the low molecular weight heparin Fragmin
in the treatment of deep vein thrombosis

AUTHORS	ALHENC-GELAS M., JESTIN-LE GUERNIC C., VITOUX J.F. et al.
REF	Thromb. Haemostasis 1994; 71: 698-702

STUDY	Multicenter, randomized, comparison of two dose regimens
CENTERS (n)	11
COUNTRY	France
PATIENTS (n)	*included* 122
	evaluated 107

OBJECTIVE

To compare efficacy and safety of fixed dose (BW) to AXa-adjusted dose in the initial treatment of recent DVT

DIAGNOSIS OF DVT

Venography within 12h after admission in symptomatic patients

INITIAL TREATMENT

At entry, all symptomatic patients received UFH in iv infusion and after diagnosis confirmation, randomization between 2 groups:

STUDY DRUG	**Dalteparin**	sc *fixed BW-adjusted doses* 100 AXa IU/kg b.i.d. non monitored
		or
	Dalteparin	sc *AXa-adjusted doses* (D2, D6 systematically) range 0.5-1 IU/ml (3 to 4h) initial doses: 100 AXa IU/kg b.i.d. treatment duration: 10 days

LONG-TERM TREATMENT	**Oral anticoagulant**	from D7

ASSESSMENTS

❏ Bilateral venography at entry and at D10±1 (Marder's score blindly evaluated).
❏ Lung scan or pulmonary angiography before and at the end of treatment.
❏ AXa monitoring.
❏ Laboratory tests
❏ Bleeding complications.

ALHENC-GELAS M. et al. 1994

	Dalteparin BW-adjusted dose x 2 100 AXa IU/kg x 2		Dalteparin AXa-adjusted dose x 2		p
Patients	58		64		
Evaluable venograms (D10)	48		59		
Recurrent DVT	0		0		
Marder's score (D0-D10):					
difference (mean value ± SD)	6.8±6.1		5.6±4.8		NS
improved	40	83.0%	44	75.0%	NS
no change	7		15		
worsened	2	4.0%	1	1.7%	NS
PE lung scan new defects	4		3		
Major hemorrhage	1 (D9)		0		NS
AXa IU/ml* below 0.5 IU	20% of patients		14% of patients		
above 1 IU	1 patient		1 patient		

* 3-4h after injection.

COMMENTS
- ❏ Dose adjustment to AXa plasma level (0.5-1 IU/ml) did not improve efficacy and safety even though the mean twice daily dosage was slightly higher (103.5±10.6 IU/kg vs 100.1±1.7 IU/kg) in this group.
- ❏ More than one-third of patients presented a PE at D0.

Comparison of once daily subcutaneous Fragmin with continuous intravenous unfractionated heparin in the treatment of deep vein thrombosis

AUTHORS	LINDMARKER P., HOLMSTRÖM M., GRANQVIST S. et al.
REF	Thromb. Haemostasis 1994; 72: 186-190

STUDY	Open-label, multicenter, randomized
CENTERS (n)	5
COUNTRY	Sweden
PATIENTS (n)	*enrolled* 204
	evaluated 180 (for efficacy)

OBJECTIVE

Comparison of dalteparin sc o.d. without monitoring, with UFH administered in infusion and APTT-adjusted

INITIAL DIAGNOSIS OF DVT

Bilateral venography

INITIAL TREATMENT		*All patients received UFH iv bolus 5000 IU followed by an infusion 800-1700 IU/h (maximum 24h)*
STUDY DRUG	**Dalteparin**	sc daily dose: 200 AXa IU/kg/24h (maximum: 18,000 IU/D) treatment duration: 5-9 days
REFERENCE DRUG	**UFH**	iv infusion: APTT-adjusted: x 1.5-3 treatment duration: 5-9 days
LONG-TERM TREATMENT	**OAC**	oral route from D1 up to 3 months minimum initial dose: 10-15mg then adjusted to INR 2-3

ASSESSMENTS

❑ Venographic changes before and after initial treatment (Marder's score).
❑ Symptomatic DVT, death, during 6-month follow-up.
❑ Bleeding complications.

LINDMARKER P. et al. 1994

	Dalteparin 200 IU/kg x 1		UFH infusion		p
Patients with DVT	Distal	Proximal	Distal	Proximal	
	33	58	38	51	
Changes in Marder's score:					
improvement	64%	59%	66%	61%	NS
no change	30%	36%	29%	29%	NS
worsening	6%	5%	5%	10%	NS
Major bleeding	0		0		
Minor bleeding	4		2		NS
Thrombocytopenia	0		1		—
Six-month follow-up					
Recurrence of DVT/PE	5		3		NS
Death	2		2		—

COMMENTS

❑ Dalteparin given sc once daily in a fixed dose body weight-adjusted, was as effective and safe as continuous infusion of UFH monitored by APTT.

❑ No correlation has been observed between AXa or APTT levels and changes in Marder's score.

Comparison of subcutaneous unfractionated heparin with a low molecular weight heparin (Fragmin®) in patients with venous thromboembolism and contraindications to coumarin

AUTHORS	MONREAL M., LAFOZ E., OLIVE A., et a.l
REF	Thromb. Haemostasis 1994; 71: 7-11

STUDY	Open-label, randomized, two parallel groups
CENTERS *(n)*	1
COUNTRY	Spain
PATIENTS *(n)*	80

with at least one (absolute or relative) contraindication to oral anticoagulant.

INITIAL DIAGNOSIS OF DVT
Bilateral venography,
B-mode ultrasonography.
Randomization at hospital discharge
after in-hospital initial treatment of DVT
with UFH

INITIAL TREATMENT	*During hospital stay*	
	UFH	intermittent iv administration leading dose 100 IU/kg, then, o.d. APTT-adjusted (x 1.5-2)
LONG-TERM TREATMENT	*Home treatment*	
STUDY DRUG	**Dalteparin**	sc daily dose: 5000 AXa IU b.i.d. treatment duration: 3-6 months
REFERENCE DRUG	**UFH**	sc daily dose: 10,000 IU b.i.d. treatment duration: 3-6 months

ASSESSMENTS

- ❑ DVT: initial bilateral venography or B-mode ultrasonography.
- ❑ PE: lung scan before hospital discharge and at 3- and 6-month follow-up.
- ❑ Recurrence of DVT: clinical observation confirmed by venography.
- ❑ Bleeding complications.
- ❑ Bone mineral density before discharge and then 3 and 6 months after.

MONREAL M. et al. 1994

	Dalteparin 5000 AXa IU x 2	UFH 10,000 IU x 2	p
Patients	40	40	
Recurrent thromboembolic events			
high probability perfusion defects (PE)	0	2	NS
probable perfusion defects (PE)	2	3	NS
DVT	2	3	NS
Bleeding complications			
major bleeding	0	0	
minor bleeding	4	6	NS
Spinal fractures	1 2.5%	6* 15%	NS (0.054)

* 2 with discontinuation of therapy.

COMMENTS
- Interesting trial regarding the effect on bone mineral density (BMD) after a long-term treatment with UFH or LMWH administered in high sc doses. The spinal fractures occurred 82-175 days after randomization and involved T10 to L5 with a predilection for T12.
- The decrease in BMD was not significantly greater for patients with spinal fractures as compared to those without.
- The difference in spinal fractures between the two treatments reached a significant difference in patients aged 80 years or more (0/11 for dalteparin vs 5/12 for UFH).

Subcutaneous low-molecular-weight heparin Fragmin versus intravenous unfractionated heparin in the treatment of acute non massive pulmonary embolism: an open randomized pilot study

AUTHORS	MEYER G., BRENOT F., PACOURET G. et al.
REF	Thromb. Haemostasis 1995; 74: 1432-1435

STUDY	Pilot, open-label, multicenter, randomized
CENTERS (n)	3
COUNTRY	France
PATIENTS (n)	*included* 60
	evaluated 55

INCLUSION CRITERIA
Symptoms suggesting acute PE within 5 days

INITIAL DIAGNOSIS
Pulmonary angiography scored according to Miller. Patients with a Miller's index > 20/34 were excluded

STUDY DRUG	**Dalteparin**	sc daily dose: 120 AXa IU/kg b.i.d.
		treatment duration: 10 days
REFERENCE DRUG	**UFH**	continuous iv infusion
		initial dose: 500 IU/kg/24h then, APTT-adjusted (x 2-3 control values)
		treatment duration: (≈ 10 days) stopped 3-4 days after INR 2-3
LONG-TERM TREATMENT	**OAC**	from D7 up to at least 3 months (INR 2-3)

ASSESSMENTS
- ❑ PE recurrence within initial treatment (10 days) based on lung scan perfusion at entry and at D10±1; in case of suspected recurrence, confirmation by angiography.
- ❑ Outcome in pulmonary scintigraphic vascular obstruction score (PVOs) between D1, D10 and 3 months.
- ❑ Bleeding complications.
- ❑ Laboratory tests.

MEYER G. et al. 1995

	Dalteparin 120 AXa IU/kg x 2	UFH infusion	p
Patients	27	28	
PVO score % (mean value ± SD)			
D0	41±19	37±18	NS
D10	26±15	22±15	NS
Absolute decrease	17±13	16±13	NS
PVO score decreased (n patients)	25 92.6%	26 92.8%	
PVO score unchanged	1	2	
AXa (IU/ml) 3-4h after injection at			
D0	0.2±0.2	0.3±0.3	
D10	1.0±0.4	0.5±0.3	
Major bleeding	0	0	
Minor hematomas	1	4	
Three-month follow-up			
death	1 (2nd month)	1 (D13)	
PVO score % (mean value ± SD)	11±12 (n=18)	10±13 (n=27)	

COMMENTS

❑ In this trial, the efficacy of a LMWH sc administered twice daily for the treatment of PE was as effective and safe as UFH administered by continuous iv infusion.

A multicenter comparison of once daily subcutaneous dalteparin (low molecular weight heparin) and continuous intravenous heparin in the treatment of deep vein thrombosis

AUTHORS	LUOMANMÄKI K., GRANQVIST S., HALLERT C. et al.
REF	J. Intern. Med. 1996; 240: 85-92

STUDY	Multicenter, double-blind, randomized
CENTERS *(n)*	7
COUNTRIES	Finland, United States, Sweden
PATIENTS *(n)*	*randomized* 330
	evaluated 248 for safety
	190 for efficacy

OBJECTIVE
Comparison of efficacy and safety of dalteparin sc fixed dose o.d. versus iv UFH in the initial treatment of DVT

INITIAL DIAGNOSIS OF DVT
Bilateral venography
When randomization occurred before venography, initial bolus of either:
• dalteparin 5000 AXa IU sc or
• UFH 5000 IU iv

STUDY DRUG	Dalteparin	sc daily dose: 200 AXa IU/kg o.d.
		first injection: at least 4h after the initial bolus (when bolus)
		treatment duration: 5-10 days
REFERENCE DRUG	UFH	iv daily dose: infusion adjusted to APTT values (x1.5-3)
		20 000- 40 000 IU/24h
		treatment duration: 5-10 days
LONG-TERM TREATMENT	OAC	oral route from D1 (INR 2-3)
		treatment duration: at the physician's discretion

ASSESSMENTS
❑ Quantitative venographic scores (Marder's score) after termination of dalteparin or UFH therapy (D6 to D10)
❑ Major bleeding
❑ 6-month follow-up for clinical recurrence of thromboembolic events.
❑ PE: lung scan or angiography if clinical symptoms   ❑ Laboratory tests.

LUOMANMÄKI K. et al. 1996

	Dalteparin 200 AXa IU/kg x 1		UFH iv infusion		p
Patients with venogram	92		98		
Marder's score:					
improvement	47	51%	61	62%	NS
no change	34	37%	30	31%	NS
worsening	11	12%	7	7%	NS
PE	1		0		
Major bleeding	0		1		
Median time to pain relief (days)	3.5		3.5		
AXa level (IU/ml) at D5 24h after injection	0.10±0.06		—		
Six-month follow-up:					
recurrence of VTE	3/97		2/103		NS
death	1/97		5/103		

COMMENTS

❑ DVT can be effectively and safely treated with fixed, o.d., subcutaneous injections of dalteparin.

❑ No correlation was observed between AXa activity and change in Marder's score nor in the occurrence of bleeding complications.

Once-daily subcutaneous dalteparin, a low molecular weight heparin, for the initial treatment of acute deep vein thrombosis

AUTHORS	FIESSINGER J.N., LOPEZ-FERNANDEZ M., GATTERER E. et al.
REF	Thromb. Haemostasis 1996; 76: 195-199

STUDY	Open-label, multicenter, randomized
CENTERS (n)	16
COUNTRIES	France, Spain, Sweden, Austria
PATIENTS (n)	*randomized* 268
	evaluated 243 for safety
	199 for efficacy

OBJECTIVE
Assessment of efficacy and safety of once daily injection for the initial treatment of acute DVT

INITIAL DIAGNOSIS OF DVT
- Bilateral venography
- When randomization occurred before venography, initial dose of either:
  — dalteparin 5000 AXa IU sc or
  — UFH 5000 IU iv

STUDY DRUG	**Dalteparin**	sc daily dose: 200 AXa IU/kg o.d. (maximum: 18,000 IU/day)
REFERENCE DRUG	**UFH**	iv infusion (20,000-40,000 IU/24h) APTT-adjusted x 1.5-3 treatment duration: at least 5 days (5-10 days)
LONG-TERM TREATMENT	**OAC**	oral route from D1 (INR 2-3) treatment duration: according to the physicians

ASSESSMENTS
- ❏ Marder's score before and after treatment (blind assessment by independent radiologist unaware of study medication).
- ❏ Major bleeding.
- ❏ PE (diagnosis not stated).
- ❏ 6-month follow-up.

FIESSINGER J.N. et al. 1996

	Dalteparin 200 AXa IU/kg x 1		UFH infusion		p
Patients	96		103		
Marder's score:					
improvement	65	67.7%	62	60.2%	NS
no change	23	24.0%	29	28.2%	NS
worsening	8	8.3%	12	11.6%	NS
Major bleeding	0		2		
Thrombocytopenia	1*		2		
Six-month follow-up:					
Recurrence of DVT	4**		2*		
Death	1 (cancer)		4 (cancer)		

* On chemotherapy.
** None of these patients was receiving OAC at the time of recurrence.

COMMENTS
- ❑ This trial showed that dalteparin 200 AXa IU/kg o.d. by subcutaneous injection, without laboratory monitoring, started without any pre-treatment with UFH was as effective and safe as conventional UFH therapy.
- ❑ No statistical correlation was found between AXa activity and changes in Marder's score, nor in the occurrence of bleeding.
- ❑ This therapeutic regimen may be suitable for treatment of DVT in outpatients.

Frequency of pulmonary embolism in patients who have iliofemoral deep vein thrombosis and are treated with once- or twice-daily low molecular weight heparin

AUTHORS	PARTSCH H., KECHAVARZ B., MOSTBECK A. et al.
REF	J. Vasc. Surg. 1996; 24: 774-782

STUDY	Open-label, randomized parallel group
CENTERS (n)	1
COUNTRY	Austria
PATIENTS (n)	*included* 140
	evaluated 140
	24% with malignancy

OBJECTIVE
To compare in ambulatory very high risk patients (with confirmed iliofemoral DVT) two different regimens of dalteparin (o.d. vs b.i.d.) on the frequency of PE

DIAGNOSIS OF DVT
Duplex ultrasonography confirmed by venography

STUDY DRUG	**Dalteparin**	• sc daily dose: 200 AXa IU/kg o.d.
		or
		• sc daily dose: 100 AXa IU/kg b.i.d.
+ Elastic bandages		treatment duration: about 11.5±4.8 days
LONG-TERM TREATMENT	**OAC**	since D7 for 3 months
		or
	Dalteparin	in 50% of patients because contraindication to coumarin (5000-10,000 AXa IU/day)
		treatment duration: 3 months

ASSESSMENTS
- ❏ Decrease in frequency of PE judged according VQ scan and chest radiography before and after 10 days of treatment.
- ❏ Bleeding complications.
- ❏ Death.

PARTSCH H. et al. 1996

	Dalteparin 200 AXa IU/kg x 1		Dalteparin 100 AXa IU/kg x 2		p
Patients	76		64		
Initial lung scan (D0)					
PE high probability	36	47.4%	29	45.3%	NS
symptomatic PE	11	14.5%	8	12.5%	NS
Second lung scan (at D10)					
PE high probability	36	47.4%	22	34.3%	
reduction in frequency		0.0%		24.1%	
totally cleared	2/36	5.5%	8/29	27.6%	
symptomatic PE*	4		1		
reduction in frequency	4/76	5.3%	1/64	1.6%	<0.05
new PE	6		2		
fatal PE	1		0		
Major bleeding complications	1		0		
Death	2		1		

* vs symptomatic PE at D0.

COMMENTS

❑ This study showed that dalteparin given b.i.d. in patients with severe iliofemoral DVT appeared to be more effective in reducing both symptomatic and asymptomatic PE (better constant antithrombotic level ?) maximal AXa activity: 1.12 ± 0.47 in o.d. group vs 0.91 ± 0.46 IU/ml in dalteparin b.i.d.

❑ 50% of patients with DVT in the inferior vena cava had PE compared with 33% when DVT is lower.

❑ Symptomatic PEs were infrequent in young patients.

❑ An extension of this study including 631 patients was published in Med. Welt. 1997; 48 : 84-90. Investigators concluded that under certain preconditions, home-therapy of DVT is feasible.

A six-month venographic follow-up in 164 patients with acute deep vein thrombosis

AUTHORS	HOLMSTRÖM M.C., LINDMARKER P., GRANQVIST S. et al.
REF	Thromb. Haemostasis 1997; 78: 803-807

STUDY	Open-label, randomized
CENTERS (n)	3
COUNTRY	Sweden
PATIENTS (n)	*included* 204
	evaluated 164 (at 6 months)

INCLUSION CRITERIA

Patients with venographic proven DVT

OBJECTIVE

To evaluate Marder's score changes, 6 months after the initial diagnosis of DVT

STUDY DRUG	**Dalteparin**	sc daily dose: 200 AXa IU/kg o.d.
		treatment duration: 5-10 days
REFERENCE DRUG	**UFH**	continuous iv infusion APTT-adjusted
		treatment duration: 5-10 days
LONG-TERM TREATMENT	**OAC**	Warfarin for both groups since D1 up to 3 months at least

+ Elastic compression stocking

ASSESSMENTS

❑ DVT: venography at entry, after 5-10 days and after 6 months, Marder's score changes.

❑ Laboratory tests.

❑ Univariate analyses (male gender/D-dimers).

HOLMSTRÖM M. et al. 1997

	Dalteparin 200 AXa IU/kg x 1		UFH iv infusion		p
Venography 1 (at D0)	101		103		
DVT D/P*	49/37		29/49		
Venography 2 (at 5-10 days)	100 (1 iliacal vein thrombus)		102 (1 thrombocytopenia)		
Six-month follow-up:					
death	2		3		
recurrent DVT	2		3		
Venography 3 (at 6 months)	86		78		
complete lysis (D/P)*	32	(24/8) 37.2%	31	(25/6) 39.7%	NS
improvement > 50%	28	(11/7) ⎤	21	(9/12) ⎤	
improvement ≤ 50%	19	(7/12) ⎦ 54.6%	21	(13/8) ⎦ 53.8%	NS
unchanged	5	(5/0)	2	(1/1)	
worsened	2	(2/0)	3	(1/2)	

* D/P= distal/proximal.

COMMENTS
- ❑ With both initial treatments, in the majority of the patients, the thrombus decreased in size or lysed completely irrespective of its localization.
- ❑ The level of d-dimer on day 5 was significantly associated with an improvement in venographic outcome after 6 months (results not shown).
- ❑ Resolution of the thrombus was enhanced in males (results not shown).

Subcutaneous low-molecular-weight heparin compared with continuous intravenous unfractionated heparin in the treatment of proximal deep vein thrombosis

AUTHORS	SIMONNEAU G., CHARBONNIER B., DECOUSUS H. et al. for the DVT Enox Study
REF	Arch. Intern. Med. 1993; 153: 1541-1546

STUDY	Open-label, multicenter, randomized
CENTERS (n)	16
COUNTRIES	France, Belgium
PATIENTS (n)	*included* 134
	evaluated 117

Patients with confirmed DVT without sign of PE (patients with recent surgery excluded)

OBJECTIVE
Efficacy of sc administration of enoxaparin in the initial treatment of DVT (based on thrombus size reduction)

INITIAL DIAGNOSIS OF DVT
Bilateral venography at D0

STUDY DRUG	**Enoxaparin**	sc daily doses: 1mg/kg b.i.d. treatment duration: 10 days no monitoring
REFERENCE DRUG	**UFH**	iv infusion 500 IU/kg, then adjusted to APTT (1.5-2.5 initial values) treatment duration: 10 days
LONG-TERM TREATMENT	**OAC**	started at D10 and continued for at least 3 months

ASSESSMENTS
- ❏ DVT: Marder's scores D0-D10 blindly evaluated.
- ❏ Lung scan at entry and on D10; if suspected new PE, angiography.
- ❏ Major/minor bleeding
- ❏ Laboratory parameters.
- ❏ Thrombocytopenia.
- ❏ Three-month follow-up for recurrent thromboembolic events.

SIMONNEAU G. et al. 1993

	Enoxaparin 1mg/kg x 2	UFH infusion	
Initial treatment			
Patients	60	57	
Marder's score D0-D10:			
improved	35	18	chi^2 test
unchanged	25	34	p=0.003
worsened	0	5	
Patients with lung scan new defects	2	4	
Major hemorrhage	0	0	
Minor hemorrhage	4	0	
Thrombocytopenia	0	1	
Death	0	0	
Three-month follow-up			
recurrent DVT/ PE	0	1	
death (not thrombosis-related)	3	2	

COMMENTS

❑ Enoxaparin administered subcutaneously b.i.d. without monitoring was at least as effective and safe as intravenously monitored UFH in the initial treatment of DVT.

❑ No correlation between AXa level and venographic outcome in enoxaparin group.

❑ No correlation between APTT values and thromboembolic recurrences in UFH group.

Low molecular weight heparin versus warfarin in the prevention of recurrences after deep vein thrombosis

AUTHORS	PINI M., AIELLO S., MANOTTI C. et al.
REF	Thromb. Haemostasis 1994; 72: 191-197

STUDY	Open-label, randomized
CENTERS (n)	1
COUNTRY	Italy
PATIENTS (n)	included 187

OBJECTIVE
To compare the efficacy of enoxaparin vs OAC after an initial conventional treatment of DVT with UFH

INITIAL DIAGNOSIS OF DVT
Venography/strain gauge plethysmography + D-dimer test

INITIAL TREATMENT
to all patients

From day 0 up to day 10
UFH   iv bolus 5000 IU then sc dose b.i.d. 250 IU/kg according to APTT (1.3-1.9) treatment duration ≈ 10 days

+ Elastic stockings

LONG-TERM TREATMENT   From day 11 until 3 months:

Enoxaparin   sc dose: 40mg o.d.- home treatment
or
OAC (Warfarin)   oral daily dose: 10mg first dose, 4 days before heparin stopped (then adjusted to INR 2.5)

ASSESSMENTS
❑ Recurrences of thromboembolic events confirmed by objective methods at 3-month follow-up.
❑ Bleeding complications
❑ 9-month follow-up.

PINI M. et al. 1994

	Enoxaparin 40mg x 1	Warfarin	p
Patients at D10	93	94	
Treatment period: D11- 3 months			
Recurrence of DVT	5	3	
PE	1 (week 1)	1 (week 7)	
Total events	6 6%	4 4%	NS
Total bleeding complications	4 4%	12 13%	0.04
Major hemorrhage	3	3	
Death	4	3	
Nine-month follow-up *			
Recurrence of DVT (at month)	5 (4, 5, 6, 9, 10)	4 (5, 7, 8, 11)	
PE (at month)	5 (4, 5, 6, 7, 11)	0	
Total events	10	4	
Death	7 (1 fatal PE)	5	

* 36% of patients in OAC group, prolonged warfarin treatment up to 6 months and 15% up to 1 year.

COMMENTS

❑ Although the 40mg dosage of enoxaparin may appear inadequate (too low) especially just after the switch from UFH administered during the initial treatment of DVT, the incidence of total events was not significantly different from OAC-treated patients.

❑ The recurrences of thromboembolic events were mainly observed in medical patients so the duration of anticoagulation in these patients should be longer than 3 months.

❑ The 3-month recurrences in OAC-group developed also in patients with a satisfactory INR.

A comparison of low-molecular-weight heparin administered primarily at home with unfractionated heparin administered in the hospital for proximal deep vein thrombosis

AUTHORS	LEVINE M., GENT M., HIRSH J. et al.
REF	N. Engl. J. Med. 1996; 334: 677-681

STUDY	Open-label, multicenter, randomized	
CENTERS (n)	14	
COUNTRY	Canada	
PATIENTS (n)	*included*	500

OBJECTIVE
To test the feasibility of enoxaparin as initial home-treatment in patients with acute proximal DVT without evidence of PE

INITIAL DIAGNOSIS OF DVT
Impedance plethysmography (IPG)

STUDY DRUG	**Enoxaparin** *In hospital and/or at home*	sc daily doses: 1mg/kg b.i.d. treatment duration: at least 5 days
REFERENCE DRUG	**UFH** *In hospital*	iv route: bolus 5000 IU then infusion daily-adjusted to APTT values (60-85 sec) for at least 5 days
LONG-TERM TREATMENT	**Warfarin**	oral route 1st dose 10mg from D2 then daily adjusted to INR (2-3) treatment duration: 3 months at least

ASSESSMENTS
- ❑ Major hemorrhage during initial treatment.
- ❑ Three-month follow-up for:
  symptomatic recurrent DVT confirmed by systematic impedance plethysmography (at D0 and once monthly), venography or duplex ultrasonography.
- ❑ Clinical PE confirmed by lung scan or angiography.

LEVINE M. et al. 1996

	Enoxaparin 1mg/kg x 2		UFH infusion	
Patients	247		253	
Initial treatment				
Patients admitted to hospital	127*	51%	253**	100%
Early discharge	29		0	
Mean hospital stay (days ± SD)	2.2±3.8		6.5±3.4	
Patients not admitted to hospital	120	49%	0	
Major hemorrhage	5		3	
Three-month follow-up with OAC				
DVT/PE recurrences	13	5.3%	17	6.7%
death	11		17 (2 fatal PE)	

Of whom 98* and 102** were hospitalized before randomization.

COMMENTS
- ❏ Patients with proven proximal DVT without signs or symptoms of PE can be safely and effectively treated at home with a LMWH (enoxaparin) self-administered subcutaneously.
- ❏ INR was in the target range for less than 2/3 of patients.

A multicenter clinical trial comparing
once or twice-daily subcutaneous enoxaparin and intravenous heparin
in the treatment of acute deep vein thrombosis

AUTHORS	SPIRO T. E. for the Enoxaparin Clinical Trial Group
REF	Thromb. Haemostasis 1997; (Supp) (Abst 1527)

STUDY	Open-label, multicenter, randomized, controlled, two parallel dosages	
CENTERS *(n)*	74	
COUNTRIES	16	
PATIENTS *(n)*	*included*	900

INCLUSION CRITERIA
Patients with symptomatic DVT confirmed by venography or ultra-sonography with or without PE

OBJECTIVE
To compare once versus twice daily sc dosage of enoxaparin in the initial treatment of DVT

STUDY DRUG	**Enoxaparin**	• 1.5 mg/kg o.d. or • 1mg/kg b.i.d. these two dosages blindly administered treatment duration: probably about 5-8 days
REFERENCE DRUG	**UFH**	iv bolus then iv continuous infusion
LONG-TERM TREATMENT	**Warfarin**	from D1 up to D90

ASSESSMENTS
- ❑ DVT: clinical symptoms confirmed by venography or ultrasonography.
- ❑ PE: clinical symptoms confirmed by lung scan.
- ❑ Recurrence of events during a 3-month follow-up (primary efficacy outcome).
- ❑ Occurrence of bleeding during initial treatment.
- ❑ Death.

SPIRO T.E. 1997

	Enoxaparin			UFH		p
	1mg/kg x 2		1.5mg/kg x 1	iv infusion		
Patients	312		298	290		
Initial period						
total hemorrhage	54	17.3%	46	15.4%	39	13.4%	NS
major hemorrhage	4	1.3%	5	1.7%	6	2.1%	NS
Three-month follow-up						
recurrence of thromboembolic events	9	2.9%	13	4.4%	12	4.3%	NS
Death	7	2.2%	11	3.7%	9	3.1%	NS

COMMENTS
- ❏ Enoxaparin sc administered once or twice daily was as effective and safe as continuous iv infusion of UFH.
- ❏ Even though the difference was non significant, the twice daily regimen (total dosage 2mg/kg) appeared to be more effective than the lower once daily one (1.5mg/kg x 1).

Early versus late switch from enoxaparin to oral anticoagulant in the treatment of acute deep venous thrombosis: ANTENOX, a multicenter randomized open study

AUTHORS	LEROYER C., ILL P., DEVILLARD A. et al.
REF	Thromb. Haemostasis 1997; (Suppl) (Abst 3081)

STUDY	Open-label, multicenter, randomized
CENTERS (n)	3
COUNTRY	France
PATIENTS (n)	*included* 223
	evaluated 216

OBJECTIVE

To evaluate 2 different strategies for introducing OAC in the initial treatment of DVT (D1 vs D10)

INITIAL DIAGNOSIS

DVT: symptomatic confirmed by bilateral venography
PE: lung scan or angiography

STUDY DRUG

Enoxaparin sc daily dose: 1 mg/kg x 2
treatment duration ≈ 8 days
+ **OAC** (fluindione 20mg) **from D1** up to D90±20 (INR 2-3)

versus

Enoxaparin sc daily dose: 1 mg/kg x 2
treatment duration ≈ 14 days
+ **OAC** (fluindione 20mg) **from D10** up to D90±20 (INR 2-3)

+ Elastic compression stockings in both groups

ASSESSMENTS

❑ Recurrences of thromboembolic events during a 3-month follow-up confirmed by venography, angiography or lung scan.

❑ Hemorrhagic complications.

❑ Death (autopsy when possible).

LEROYER C. et al. 1997

	Enoxaparin 1mg/kg x 2 + OAC D1		Enoxaparin 1mg/kg x 2 + OAC D10		p
Patients	112		111		
Three-month follow-up					
Clinically suspected recurrent events	12	11%	8	7%	
Validated recurrence of thromboembolic events	0	0%	1 (PE)	0.9%	NS
Major hemorrhage	5	4%	2	2%	NS
Minor hemorrhage	7	6%	7	6%	
Death	5	4%	2	2%	NS

COMMENTS

❑ Interesting study showing that the early addition on D1 of oral anticoagulant to LMWH was as effective and safe as late switch (D10) in preventing thromboembolic events.

❑ This therapeutical approach reduces hospital length stay: 10.9±5.7 days vs 15.0±8.3.

A randomized trial of subcutaneous low molecular weight heparin (CY216) compared with intravenous unfractionated heparin in the treatment of deep vein thrombosis

AUTHORS	A Collaborative European Multicentre Study
REF	Thromb. Haemostasis 1991; 65 : 251-256

STUDY Open-label, multicenter, randomized, two parallel groups

CENTERS (n) 17
COUNTRIES France, Italy, Spain, Switzerland

PATIENTS (n) enrolled 166
evaluated 148 (for efficacy)

OBJECTIVE
Efficacy of initial treatment based on thrombus evolution (Arnesen's and Marder's scores) in medical or surgical patients.

DIAGNOSIS OF DVT
Bilateral venography blindly evaluated

STUDY DRUG **Nadroparin** sc daily dose: 450 AXa ICU/kg (170 AXa IU) subdivided in 2 injections (≈ 85 IU/kg x 2)

0.5ml x 2 for BW 50-59 kg   0.7ml x 2 for BW 70-79 kg
0.6ml x 2 for BW 60-69 kg   0.8ml x 2 for BW 80-89 kg
treatment duration: 10 days

REFERENCE DRUG **UFH** iv infusion; initial dose 20 IU/kg/h then, daily APTT-adjusted (x 1.5-2)
treatment duration: 10 days

LONG-TERM TREATMENT **sc heparin or oral anticoagulant** — duration non stated

ASSESSMENTS

❑ Quantitative/qualitative evaluation: venographic changes between D0-D10.
❑ Lung scans at D0 and D10 confirmed by angiography if abnormal findings.
❑ Major hemorrhage requiring premature termination of treatment.
❑ 3-month follow-up for recurrent thromboembolisms.

A collaborative European Multicentre Study. 1991

	Nadroparin $\approx$ 85IU/kg x 2	UFH iv infusion	
Patients (evaluable venograms)	77	71	
Initial treatment			
Venographic score (Arnesen)			
substantial lysis	34 44.0%	21 28.0%	chi^2
moderate lysis	23 29.0%	23 32.0%	
unchanged or increased	20 27.0%	27 40.0%	p=00.3
Pulmonary scan			
Pulmonary defect D0	12.7%	8.3%	
D10	8.3%	6.3%	
Major hemorrhage	2 2.3%	4 5%	
Three-month follow-up			
Patients	78	73	
Thromboembolic events (DVT/ PE)	2 (1 DVT/ 1 fatal PE)	0	
Death	3	3	

COMMENTS
- ❏ Nadroparin at fixed body weight sc dose was at least as effective as conventional intravenous UFH regimen, in particular without increased risk of PE, thrombus extension or hemorrhagic complication.
- ❏ The improvement in the nadroparin group according to Arnesen and/or Marder's score (not shown here) was significantly better than in UFH group.
- ❏ Simplified therapy without laboratory monitoring.

Comparison of subcutaneous low molecular weight heparin with intravenous standard heparin in proximal deep vein thrombosis

AUTHORS	PRANDONI P., LENSING A.W., BULLER H. et al.
REF	Lancet. 1992; 339: 441-445

STUDY	Open-label, randomized
CENTERS (n)	1
COUNTRY	Italy
PATIENTS (n)	*randomized* 170
	evaluated 168 (at D10)

OBJECTIVE

Efficacy of initial treatment with nadroparin or UFH on thromboembolic disorder recurrences observed at D10 and at 6-month

INITIAL DIAGNOSIS OF DVT

Venography, lung scan, chest radiograph at D0 and D10

STUDY DRUG	**Nadroparin**	sc daily doses ≈ 85 AXa IU/kg x 2
		2 x 0.5ml < 55kg, 0.6ml for 55-80kg, 0.7ml for > 80kg
		treatment duration: 10 days
REFERENCE DRUG	**UFH**	iv bolus (100 IU/kg) then infusion of a total daily dose of ≈ 35 000 IU, APTT-adjusted (x 1.5-2)
		treatment duration: 10 days
LONG-TERM TREATMENT	**Warfarin**	oral route
		initial dose: 5mg then weekly adjusted to INR = 2-3
		treatment duration: from D7 up to at least 3 months

ASSESSMENTS

❏ DVT, PE: venography, lung scan at D0 and D10 (blind evaluation).

❏ Clinical assessment at 1, 3, 6 months for recurrent DVT and PE.

PRANDONI P. et al. 1992

	Nadroparin 85 AXa IU/kg x 2		UFH iv infusion		p
Initial treatment (D0-D10)					
Patients with venograms	83		85		
• improved	50	60% ⎤	36	42% ⎤	chi²
• unchanged	28	34% ⎥	35	41% ⎥	0.017
• worsened	5	6% ⎦	14	16% ⎦	
Lung scan new defects	4/79	5%	15/81	19%	<0.02
Severe hemorrhage	1	1%	3	4%	
Thromboembolic events	1 (fatal PE)		4*		
6-month follow-up					
Thromboembolic events					
DVT/PE (fatal)	2/4 (3 fatal PE)		5/7 (3 fatal PE)		
Total thromboembolic events (D0-6 months)	6	7%	12	14%	NS
Other death	3		9		
Death in cancer patients	1/15	7%	8/18	44%	0.02

* 1 PE, 3 DVT recurrences.

COMMENTS
- ❏ Despite the large mean interval between onset of symptoms and initiation of treatment (10 days), the changes in venographic score showed a significant difference in favor of nadroparin.
- ❏ No significant difference in thromboembolic events during the 6-month follow-up, but less pulmonary defects in nadroparin group.
- ❏ Unexpected mortality reduction in cancer patients treated with nadroparin.
- ❏ Home-treatment appeared possible since nadroparin was administered without monitoring.

Subcutaneous low molecular weight heparin versus subcutaneous unfractionated heparin in the treatment of deep vein thrombosis: a Polish multicentre trial

AUTHORS	LOPACIUK S., MEISSNER J., FILIPECKI S. et al.
REF	Thromb. Haemostasis. 1992; 68: 14-18

STUDY	Open-label, multicenter, randomized
CENTERS (n)	6
COUNTRY	Poland
PATIENTS (n)	included 149
	evaluated 134

OBJECTIVE
Efficacy of initial treatment with nadroparin or UFH based on thrombus changes (Arnesen's score)

DIAGNOSIS OF DVT
Bilateral venograms blindly evaluated at D1 and D10

STUDY DRUG	Nadroparin	sc daily doses ≈ 85 AXa IU/kg x 2 (corresponding to 225 AXa ICU/kg b.i.d.) treatment duration: 10 days
REFERENCE DRUG	UFH	iv bolus (5000 IU), then sc daily dose 500 IU/kg as 2 injections adjusted thereafter according to APTT or recalcification clotting time treatment duration: 10 days
LONG-TERM TREATMENT	Acenocoumarol	oral dose adjusted to INR 2-3 treatment duration ≥ 3 months - started at D7

ASSESSMENTS
- ❏ Venographic changes D0-D10 with blind evaluation.
- ❏ PE: clinical symptoms confirmed by lung scan or angiography
- ❏ Major hemorrhage.
- ❏ 3-month follow-up.

LOPACIUK S. et al. 1992

	Nadroparin 85 AXa IU/kg x 2		**UFH** sc APTT-adjusted doses x 2		
Initial treatment					
Patients	74		75		
Evaluable venograms	68		66		
Venographic score (Arnesen):					
improved (completely or partially)	45	66.0%	32	48.5%	chi^2
unchanged	13	19.0%	22	33.5%	
worsened	10	15.0%	12	18.0%	p=0.05
PE (symptomatic)	0		1		
Major hemorrhage	0		1		
Three-month follow-up with OAC					
Patients	74		72		
DVT recurrences	0		2		
PE (symptomatic)	0		0		
Death	0		1		

COMMENTS

- Improvement in Arnesen's score was better in nadroparin-treated patients than in UFH group.
- Without initial intravenous bolus administration, treatment directly with sc nadroparin was at least as effective as heparin given in initial iv bolus then by sc route monitored daily.
- Very few bleeding complications.

Randomized trial of subcutaneous low molecular weight heparin CY216 (Fraxiparine) compared with intravenous unfractionated heparin in the curative treatment of submassive pulmonary embolism. A dose-ranging study

AUTHORS	THERY C., SIMONNEAU G., MEYER G. et al.
REF	Circulation. 1992; 85: 1380-1389

STUDY	Open-label, multicenter, randomized
CENTERS (n)	12
COUNTRY	France
PATIENTS (n)	*included* 101
	evaluated 94 (ITT)

OBJECTIVE

Determination of the optimal nadroparin dosage for the treatment of submassive PE in patients with recent (within 3 days) proven pulmonary embolism with vascular obstruction of 15-55%

DIAGNOSIS OF PE/DVT

Lung angiography and bilateral venography blindly evaluated at D0 and

STUDY DRUG	**Nadroparin**	3 tested sc daily doses (in 2 injections) :
		• 400 AXa ICU/kg (≈ 150 AXa IU/kg)
		• 600 AXa ICU/kg (≈ 230 AXa IU/kg)
		• 900 AXa ICU/kg (≈ 340 AXa IU/kg)
		treatment duration: 14 days
REFERENCE DRUG	**UFH**	iv bolus 50 IU/kg then infusion 600 IU/kg adjusted to APTT (x 2.5-3)

ASSESSMENTS

❏ Pulmonary angiogram (Miller's score at D0 and D8±1).
❏ DVT: bilateral venography at D0 and D8.
❏ Bleeding complications.
❏ Adverse events.

THERY C. et al. 1992

	Nadroparin AXa ICU/kg			**UFH**	**p**
sc daily dose AXa ICU/kg	400	600	900*	iv infusion	
Patients	35	26	7	33	
Pulmonary angiograms (D8):	31	18	6	21	
improved	29 (93.5%)	17 (94.4%)		21 (100%)	
unchanged	0	1		0	
worsened	2	0	0	0	
Reduction in vascular obstruction					
(D0-D8)	20.5±2.3%	21.0±3.4%		23.7±2.3%	NS
Patients with DVT (D0)	30	17		25	
Patients assessed at D8	29	15		15	
DVT improved	22	14		13	NS
unchanged	5	0		1	
worsened	2	1		1	
Major hemorrhage leading to interruption of treatment	0	5 (19%)	4 (57%)	2 (6%)	
Death	1(septic shock)	0	4 (AMI)	1 (AMI)	

* Discontinued regimen.

COMMENTS

❑ In this trial, the best dose regimen for efficacy/risk ratio (400 AXa ICU/kg) was very close to the dosage used for the treatment of DVT (450 AXa ICU/kg corresponding to ≈ 170 AXa IU/kg).

❑ A submassive PE can effectively be treated by sc LMWH.

❑ No correlation between dosage (and AXa activity) and relative angiographic or venographic improvement.

❑ Good correlation between dosage (but not necessarily with AXa level) and major hemorrhage.

Treatment of venous thrombosis with intravenous unfractionated heparin administered in the hospital as compared with subcutaneous low molecular weight heparin administered at home

AUTHORS	KOOPMAN M.M.W., PRANDONI P., PIOVELLA F. et al. for the TASMAN Group
REF	N. Engl. J. Med. 1996; 334: 682-687

STUDY	Open-label, multicenter, randomized
CENTERS *(n)*	10
COUNTRIES	Europe, Australia, New Zealand
PATIENTS *(n)*	400

OBJECTIVE
To test the feasibility of home treatment in patients with symptomatic confirmed proximal DVT without symptomatic PE

INITIAL DIAGNOSTIC OF DVT
Venography or ultrasonography

STUDY DRUG	**Nadroparin** *At hospital and/or at home*	sc twice daily dose B.W. adapted ($\approx$ 85AXa IU/kg x 2) treatment duration: about 6 days (6.5 ± 2.2)
REFERENCE DRUG	**UFH** *At hospital*	iv initial bolus 5000 IU then continuous infusion 1250 IU/h APTT-adjusted (x 1.5-2 above control values)
LONG-TERM TREATMENT	**OAC**	from first day up to at least 3 months (INR 2-3)

ASSESSMENTS
- Blind assessment commitee for all diagnoses and outcomes.
- Symptomatic recurrent DVT confirmed by venography or Doppler ultrasonography during a 6-month follow-up.
- Lung scan or angiography for suspected PE.
- Major bleeding.
- Thrombocytopenia.
- Quality of life.

KOOPMAN M.M.W. et al. 1996

	Nadroparin 85 IU/kg x 2		UFH iv infusion	
Total patients	202		198	
Initial treatment				
Admitted to hospital	130	64.4%	198	100%
Treated entirely in hospital	50	24.7%	198	100%
Not admitted to hospital	72	35.6%	0	0%
Early discharge	80	39.6%	0	0%
Average hospital stay (D)	2.7		8.1	
Major bleeding	1 (D6)	0.5%	2 (D1,D2)	1%
Thrombocytopenia with spontaneous recovery	3		5	
6-month follow-up				
DVT recurrences	10		12	
PE	4 (2 fatal)		5 (1 fatal)	
Total thromboembolic events	14	6.9%	17	8.6%
Major bleeding	0		2 (fatal)	
Death	14	6.9%	16	8.1%

COMMENTS

❏ These results suggest that a large proportion of patients with established proximal DVT can be safely and effectively treated at home using sc nadroparin self-administered.

❏ Physical activity and social functioning was better in patients assigned to nadroparin.

❏ This medical strategy strongly reduces the cost of therapy; reduction of 67% in duration of hospitalization.

Comparison of a once daily with a twice daily subcutaneous nadroparin calcium regimen in the treatment of deep vein thrombosis: the FRAXODI study

AUTHORS	CHARBONNIER B.A., FIESSINGER J.N., BANGA J.D. et al.
REF	Thromb. Haemostasis 1998; 7-9: 897-901

STUDY	Multicenter, randomized, double-blind, two parallel groups
CENTERS (n)	70
COUNTRIES	11 European countries
PATIENTS (n)	included 651
	evaluated 651

OBJECTIVE

To assess if a single daily injection using a concentrated formulation is at least as effective and well tolerated as the same daily dose divided in two injections of the standard concentration in the initial treatment of symptomatic proximal DVT.

STUDY DRUG **Nadroparin** sc daily dose: 170 AXa IU/kg administered
• **in two injections** using a standard concentration of 9500 AXa IU/ml ≈ 0.1ml/10kg x 2
• **in one injection** using a concentrated formulation of 19,000 AXa IU/ml ≈ 0.1ml/10kg x 1
treatment duration: 4 to 10 days

LONG-TERM TREATMENT **OAC** from D1 up to at least 3 months (INR 2-3)

ASSESSMENTS

❑ Symptomatic proximal DVT: worsening or recurrence of initial DVT or onset of a DVT in the contralateral leg confirmed by venography.

❑ Symptomatic PE confirmed by lung scan and/or angiography.

❑ Combined end-point: DVT recurrence/PE/death thrombosis-related at 3 months.

❑ Major, minor hemorrhage.

❑ Adverse events.

CHARBONNIER B.A. et al. 1998

| | Nadroparin 170 AXa IU/kg | | | p |
	in 1 injection		subdivided in 2 injections	
Patients	316		335	
Three-month follow-up				
DVT recurrences	8		13	
Non fatal PE	3	0.9%	4	1.2%
Total thromboembolic events	11	3.5%	17	5.1%
Death (possible PE)	2	0.6%	6	1.8%
Combined outcome*	13	4.1%	24	7.2%	<0.001
Total death	9	2.8%	13	3.9%
Major hemorrhage during initial treatment with OAC alone	4 (2 fatal) 1.3% 5 (1 fatal) 1.6%		4 (1 fatal) 1.2% 4 (1 fatal) 1.2%	
Thrombocytopenia	3	0.9%	2	0.6%

* Primary end-point.

COMMENTS

❑ The initial treatment of symptomatic proximal DVT with a single daily injection of nadroparin (body weight adjusted dose) was as effective and safe as the same dosage administered twice daily.

❑ The combined primary end-point was significantly reduced in nadroparin once daily-treated patients (each of the outcomes DVT recurrences, fatal and non fatal PE was reduced).

Low molecular weight heparin in the treatment of patients with venous thromboembolism

AUTHORS	The Columbus Investigators
REF	N. Eng. J. Med. 1997; 337: 657-662

STUDY	Multicenter, open-label, randomized
CENTERS (n)	>30
COUNTRIES	Canada, Europe
PATIENTS (n)	randomized 1021
	evaluated 1021

INCLUSION CRITERIA
Patients with acute symptomatic DVT or PE or both. About one third with associated PE and DVT

OBJECTIVE
Can treatments of both be the same?

STUDY DRUG	Reviparin	sc daily doses: • 6300 AXa IU b.i.d. for BW > 60kg
		• 4200 AXa IU b.i.d. for BW 46-60kg
		• 3500 AXa IU b.i.d. for BW < 45kg
		at home or in-hospital treatment: duration at least 6 days

REFERENCE DRUG	UFH	iv bolus 5000 IU then
		iv infusion 1250 IU/h adjusted to APTT x 1.5-2.5 control values
		in-hospital treatment duration: at least 6 days

LONG-TERM TREATMENT	Oral anticoagulant for both groups from D1/D2 up to 12 weeks

ASSESSMENTS
- ❏ Confirmation of DVT and PE by venography or compression ultrasonography (CUS), pulmonary angiogram or lung scan.
- ❏ Daily clinical examination.
- ❏ Primary end point: recurrence of confirmed symptomatic DVT or PE plus major bleeding within 12-week follow-up.
- ❏ Death.

The Columbus Investigators, 1997

	Reviparin BW-adjusted dose x 2		UFH iv infusion		p
Patients (total number)	510		511		
With DVT only	372	73.0%	378	74.0%	
With PE	138	27.0%	133	26.0%	
Recurrent thromboembolism					
D0-D14	16		15		
D0-D84:	27*	5.3%	25**	4.9%	NS
in patients with PE	8		8		
in patients with DVT	19		17		
Major bleeding					
D0-D14	10	(0 fatal)	8	(2 fatal)	
D0-D84	16	3.1%	12	2.3%	NS
Death					
D0-D14	5 (2 PE)		4 (2 PE)		
D0-D84	36 (3 PE)	7.1%	39 (3 PE)	7.6%	

* Symptomatic DVT in 17 patients.
** Symptomatic DVT in 15 patients.

COMMENTS
❏ First trial in which patients with thromboembolism (DVT and/or PE) were evaluated after receiving the same treatment regimen.
❏ Reviparin and UFH regimens (≈ 29.000 ± 7800 IU/24h) were not significantly different regarding effectiveness and safety.
❏ In cancer patients, the recurrences were twice higher than in non cancer patients (data not shown).
❏ 69% of recurrent PE occurred in the same territory where first diagnosed (lung) and 31% in patients with previous DVT.
❏ All six fatal PE occurred in patients with PE at presentation.

Subcutaneous low molecular weight heparin compared with continuous intravenous heparin in the treatment of proximal vein thrombosis

AUTHORS	HULL R.D., RASKOB G.E., PINEO G.F. et al.
REF	N. Eng. J. Med. 1992; 326: 975-982

STUDY	Multicenter, randomized, double-blind
CENTERS (n)	15
COUNTRIES	United States, Canada
PATIENTS (n)	enrolled 432
	evaluated 432

INCLUSION CRITERIA
- Patients with symptomatic DVT confirmed by venography/impedance plethysmography or B-mode
- Lung scan within 48h of the study entry

OBJECTIVE
Evaluation of thromboembolic recurrency, 3 months after initial therapy

STUDY DRUG	Tinzaparin	sc daily dose: 175 AXa IU/kg o.d. plus iv bolus and infusion of saline treatment duration: 5-6 days
REFERENCE DRUG	UFH	iv route bolus 5000 IU then continuous infusion of 40,320 IU/24h or 29,760 IU/24h according to risk factors, thereafter based on daily APTT values (x 1.5-2.5) sc injection of placebo o.d. treatment duration: 5-6 days
LONG-TERM TREATMENT	Warfarin	oral initial daily dose: 10mg started on D2 of initial therapy, thereafter adjusted to an INR 2-3 for at least 3 months

ASSESSMENTS
- During the initial treatment, daily clinical examination for recurrent DVT, PE and hemorrhage.
- 3-month follow-up for recurrent venous thromboembolisms confirmed by venography, IPG, lung scan, angiography.

HULL R.D. et al. 1992

	Tinzaparin 175 AXa IU/kg x 1		UFH iv infusion		p
Patients	213		219		
Three-month follow-up					
Recurrent DVT	3		9		
PE	3	(1 fatal)	6	(4 fatal)	
Total thromboembolism (new episodes)	6	2.8%	15**	6.9%	0.07
Major hemorrhage during initial therapy	1	0.5%	11	5.0%	0.001
Thrombocytopenia*	6	2.8%	3	1.4%	
Total death	10	4.7%	21	9.6%	0.05

* Platelet counts <150,000/mm^3.
** APTT was in therapeutic range in 13 patients and subtherapeutic in 2, during initial heparin treatment.

COMMENTS

❑ This pioneering trial showed that a LMWH subcutaneously administered o.d. without monitoring is at least as effective and safe as conventional intravenous monitored UFH regimen for the initial treatment of DVT.

❑ The initial treatment of DVT with tinzaparin was associated with fewer death during the 3-month follow-up. This observation has been reported for other LMWHs but the reason for these differences remains obscure.

A comparison of low molecular weight heparin with unfractionated heparin for acute pulmonary embolism

AUTHORS	SIMONNEAU G, SORS H, CHARBONNIER B, BEAU B for the THESEE Group
REF	N. Engl. J. Med. 1997; 337: 663-669

STUDY	Open-label, multicenter, randomized, two parallel groups
CENTERS (n)	57
COUNTRY	France
PATIENTS (n)	*included* 612
	evaluated 612

INCLUSION CRITERIA
Symptomatic PE documented by VQ lung scan or angiography or inconclusive VQ lung scan + DVT (documented by venography or ultrasonography)

EXCLUSION CRITERIA
PE requiring thrombolysis or surgery

STUDY DRUG	**Tinzaparin**	sc daily dose: 175 AXa IU/kg o.d. treatment duration: at least 5 days (7.3±2.3)
REFERENCE DRUG	**UFH**	iv infusion APTT-adjusted (x 2-3 above control value) treatment duration: at least 5 days (7.0±2.4) *69% of included patients received therapeutic doses of UFH before randomization (during 18±6h)*
LONG-TERM TREATMENT		Oral anticoagulant for both groups from D1-D3 to at least 3 months (INR 2-3)

ASSESSMENTS
❏ Primary outcomes: combined end point defined as:
  • symptomatic recurrent venous thromboembolism objectively documented,
  • major bleeding
  • and death from D1 to D8 (and from D1 to D90).
❏ Secondary outcome:
  • change in pulmonary vascular obstruction from D1 to D8.

SIMONNEAU G. et al. 1997

	Tinzaparin 175 AXa IU/kg x 1		UFH iv infusion		p
Patients	304		308		
Recurrent thromboembolism D1-D8 Total D1-D90	3 5	 1.6%	2 6	 1.9%	 NS
Major bleeding (MB) D1-D8 Total * D1-D90	3 6	 2.0%	5 8	 2.6%	 NS
Death D1-D8 Total D1-D90	4 (2 PE) 12 (3 PE, 1 MB)	 3.9%	3 (2PE, 1MB) 14 (3 PE, 2 MB)	 4.5%	 NS
Primary combined endpoints D1-D8 Total* D1-D90	9 18	3.0% 5.9%	9 22	2.9% 7.1%	NS NS
Secondary endpoint Lung scan: vascular obst. % D1 (patients) D8 (patients)	(273) (258)	47±20% 18.4±13.5%	(274) (260)	46±21% 19±13.9%	NS NS

* Patients who experienced event both between D1-D8 and D9-D90 were counted only once.

COMMENTS

❑ Both treatments tinzaparin and UFH were similar in terms of efficacy and safety.

❑ This study clearly showed that patients with acute PE (except for those with impaired hemodynamics) can be treated effectively and safety with o.d. sc tinzaparin, without laboratory monitoring.

❑ The effective dose of tinzaparin for treatment of PE and/or for treatment of DVT is identical.

Expert comments

RUSSELL HULL. *Treatment of venous thromboembolism: advantages of LMWHs*

Unfractionated heparin has been used extensively in the prevention and treatment of venous thromboembolism. Recently, various low-molecular-weight heparins have been evaluated against a number of different controls for these same clinical problems. In a number of countries, the low-molecular-weight heparins have replaced unfractionated heparin for both the prevention and the treatment of venous thromboembolism.

The anticoagulant response to a standard dose of heparin varies widely among patients. Heparin is poorly absorbed from a subcutaneous site, especially at lower doses (1).

Unless a prescriptive heparin nomogram is used, many patients receive inadequate heparin in the initial 24 - 48 hours of treatment (2-4). This inadequate therapy has been shown to increase the incidence of venous thromboembolism during follow up (5-7). Treatment is further complicated by the fact that there is diurnal variation in the APTT response in patients on a constant infusion of intravenous heparin (8). A peak response is seen at 3 AM, and a reduction of heparin infusion in response to the high APTT could result in subtherapeutic levels later in the day (8). There is a wide variation in the sensitivity of various thromboplastins used in performing the APTT, and even with the same thromboplastin, different coagulometers may yield different results (8). It is necessary for each laboratory to define a therapeutic range with respect to their APTT in terms of heparin blood levels (therapeutic range 0.2 - 0.4 U per ml of heparin) (8).

Although there is a strong correlation between subtherapeutic APTT values and recurrent thromboembolism, the relationship between supratherapeutic APTT and bleeding (APTT ratio 2.5 or more) is less definite (8). Indeed, bleeding during heparin therapy is more closely related to underlying clinical risk factors than to APTT elevation above the therapeutic range (10,11).

The low-molecular-weight heparins are different compounds with distinct pharmacologic properties (12,13), and because different regimens have been used in clinical trials, it is considered inappropriate to use meta-analyses for comparing the effects of low-molecular-weight heparin with placebo, unfractionated heparin, or other active agents.

Despite the various differences between the low-molecular-weight heparins, clinical outcomes in clinical trials are very similar, particularly in prophylactic studies using lower doses. In the higher doses used in treatment of thrombotic disorders, it is possible that differences in outcomes may become apparent.

In the treatment of established venous thromboembolism, low-molecular-weight heparin given by subcutaneous injection has a number of advantages over continuous intravenous unfractionated heparin. It can be given by once- or twice-daily subcutaneous injection, and the antithrombotic response to low-molecular-weight heparin is highly correlated with body weight, permitting administration of a fixed dose without laboratory monitoring.

In a number of early clinical trials (some of which were dose-finding phase I-II studies), low-molecular-weight heparin given by subcutaneous or intravenous injection was compared with continuous intravenous unfractionated heparin, with repeat venography at day 7-10 being the primary endpoint (14-18). These studies demonstrated that low-molecular-weight heparin was at least as effective as unfractionated heparin in preventing extension or increasing resolution of thrombi on repeat venography (14-18). More recently, the more relevant clinical endpoints of recurrent venous thromboembolism or death during follow up have been assessed (19-23, 24-26). These studies are not all comparable because (a) different regimens of low-molecular-weight heparins were used, (b) not all studies ensured that adequate intravenous heparin therapy was given or properly monitored, and (c) some studies included patients with distal as well as proximal deep vein thrombosis. Only one study (19) was double blinded, although others used blinded assessment of outcome measures for both efficacy and safety. Low-molecular-weight heparin was given for 6-14 days, with warfarin therapy starting either on day 2 (19) or day 7-10 (20-23). Warfarin was continued for three months with the target INR range between 2.0 - 3.0. Consequently meta-analysis should not be used to assess efficacy and safety. The outcomes in terms of recurrent venous thromboembolism, major bleeding, and mortality for five clinical trials using clinical endpoints are summarized in Table 1.

One clinical trial was a double-blind randomized study of 432 patients who received either once-daily subcutaneous low-molecular-weight heparin (tinzaparin) or unfractionated heparin by continuous intravenous infusion using a heparin nomogram to ensure adequate heparinization (19). Warfarin was started on day 2 and was continued for three months, with a targeted INR of 2-3. Patients on low-molecular-weight heparin had fewer recurrent events (non significant), and the rates of major bleeding and death were significantly lower when compared with the unfractionated heparin group. None of the other clinical trials demonstrated a significant decrease in any of these clinical events. When the result of this trial and that of Prandoni et al (20) were pooled, there was a striking decrease in mortality in the patients receiving low-molecular-weight heparin, particularly for patients with cancer (27). Most of the abrupt deaths could not be attributed to thromboembolic events, suggesting that the benefits of low-molecular-weight heparin may not be entirely related to thrombotic events.

A cost-effectiveness analysis indicated that low-molecular-weight heparin was cost-effective when compared with continuous intravenous heparin under the study protocol conditions, because monitoring was not necessary and there were fewer complications requiring rehospitalization and treatment (28). These findings were verified by a sensitivity analysis. It was estimated that 37% of patients on low-molecular-weight heparin could have been discharged on day 2, which would have further increased the cost-effectiveness of the low-molecular-weight heparin (28).

REFERENCES	TREATMENT	RECURRENT VENOUS THROMBOEMBOLISM N. (%)	MAJOR BLEEDING n. (%)	MORTALITY n. (%)
Prandoni et al (20)	Nadroparin	6/85 (7.1)	1/85 (1.2)	6/85 (7.1)
	Heparin	12/85 (14.1)	3/85 (3.8)	12/85 (14.1)
Hull et al (19)	Tinzaparin	6/213 (2.8)	1/213 (0.5)[a]	10/213 (4.7)[a]
	Heparin	15/219 (6.8)	11/219 (5.0)	21/219 (9.6)
Lopaciuk et al (21)[b]	Nadroparin	0/74 (0)	0/74	0/74
	Heparin	3/72 (4.2)	1/72 (1.4)	1/72 (1.4)
Lindmarker et al (23)[c]	Dalteparin	5/101 (5.0)	1/101	2/101 (2.0)
	Heparin	3/103 (2.9)	0/103	3/103 (2.9)
Simonneau et al (22)	Enoxaparin	0/67	0/67	3/67 (4.5)
	Heparin	0/67	0/67	2/67 (3.0)
Levine et al (24)	Enoxaparin	13/247 (5.3)	5/247 (2.0)	11/247 (4.5)
	Heparin	17/253 (6.7)	3/253 (1.2)	17/253 (6.7)
Koopman et al (25)	Nadroparin	14/202 (6.9)	1/202 (0.5)	14/202 (6.9)
	Heparin	17/198 (8.6)	4/198 (2.0)	16/198 (8.1)
Columbus Investigators (26)	Clivarin	27/510 (5.3)	16/510 (3.1)	36/510 (7.1)
	Heparin	25/511 (4.9)	12/511 (2.3)	39/511 (7.6)

(a) p<0.05 vs heparin   (b) 19.5% had calf vein deep vein thrombosis (involvement of the popliteal).   (c) 42.6% distal deep vein thrombosis only.

Table 1   Randomized trials of low-molecular-weight heparin vs unfractionated heparin for the treatment of proximal deep vein thrombosis: results of long-term follow up

Two recently reported studies indicate that, in selected patients, low-molecular-weight heparin treatment can be administered safely outside the hospital (24,25). Patients who met the entry criteria were randomized to receive twice-daily low-molecular-weight heparin either entirely outside of the hospital or with early discharge, or continuous intravenous heparin in the hospital. Warfarin was started on day 1 or 2 and was continued for three months. All studies showed equivalence with respect to the incidence of recurrent venous thromboembolism, major bleeding, and mortality rates (24,25). Whether or not out-of-hospital treatment can be more widely applied in the treatment of proximal venous thrombosis awaits further study.

Evidence is accumulating that low-molecular-weight heparins can be used safely for the treatment of acute, submassive pulmonary embolism as well. One recent study reported that initial therapy of subcutaneous LMWH is as safe and effective as unfractionated intravenous heparin in acute pulmonary embolism patients (29). Studies are currently underway to assess the effectiveness and safety of treatment with low-molecular-weight heparin for three months compared with standard heparin followed by warfarin therapy, and for the treatment of proximal venous thrombosis in pregnancy comparing administration of once-daily low-molecular-weight heparin with twice-daily, adjusted-dose, subcutaneous unfractionated heparin.

REFERENCES

(1) Bara L. Billaud E. Gramond G. et al. Comparative pharmacokinetics of low molecular weight heparin (PK 10169) and unfractionated heparin after intravenous and subcutaneous administration. Thromb Res 1985; 39:631-636.

(2) Fennerty A. Thomas P. Backhouse G. et al. Audit of control of heparin treatment. BMJ 1985; 290:27-28.

(3) Wheeler AP. Jaquiss RD. Newman JH. Physician practices in the treatment of pulmonary embolism and deep-venous thrombosis. Arch Intern Med 1988; 148:1321-1325.

(4) Cruickshank MK. Levine MN. Hirsh J. et al. A standard nomogram for the management of heparin therapy. Arch Intern Med 1991; 151: 333-337.

(5) Hull RD. Raskob GE. Hirsh J. et al. Continuous intravenous heparin compared with intermittent subcutaneous heparin in the initial treatment of proximal-vein thrombosis. N Engl J Med 1986; 315:1109-1114.

(6) Raschke RA. Reilly BM. Guidry JR. et al. The weight-based heparin dosing nomogram compared with a standard care nomogram. Ann Intern Med 1993; 119:874-881.

(7) Hull RD. Raskob GE. Brant RF. Pineo GF. Valentine KA. Relation Between the Time to Achieve the Lower Limit of the APTT Therapeutic Range and Recurrent Venous Thromboembolism During Heparin Treatment for Deep Vein Thrombosis. Arch Intern Med December 1997 Vol 157 2562-2568.

(8) Hull RD. Raskob GE. Rosenbloom DR. et al. Optimal therapeutic level of heparin therapy in patients with venous thrombosis. Arch Int Med 1992; 152:1589-1595.

(9) Brill-Edwards P. Ginsberg S. Johnston M. et al. Establishing a therapeutic range for heparin therapy. Ann Intern Med 1993; 119:104-109.

(10) Hull RD. Raskob GE. Rosenbloom D. et al. Heparin for 5 days as compared with 10 days in the initial treatment of proximal venous thrombosis. N Engl J Med 1990; 322:1260-1264.

(11) Campbell NR. Hull RD. Brant RF. Hogan DB. Pineo GF. Raskob GE. Aging & Heparin Related Bleeding. Arch Intern Med 1996; 156: 857-859.

(12) Fareed J. Walenga JM. Hoppensteadt D. et al l. Comparative study on the in vitro and in vivo activities of seven low-molecular-weight heparins. Haemostasis 1988; 18(Suppl.3):3-15.

(13) Barrowcliffe TW. Curtis AD. Johnson EA. et al. An international standard for low molecular weight heparin. Thromb Haemost 1988; 60:1-7.

(14) Holm HA. Ly B. Handeland GF. et al. Subcutaneous heparin treatment of deep venous thrombosis. A comparison of unfractionated and low molecular weight heparin. Haemostasis 1986; 16:30-37.

(15) Albada J. Nieuwenhuis HK. Sixma JJ. Treatment of acute venous thromboembolism with low molecular weight heparin (Fragmin): results of a double-blind randomized study. Circulation 1989; 80:935-940.

(16) Bratt G. Aberg W. Johansson M. et al. 1990. Two daily subcutaneous injections of Fragmin as compared with intravenous standard heparin in the treatment of deep venous thrombosis (DVT). Thromb Haemost 1990; 64:506-510.

(17) Harenberg J. Hulk K. Bratsch H. et al. Therapeutic application of subcutaneous low-molecular-weight heparin in acute venous thrombosis. Haemostasis 1990; 20(Suppl.1):205-219.

(18) Siegbahn A. Hassan S. Boberg J. et al. Subcutaneous treatment of deep venous thrombosis with low molecular weight heparin. A dose finding study with LMWH-Novo. Thromb Res 1989; 55:267-278.

(19) Hull RD. Raskob GE. Pineo GF. et al. 1992. Subcutaneous low-molecular-weight heparin compared with continuous intravenous heparin in the treatment of proximal-vein thrombosis. N Engl j Med 1992; 326:975-988.

(20) Prandoni P. Lensing AW. Buller HR. et al. Comparison of subcutaneous low-molecular-weight heparin with intravenous standard heparin in proximal deep-vein thrombosis. Lancet 1992; 339:441-445.

(21) Lopaciuk S. Meissner AJ. Filipecki S. et al. Subcutaneous low-molecular-weight heparin versus subcutaneous unfractionated heparin in the treatment of deep vein thrombosis: a Polish multicentre trial. Thromb Haemost 1992; 68:14-18.

(22) Simonneau G. Charbonnier B. Decousus H. et al. Subcutaneous low-molecular-weight heparin compared with continuous intravenous unfractionated heparin in the treatment of proximal deep vein thrombosis. Arch Int Med 1993; 153:1541-1546.

(23) Lindmarker P. Holmstrom M. Granqvist S. et al 1994. Comparison of once-daily subcutaneous Fragmin with continuous intravenous unfractionated heparin in the treatment of deep vein thrombosis. Thromb Haemost; 72:186-190.

(24) Levine M. Gent M. Hirsh J. et al. A comparison of low molecular weight heparin administered primarily at home with unfractionated heparin administered in the hospital for proximal deep vein thrombosis. N Englj Med 1996; 334:677-681.

(25) Koopman MMW. Prandoni P. Piovella F. et al. Treatment of venous thrombosis with intravenous unfractionated heparin administered in the hospital as compared with subcutaneous low-molecular-weight heparin administered at home. N Engl J Med 1996; 334:682-687.

(26) The Columbus Investigators. Low-molecular-weight heparin in the treatment of patients with venous thromboembolism. N Engl J Med 1997; 337: 657-662.

(27) Green D. Hull RD. Brant R. Pineo GF. Lower mortality in cancer patients treated with low-molecular-weight versus standard heparin. Lancet 1992; 339:1476.

(28) Hull RD. Raskob GE. Rosenbloom D. Treatment of proximal vein thrombosis with subcutaneous low-molecular-weight heparin vs. intravenous heparin; An economic perspective. Arch Intern Med Feb 10 1997; 157: 289-94.

(29) Simmoneau G. Sors H. Charbonnier B. et al. A comparison of low-molecular-weight heparin with unfractionated heparin for acute pulmonary embolism. N Engl J Med 1997; 337:663-669.

PAOLO PRANDONI. *Comments on treatment of venous thromboembolism*

Low molecular weight heparins (LMWHs) are a relatively new group of anticoagulants that are being used in place of unfractionated heparin (UFH) for various indications, including the treatment of patients with acute venous thromboembolism (VTE). These compounds offer the advantage of a higher bioavailability coupled with a longer half-life when compared with UFH. This results in a more predictable dose response, allowing administration of LMWHs without the dose adjustment and monitoring procedures required for UFH.

A summary of existing literature, using a systematic approach, is provided in this comprehensive overview. In the last decade, an impressive number of adequate studies have been performed that have compared LMWHs with UFH in the initial treatment of both deep vein thrombosis (DVT) and pulmonary embolism (PE). In the majority of early clinical studies addressing the treatment of DVT, the effect of therapy on thrombus size was assessed by comparing pre-treatment venograms with those obtained after 5 to 10 days of therapy. On the basis of a few meta-analyses of theses studies, LMWHs prevented thrombus growth at a greater extent than UFH (1,2).

More recently, several comparative trials have been performed that have included the prospective assessment of relevant clinical outcomes, that is, symptomatic recurrent VTE, major bleeding, and mortality. In all studies, LMWHs were administered subcutaneously once or twice daily in fixed doses adjusted to body weight. Pooled analyses of trials published until the end of 1995 suggested a superiority of LMWHs over UFH for prevention of recurrent thromboembolism (1,2). In each single study the heparin fraction was at least as effective as UFH, with a trend in favor of LMWHs when the investigated compound was nadroparin, tinzaparin or enoxaparin, and in favor of UFH when the investigated drug was dalteparin. These analyses also suggested a greater safety of LMWHs in comparison with UFH (1,2). It is to be specified, however, that a statistically significant reduction of major bleeding was observed in the only North American study by Hull et al. using tinzaparin, whereas in all the other studies no appreciable differences in terms of tolerability were recorded between LMWHs and UFH when the investigated compound was nadroparin, enoxaparin or dalteparin. As an interesting side note, the pooled long-term mortality was lower in patients treated with LMWHs. This effect was almost entirely attributable to differences in the subgroup of patients with cancer.

The observation that LMWHs are at least as effective and safe as UFH when administered by fixed-dose subcutaneous injections, stimulated the hypothesis that it might be possible to use LMWH preparations to treat selected patients with DVT in an out-of-hospital setting. To test this fascinating hypothesis, two muticenter clinical trials have been recently performed (Koopman et al 1996; Levine et al 1996) with the use of nadroparin and enoxaparin respectively. Their conclusions consistently supported the feasibility, efficacy and safety of home-treatment of uncomplicated patients with DVT with subcutaneous fixed doses of LMWHs. Furthermore, this strategy was associated with an improvement of quality of life, and a relevant reduction of health care costs.

To test the hypothesis that LMWH treatment might be extended to cover the entire spectrum of patients presenting with acute VTE (thus including also patients with non-critical pulmonary embolism), two multicenter clinical trials have been recently performed (Columbus study 1997; Simonneau et al 1997). In the first investigation, all consecutive patients with acute VTE were enrolled in the study, irrespective of the modality of clinical presentation, whereas in the second, only patients with symptomatic PE were eligible for the study. In both studies, the investigated LMWH (reviparin and tinzaparin respectively) proved to be at least as effective and safe as UFH, thus suggesting that under some circumstances, non critical patients with symptomatic PE might be treated safely at home with LMWHs.

Recently, an updated meta-analysis of all comparative investigations with high methodological quality published until the end of 1997 has become available (3). The results of this meta-analysis showed no statistically significant differences in recurrent VTE or bleeding between LMWH and UFH. Once again, a statistically significant difference could be found in favor of LMWHs for total mortality. This effect was mainly attributable to differences in the subgroup of patients with cancer. This finding suggests the hypothesis that LMWHs might exert an inhibitory effect on tumor growth that is not apparent with UFH.

Although preliminary, the results of a few studies described in this overview suggest that LMWH preparations might be used in place of oral anticoagulants for the long-term prophylaxis of recurrent thromboembolism in patients suffering an episode of acute VTE. Besides the practical advantage of a single daily subcutaneous injection without the need for laboratory monitoring, there is the advantage of a lower incidence of thrombocytopenia and (possibly) osteoporosis.

REFERENCES
(1) LENSING A.W.A., PRINS M.H., DAVIDSON B.L., HIRSH J. Treatment of deep venous thrombosis with a low molecular weight heparin: a meta-analysis. Arch. Intern. Med. 1995; 155 : 601-607
(2) SIRAGUSA S., COSMI B., PIOVELLA F., HIRSH J., GINSBERG J.S. Low molecular weight heparins and unfractionated heparin in the treatment of patients with acute venous thromboembolism: results of a meta-analysis. Am. J. Med. 1996; 100 : 269-277
(3) DOLOVICH J., GINSBERG J.S. Low molecular weight heparins in the treatment of venous thromboembolism. Vessels 1997; 3 : 4-11

JEAN-NOËL FIESSINGER. *Treatment of venous thromboembolism with LMWHs*

Development of low molecular weight heparins (LMWHs) in the treatment of venous thromboembolism was the result of the success these compounds achieved in the prophylaxis of venous thromboembolic disease. The efficacy and safety of this approach as evidenced by results presented in this chapter quickly made LMWHs the reference therapy during the initial period of an established deep venous thrombosis. These results logically led to an extension of indications to include pulmonary embolism and the favorable results obtained in the first studies justified considering thromboembolic disease as a single clinical entity.

Thus, for the outside observer, LMWHs appear to have gone from one success to another in many prestigious clinical trials. The continuing discussions on the true benefit of LMWHs compared to unfractionated (standard) heparin (1) often appear mainly of academic interest, as seen by medical practitioners faced with the real problem of treating patients, far removed from the comforting restrictions of a clinical trial. And yet, those of us who have witnessed the development of this therapeutic class of agents sometimes feel that much still remains to be done, that other, and more constructive actions could have been taken.

Starting with the first trials, physicians were preoccupied with the example of unfractionated heparin: the aim was to reproduce a biological activity comparable to that of unfractionated heparin. This led researchers to give preference to the subcutaneous route of administration every twelve hours and a dosage of 100 to 120 anti-factor Xa International Units (IU) to obtain maximum plasma activity between 0.5 and 1 IU (2). Favorable results of study protocol in which a fixed dose adjusted to body-weight was used gradually, led to the conclusion that dosage adjustment was unnecessary (3). But the truly revolutionary finding came with the experience of treatment with a single injection (4). The efficacy and, even more, the safety with regard to the risk of bleeding with use of a single injection of 175 IU/kg, fully confirmed the fact that anti-Xa activity was only a far-removed illustration of the effectiveness of LMWH. Comparison of the two sc frequencies of injection (5) for a given heparin compound clearly established treatment with LMWH as the reference therapy but a trend showing the superiority of a single injection also showed the limits of current development. Without clinically significant biological parameters or dose-finding studies, the dosage of LMWH to be used remained empirical. Current studies tend to give priority to the lowest effective dose (6), but, on the contrary, should not emphasis be given to determining the highest dose which does not enhance the risk of bleeding?

LMWHs have their own specific characteristics, e.g. tinzaparin, which appeared as a promising treatment in one daily injection has a lower anti-Xa to anti-IIa ratio than other LMWHs. The clinical consequences of such differences have been little investigated and only in prophylaxis after general or orthopedic surgery (7). This is even more evident because dosage regimens used as prophylactic management differ from one heparin compound to another, and also, probably as a precautionary measure, dosages used for treatment are similar and very few dose-ranging studies have been conducted (8).

Thus, the results presented in this chapter are proof of this finding, i.e. that LMWHs are a major advance in the treatment of venous thrombosis and probably of pulmonary embolism. They have led to the development of ambulatory treatment of uncomplicated forms. But, such success owes much to the pragmatic approach of investigators. The mechanisms of action of LMWHs are still incompletely understood, anti-Xa activity reflects the clinical effect poorly and among other considerations, no biological marker (of safety/efficacy) stands out. The dose which most often provides the best benefit to risk ratio has not been investigated. Hence, many uncertainties remain. Let us hope that future studies will provide the key elements of answers to these and other questions.

REFERENCES

(1) THOMAS D.P. Does low molecular weight heparin cause less bleeding. Thromb. Haemostasis 1997; 78 : 1422-1425

(2) BRATT G., TÖRNEBOHM E., GRANQVIST S., ABERG W., LOCKNER D. A comparison between low molecular weight heparin (Kabi 2165) and standard heparin in the intravenous treatment of deep venous thrombosis. Thomb. Haemostasis 1985; 54 : 813-817

(3) ALHENC-GELAS M., JESTIN-LE GUERNIC C., VITOUX J.F. et al. Adjusted versus fixed doses of the low molecular weight heparin Fragmin in the treatment of deep vein thrombosis. Thomb. Haemostasis 1994; 71 : 698-702

(4) HULL R.D., RASKOB G.E., PINEO G.F. et al. Subcutaneous low molecular weight heparin compared with continuous intravenous heparin in the treatment of proximal vein thrombosis. N. Engl. J. Med. 1992; 326 : 975-982

(5) CHARBONNIER B.A., FIESSINGER J.N., BANGA J.D. et al. Comparison of a once daily with a twice daily subcutaneous low molecular weight heparin regimen in the treatment of deep vein thrombosis. Thromb. Haemostais 1998; accepted for publication

(6) TENCATE J.W., BULLER H.R., GENT M. et al. Low molecular weight heparin in the treatment of patients with venous thromboembolism, by the Columbus Investigators. N. Engl. J. Med. 1997; 337 : 657-662

(7) PLANES A., CHASTANG C., VOCHELLE N., DESMICHELS D., AIACH M., FIESSINGER J.N. Comparison of antithrombotic efficacy and hemorrhagic side effects of clivarin versus enoxaparin in patients undergoing total hip replacement surgery. Blood Coagul. Fibrinol. 1993; 4 : S33-S35

(8) THERY C., SIMONNEAU G., MEYER G. et al. Randomized trial of subcutanous low molecular weight heparin CY216 (Fraxiparine) compared with intravenous unfractionated heparin in the curative treatment of submassive pulmonary embolism. A dose ranging study. Circulation 1992: 85 : 1380-1389

GYÖRGY BLASKO. *Treatment of DVT in outpatients*

The controlled studies reported in this review in patients with acute deep venous thrombosis have satisfactorily demonstrated the advantages of home treatment of DVT with sc fixed body-weight adjusted doses of LMWHs.

In fact, the process of DVT has already been triggered days or even weeks prior to the randomization of patients in outpatients in a relatively large number of cases; the frequency of pulmonary embolism was not higher in the early-mobilized patients as compared to those who were treated on the basis of identical criteria, but bed rest. So it can be thought that proximal DVT does not need immobilization. The administration of LMWHs gave the opportunity for the ambulatory treatment besides improving the possibilities of rehabilitation and quality of life. These result in a reduction of cost. The economic evaluations of the Koopman and Levine's studies suggested that the outpatient management with LMWHs in patients with proximal venous thrombosis reduced resource utilization and total treatment cost.

However, diagnostic and therapeutic traditions differ in various countries. Deep vein thrombosis (DVT) is a potentially serious disease requiring a specialist for diagnosis and care as far as the underlying disease and the potential consequences are concerned. These may require hospital admission. The correct diagnosis requires up-to-date, sophisticated investigations, and sometimes a search for the underlying disease, first of all malignancies (we have to note that gastric, pancreactic, and pulmonary cancers may coexist and the background for acute DVT in 35-55% of the cases, which need detailed clinical investigations). Therefore, establishing the diagnosis requires an institutionalized investigation. Hospitalization may be indicated if administration of injections, visits, regular INR determinations, a 24-hour on-call service for emergencies or professional domiciliary if required, cannot be guaranteed within outpatient setting. If a hospital remains the center of care, the burden to the general practitioners (GP) can be low. On the contrary, if the patient is fully investigated, the possibility of the malignant comorbidities are excluded, the responsibility of the GP is restricted to the administration of the medication and onto the consecutive control of the oral anticoagulant therapy.

On the other hand, if the patient gets treated only, without having been examined thoroughly in order to clarify the underlying disease(s), the delayed diagnosis might be life-threatening for the patient. If the general condition of the patient allows home-treatment, performance of the diagnosis algorhithm is obligatory in a very close, acceptably near future after the mobilization. Frequently, the observed bleeding complications attributed to the oral anticoagulation shift our attention to the detailed endoscopic, gastrointestinal investigations: these situations, however, should be prevented.

As far as the cost of the treatment is concerned, patients with medical indication for hospital admission are likely to be more costly than patients with the home-care system. If hospital budget is based on a disease related group-guided reimbursement system, costs for the hospital may be insufficiently compensated for. Therefore the reimbursement system should keep open the possibility, allowing for hospital as well as home care in the reimbursement.

The absolute prerequisite of the home treatment is the exact and anatomically correct diagnosis (regarding the extension of the thrombus as well). In Eastern European countries, technical conditions are guaranteed mainly under institutional circumstances (imaging techniques, etc.). In developed countries, the so-called thrombosis centers have enough sophisticated facilities for obtaining the correct diagnosis. The technique is not omnipotent per se, the well-organized team-work of experts having similar expertise and following very strict and efficient procedures has as much importance. According to our practical experience, the investigations supportive of the first clinical diagnosis could be performed within 2-5 hours (depending on the complications, duties, laboratory and imaging techniques as well).

We have to emphasize the primary role of GPs—the changes in their attitudes; their education with respect to finding an early, correct diagnosis and not to lose the patients—to organize the final, clinical investigation in order to determine the underlying disease(s).

Another crucial question is the timing of the beginning of the treatment. Rapid treatment after a rapid diagnosis makes it possible to improve the number of recanalizations indicating the fibrinolytic treatment in the appropriate cases. To prevent early pulmonary embolization (PE) it is important to point out that no doctor has caused any danger to a patient by introducing an iv injection of a single dose of heparin even in the case of a flat-foot (as would be demonstrated later), but delays in starting anticoagulation caused a hazard of PE in many patients.

On the basis of the aforementioned, the physician indicating a home treatment of DVT with LMWHs navigated bet-ween the Scylla of early effective treatment, sometimes not without being properly informed about the underlying diseases, and the Charybdis of a delayed, and—with respect to the far future—less effective treatment and a more costly but correctly diagnosed patient.

The use of LMWHs in home treatment of DVT with early diagnosis will result in an increase in the number of distal DVTs treated in time, and will account for a definite reduction of costs based on this limited number of controlled trials. However, as far as the long-term patency of the vessels and the rate of late complications are concerned, we have to emphasize the importance of the duration time of the proper oral anticoagulant treatment in these patients, which should follow the LMWH home-treatment. The data are very controversial, with majority of the controlled clinical trialists arguing for a definite duration of time for oral anticoagulation, i.e. most of them advise it to continue for a time period between 3 and 6 months, depending on the severity and the nature of the underlying disease. In cases of multiple pulmonary embolism and serpin deficiencies, APC resistance, etc. and most of all in cases of mechanical heart valve prostheses, a life-long maintenance of an effective oral anticoagulation is mandatory. On the other hand, the uncomplicated cases of distal DVTs do not need life-long anticoagulation.

A large, pharmacoeconomically-focused, prospective study would be very important in order to come to a decision regarding this question. The anecdotic case-reports, small-size studies result in very subjective decisions regarding this issue, with the danger of facing an increased number of bleeding complications as a sequel of the treatment. The emerged role of the well-educated general practitioners is of utmost importance in this issue, since it is their effective work that could only help in decreasing all the complications of thromboembolic diseases.

We can summarize the issue with the adage of Professor K. Rak (Hungary): (The heparin treatment) "might be a mistake if it is unrequired, but what is worse, if it does not happen in the very neccessary cases".

6

Low molecular weight heparins

Anti-Xa activity
monitoring

Do plasma anti-Xa levels reflect the clinical antithrombotic activity and/or hemorrhage effects of a low molecular weight heparin?

BERNARD BONEU

The above question has been often debated in meetings devoted to low molecular weight heparins (LMWHs). In a previous publication (1) we discussed why anti-Xa monitoring is not mandatory for the management of patients treated with a LMWH, except in some situations such as a bleeding and/or renal insufficiency. We discuss below other arguments indicating the correlation between plasma anti-Xa activity and the antithrombotic/prohemorrhagic effect of LMWHs is poor.

1 - LMWHs are heterogeneous compounds having several biological activities; the anti-Xa potential reflects only one of these activities

There is no method currently available to directly determine plasma heparin concentration. After administration of a given dose, the magnitude of the pharmacological effect is indirectly evaluated by measuring the APTT prolongation and/or the inhibitory effect upon exogenous factor Xa or factor IIa added to the plasma. The APTT prolongation reflects the delay in the onset of thrombin generation. It is independent of the total amount of thrombin generated, a parameter which could be more relevant to the antithrombotic effect (2).

The ability of heparin to prolong the APTT is related to its anti-factor IIa potency. Thus LMWHs which have a lower antithrombin activity than unfractionated heparin (UFH) induce a modest APTT prolongation in comparison with UFH. The synthetic pentasaccharide, a pure anti-Xa compound, does not prolong the APTT but nevertheless exerts an antithrombotic effect.

Heparins are a mixture of polysaccharidic chains having a wide distribution of molecular weights (MW). One third of them bind to antithrombin via the pentasaccharidic sequence. The ability of these polysaccharidic chains to inhibit factor Xa is independent of their MW, while the inhibition of factor IIa requires a minimum MW of 5400 Da (17 sugar units). UFH being composed of polysaccharidic chains with a MW essentially > 5400 inhibits both factor Xa and factor IIa. Its anti-Xa/anti-IIa ratio has been arbitrarily set at 1. In contrast, LMWHs, which are prepared from UFH with different technical procedures, have a variable and lower percentage of chains with a MW > 5400. Thus the ability of a LMWH to catalyse thrombin inhibition varies widely among the different preparations, accounting for different anti-Xa/anti-IIa ratios, which range from 1.5 to more than 4.

The doses of LMWH are currently expressed in anti-Xa units. When an equal dose of two distinct LMWHs having different anti-Xa/anti-IIa ratios are delivered to a patient, the number of chains supporting an antithrombin activity which is delivered may be different. Thus the anti-Xa activity generated during a LMWH treatment reflects only one of these two activities. In other words, it may be conceivable that identical anti-Xa levels generated by two LMWHs having different anti-Xa/anti-IIa ratios may produce different antithrombotic effects.

2 - The anti-Xa activities reported in some clinical trials may be questionable

The overview of the anti-Xa data in the previous pages indicated that the same dose of the same LMWH may generate different anti-Xa levels. This suggests that the anti-Xa assays are not sufficiently standardized, as has been shown by quality control programs. It then becomes difficult to compare anti-Xa activity and clinical outcomes among different trials.

...he plasma anti-Xa activity generated after an administration of the same dose expressed ...nti-Xa units of two different LMWHs may vary significantly

In the report of Planes et al. enoxaparin and reviparin were delivered at the dose of 4000 and 4200 anti-Xa U respectively to prevent deep vein thrombosis after total hip replacement. The mean circulating anti-Xa activities determined in the same expert laboratory were 0.46 ± 0.10 and 0.36 ± 0.17 anti-Xa U/ml respectively. In the trials where tinzaparin was delivered at the dose of 2500 and 3500 anti-Xa U to prevent postoperative deep vein thrombosis in general surgery, the anti-Xa activities generated were surprisingly low (0.09 ± 0.003 and 0.15 ± 0.04 anti-Xa U-ml respectively) in comparison with the activities usually obtained with other LMWHs (4). In the Fraxodi trial, nadroparin was delivered once a day at the dose of 170 anti-Xa U/kg. In a satellite study where the same preparation (nadroparin) was delivered at the same dose to healthy volunteers, the mean Cmax of the anti-Xa activity was 1.3 U-ml (5). This value is considerably higher than the anti-Xa activity reached after an injection of tinzaparin at the same dose (0.83 anti-Xa U/ml) (JJ. Heilman, Léo Laboratory, personal communication). In spite of this discrepancy, the clinical outcomes were favorable in both trials.

4 - Does this mean that the anti-Xa activity is irrelevant in the development of a LMWH and in clinical practice?

From our point of view, the answer is no. For a given LMWH there is a good correlation between the dose delivered, the anti-Xa activity generated and the clinical outcome. For example, in the pioneering studies performed with dalteparin (6,7) it became evident that too high doses were associated with too high plasma anti-Xa activites and an unacceptable hemorrhagic risk. The same observations were made with other LMWHs. This suggests that determination of the plasma anti-Xa activity may be helpful in the development of a LMWH.

LMWHs are essentially cleared by the kidneys. Thus, after delivery of high doses of LMWHs (curative regimen), there is a risk of accumulation in the elderly who have physiologically reduced renal function. Circulating anti-Xa activity may be an indicator of the risk of overdose. It is difficult to precisely determine the upper limit that must not be exceeded. The value of 1.5 anti-Xa U/ml seems reasonable. However, we do not know if, for a given circulating anti-Xa activity, the hemorrhagic potential of different LMWHs may differ according to variable associated anti-IIa activities, molecular weight distribution, and degree of sulfation of the molecules.

In conclusion, as far as the actual generation for LMWH is concerned, circulating anti-Xa activity cannot be considered as a universal predictor of their efficacy. Due to their different method of preparation, physiochemical properties and anti-Xa/anti-IIa ratio, individual LMWHs must be considered as original compounds requiring specific clinical trials to determine the best benefit/risk ratio for a given indication.

REFERENCES

(1) BONEU B. Low molecular weight heparin therapy: is monitoring needed? Thromb. Haemostasis 1994; 72 : 330-334

(2) WIELDERS S., MUKHERJEE M. MICHIELS J., RIJKERS D.T.S., CAMBUS J.P. KNEBEK R.W.XC., KAKKAR V. HEMKER H.C., BEGUIN S. The routine determination of the endogenous thrombin potential, first results in different forms of hyper- and hypocoagulability. Thromb. Haemostasis 1997; 77 : 629-636

(3) PLANES A., CHASTANG C. VOCHELLE N. et al. Comparison of antithrombotic efficacy and hemorrhagic side effects of reviparin sodium versus enoxaparin in patients undergoing total hip replacement surgery. Blood Coag. Fibrinol. 1993; 4 : S33-S35

(4) BARA L. LEIZOROVICZ A., PICOLET H., SAMAMA M. Correlation between anti-Xa and occurrence of thrombosis and hemorrhage in post-surgical treated with either logiparin (LMWH) or unfractionated heparin. Thromb. Res. 1992; 65 : 641-650

(5) BONEU B., NAVARRO C., CAMBUS J.P., CAPLAIN H., D'AZEMAR P., NECCIARI J., DURET J.P., GAUD C., SIE P. Pharmacodynamics and tolerance of two nadroparin formulations (10,250 and 20,500 anti-Xa IU.ml-1) delivered for 10 days at therapeutic dose. Thromb. Haemostasis 1998; 79 : 338-341

(6) KOLLER M., SCHOCH U., BUCHMANN P. et al. Low molecular heparin (Kabi 2135) as thromboprophylaxis in elective visceral surgery. A randomized, double-blind study versus unfractionated heparin. Thromb. Haemostasis 1986; 56 : 243-246

(7) BRATT G., TÖRNEBOHM E., GRANQVIST S. et al. A comparison between low molecular weight heparin (Kabi 2165) and standard heparin in the intravenous treatment of deep vein thrombosis. Thromb. Haemostasis 1985; 54 : 813-817

Heparins and monitoring

FRANCIS TOULEMONDE

To monitor means to modulate the dosage of a drug according to the supposed needs of the patient, using one or several tests (bio-assays) regularly.

This attitude is strongly different from making investigations when an unusual situation occurs: the first attitude is prospective and systematic, the second is not.

Is monitoring justified for LMWH, like it was for UFH, even though monitoring is required for so few medications, knowing that we have only APTT for UFH and anti-Xa for LMW (*see B. Boneu p. 326)*?

Should prophylaxis therapy be monitored?

The high incidence of venous thromboembolism (especially postoperatively), mainly asymptomatic, requires a large scale method of prophylaxis which should be simple, safe and effective, to be used for a large number of patients (high and medium risks). Since the term " low dose heparin " (Kakkar 1972) was first used, the term prophylaxis monitoring disappeared: it is not found at all in Kakkar's latest 24 pages general review on "Prophylaxis of DVT" in 1997 (1).

But practice does not mean research and development of a new antithrombotic where investigations (different from monitoring) have to be done to learn more about the product. Experience, in fact, showed a rather poor yield of such practice compared to clinical observation (2). Many investigations (for example, Ref. 3) showed that there are poor correlations between AXa inhibition and occurrence of thrombosis and hemorrhages; this is a very major point: the tool is inaccurate for monitoring (4).

It is interesting to note that one of the rare studies concluding some existence of correlation between AXa and bleeding, used a dosage (60 mg enoxaparin/day) which had been rejected two years previously in light of the simple clinical observation of excessive instances of bleeding (5).

Thus it is readily accepted — and has long been recognized — that prophylactic therapy does not (and must not) require laboratory monitoring in 99% of cases — as mentioned just previously by B. Boneu.

Should treatment therapy be monitored?

The situation is, in this case, quite different: UFH experience was conducted using true monitoring so, why not the same for LMWH? Moreover, the drug is given in larger dosages than for prophylaxis, increasing the risks — at least theoretically.

In the field of UFH, the situation is far from clear. Here are two examples:

— Is efficient monitoring absolutely mandatory in order to reach the desired range quickly and thus avoid bleedings and recurrences two or three months later when OA is given to the patient?

Using almost same reports, one investigator (6) says yes, others (7) no.

— To improve UFH treatments, different complex nomograms are proposed: almost all of them result in recommending an increase in usual dosages. The results are quite good but is there any future for these rather complicated methods?

With regard to LMWH (so simple now), opinions have varied widely since the first paper (1985). LMWH management indeed began exactly as with UFH (continuous infusion monitored with APTT) but starting in 1991 (8), the mention of monitoring using AXa activity disappeared slowly probably as the result of evidences in many cases (see pages 275, 281, 283, 289, 305, 383) of the absence of correlation (once more) as previously mentioned for UFH (9) as for LMWH (10, 11). It is true that, at this time, the much more stable activity of LMWH compared to UFH was not yet highlighted.

In these conditions, it may be that what remains is the simple goal of achieving an AXa activity >0.7 IU/ml (and less than 1 IU) to obtain the best possible reduction of Marder's score (8). Unfortunately, this criterion was rapidly dropped thereafter, perhaps losing its significance.

Thus the treatment by subcutaneous route of LMWH has not been subject to monitoring since 1991 and the results showed monitoring to be useless.

Conclusion

Monitoring practice shows that UFH + APTT is now outdated and should be abandoned whenever possible (12). Now LMWH without monitoring is the actual practice with excellent results. That does not mean that the situation is fixed definitely: new tools or new concepts could appear (13) and, possibly, could modify the actual practice.

Thus UFH monitoring used to be a burden, also a source of appreciable cost with a low benefit (Agildgaard). To a certain extent, in a manner similar to thrombolytic agents, which were so closely controlled using bio-assays (not monitored) at their beginning, such constraints have now disappeared with the use of LMWH.

REFERENCES

(1) Kakkar V.V., Low molecular weight heparin : prophylaxis of DVT in New Therapeutic agents in thrombosis and thrombolysis, 1997, 103-127.

(2) Toulemonde F., Strategy for the development of the LMWH fraction CY216 in the prevention of postoperative deep vein thrombosis in general surgery, Semin Thromb Haemost 1989, 15, 395-400.

(3) Leizorovicz A., Bara L., Samama M. et al., Factor Axa inhibition : correlations between the plasma levels and occurrence of thrombosis and haemorrhage, Haemost 1993, 23, suppl. 1, 89-98.

(4) Walenga J.M., Hoppensteadt D., Fareed J., Laboratory monitoring of the clinical effects of L.M.W. heparins, Thromb Res. 1991, suppl. XIV, 49-62.

(5) Levine M.N., Planes A., Hirsh J. et al., Relationship between Axa levels and clinical outcome in patient receiving Enoxaparin a LMWH to prevent deep vein thrombosis after hip replacement, Thromb Haemost 1989, 62, 940-44.

(6) Hull R.D., Raskob G.E., Hirsh J. et al., Continuous IV heparin compared with intermittent subcutaneous heparin in the initial treatment of proximal vein thrombosis, N. Engl. J. Med. 1986, 315, 1109-14.

(7) Anand S., Ginsberg J.S., Kearon C. et al., The relation between the APTT response and recurrence in patients with venous thrombosis treated with continuous intravenous heparin, Arch Intern Med 1996, 156, 1677-81.

(8) Aiach M., Should deep venous thrombosis treatment with LMWH fragmin be monitored or not?, Thromb Haemost 1991, 65, 6 Abst 307.

(9) Villain P., Bouvier J.L., Le Corf et al., Do APTT and AIIa activity permit the prediction of the efficiency of heparin in patients with proximal deep vein thrombosis, Thromb Haemost 1987, 1, 58, Abst 1372.

(10) Juhan-Vague I., Delahousse B., Vergnes D et al., Irrelevance of Axa measurement in predicting the outcome of LMWH fragment (CY 222) treatment of established thrombo-embolic diseases, Thromb Haemost 1989, 1, 62, Abs 396.

(11) Toulemonde F., Strategy behind the development of the first ultra-low molecular weight heparin fragment for the treatment of thrombo-embolic diseases, Acta Therapeutica 1990, 16, 197-215.

(12) Toulemonde F., Kher A., Monitoring of heparin in the deep venous thrombosis treatment. An obsolete question?, Ann Cardiol Angeiol (F) 1995, 44, 3, 151-9.

(13) Kehr A., Aldieri R., Hemker H.C., Beguin S., Laboratory assessment of antithrombotic therapy: what tests, and if so why?, Haemost, 1997, 27, 5, 211-218.

7

Synoptic tables:
clinical trials in prophylaxis
and treatment
of venous
thromboembolism

Selected abbreviations used throughout tables

BW	body weight
D	day
DB	double-blind
DVT	deep vein thrombosis
F	number of fatal PE
FUT	fibrinogen uptake test
h	hours
Imp	improvement outcome
IPG	impedance plethysmography
iv	intravenous route
LS	lung scan
MB	major bleeding
MC	multicenter
n	number of evaluable patients
NR	not reported
OAC	oral anticoagulant
OP	open-label
PA	pulmonary angiography
PE	pulmonary embolism
RD	randomized
SB	single-blind
sc	subcutaneous route
TE	thromboembolic event
T/F	total/ fatal
UFH	unfractionated heparin
US	ultrasonography
V	venography
wors	worsened outcome
x	number of daily doses

Ardeparin (A) in prophylaxis of DVT in orthopedic surgery

First author year	Design (surgery)	n	Treatment regimen sc route daily dose	First dose preop– postop + (hours)	Duration therapy (days)	Detection method	DVT prox/total %	PE T/F (n)
Placebo comparison								
Levine, 1996	MC, RD, DB (knee)	199	A 50 IU/kg x 2 placebo	+12/+24	14	V	2/29 15.5/58	1/0 1/1
Drug and dosage comparisons								
RD group, 1994	OP, MC, RD (hip)	969 (523)	A IU/kg: 50 x 2 90 x 1 Warfarin 5mg	+8/+12	4/10	IPG, Doppler, V	3/7 7/13 6/11	0
	(knee)	(446)	A IU/kg: 50 x 2 90 x 1 Warfarin 5mg				6/25 5/28 10/41	0 1/0 1/0
Heit, 1997	MC, RD, DB (knee)	680	A IU/kg: 25 x 2 35 x 2 50 x 2 Warfarin 5mg	+12	14		NR/36 NR/28 6/27 7/38	1/0 0 1/0 0

Certoparin (C) in major abdominal surgery (MA) and gynecological surgery (GY)

First author year	Design (surgery)	n	Treatment regimen sc route daily dose	First dose preop– postop + (hours)	Duration therapy (days)	Detection method	DVT total %	PE T/F (n)
Drug comparisons								
Koppenhagen, 1992	MC, RD, DB (MA)	653	C 3000 IU x 1 UFH 5000 IU x 2	–2	?	FUT/V	7.4 7.9	0 1/1
Heilmann, 1997	RD, DB (GY)	324	C 3000 x 1 UFH 5000 IU x 3	–2	7	IPG/V	6.3 6.1	7/1 14/0

Certoparin (C) in orthopedic surgery (hip fracture- HF) and traumatology (T)

First author year	Design (surgery)	n	Treatment regimen sc route daily dose	First dose preop– postop + (hours)	Duration therapy (days)	Detection method	DVT prox/total %	PE T/F (n)
Drug comparisons								
Oertli, 1992	OP, RD (HF)	198	C 3000 IU x 1 Dextran iv	preop	10	FUT/V	15.5 32.6	2/1 2/2
Kock, 1995	OP (T)	339	C 3000 IU x 1 control group	after immobilization	up to removal of plaster cast	IPG/US	0 4.3	NR

Certoparin (C) in treatment of DVT

First author year	Design	n	Treatment regimen iv/sc route daily dose	Duration therapy (days)	Dosage adjustment	Detection method	Outcomes (%pts)		
							imp %	wors %	PE T/F
Kirchmaier, 1994	OP (pilot)	25	C ≈ 15 IU/kg/h iv	7-29	Heptest	V	68	0	NR
Kirchmaier, 1998	MC, RD, CT	309	C ≈ 15 IU/kg/h C 4000 IU x 2 UFH iv infusion	≥ 14	Heptest	V	34* 34* 32*	NR NR NR	0 0 0

* improvement greater than 30%.

Certoparin (C) in medicine

First author year	Design	n	Treatment regimen sc route daily dose	Duration therapy (days)	Detection method	DVT total (%)	PE T/F (n)
Drug comparisons							
Harenberg, 1990	MC, RD, DB	166	C 3000 IU x 1 UFH 5000 IU x 3	7-12	IPG Doppler, V	3.5 4.8	0 0

Dalteparin (D) in major abdominal (MA), cancer (C) and gynecological (GY) surgery

First author year	Design (surgery)	n	Treatment regimen sc route daily dose	First dose initiated (h preop)	Duration therapy (days)	Detection method	DVT total (%)	PE T/F (n)
Dosage comparisons								
Kakkar, 1986	OP (MA)	206	D 2500 IU x 1 D 2500 IU x 2	1-2	≥ 6	FUT, V	7.4 2.6	1/0 0
Bergqvist, 1995	RD, DB, MC (MA)	2097	D 2500 IU x 1 D 5000 IU x 1	8-16	8	FUT, V	12.7 6.6	7/2 5/2
Placebo comparison								
Ockelford, 1989	RD, DB, MC (MA)	183	D 2500 IU x 1 placebo	2 2	5-9 5-9	FUT	4.2 15.9	0 2/0
Drug comparisons								
Bergqvist, 1986	RD, DB, MC (MA)	432	D 5000 IU x 1 UFH 5000 IU x 2	2	5-7	FUT	6.4 4.3	0 0
Koller, 1986	RD, DB (MA)	138	D 2500 IU x 1 UFH 5000 IU x 2	1	≥ 5	FUT, V	2.9 2.9	0 1/0
Fricker, 1988	RD, OP (C)	80	D 5000 IU x 1 UFH 5000 IU x 3	2	10	FUT, V	0 0	0 2/0
Caen, 1988	RD, DB, MC (MA)	385	D 2500 IU x 1 UFH 5000 IU x 2	2	7	FUT	3.1 3.7	0 0
Bergqvist, 1988	RD, DB, MC (MA)	1002	D 5000 IU x 1 UFH 5000 IU x 2	18 and 2 18 and 2	5-8	FUT, V	5.0 9.2	0 4/1
Borstad, 1988	RD, DB (GY)	215	D 2500 IU x 1 UFH 5000 IU x 2	1	≥ 7	V	0 0	0 0
Hartl, 1990	RD, DB (MA)	227	D 2500 IU x 1 UFH 5000 IU x 2	2	≥ 7	FUT, V	5.2 5.3	1/1 1/1
Kakkar, 1993	RD, MC (MA)	3809	D 2500 IU x 1 UFH 5000 IU x 2	1-4	≥ 5	V	0.6 0.6	13/5 14/3
Bounameaux, 1993	RD, SB (MA)	185	D 2500 IU x 1 N 2850 IU x 1	2	9	V	32.3 16.3	NR NR

N: nadroparin.

Dalteparin (D) in total hip replacement and hip fracture (HF)

First author year	Design (surgery)	n	Treatment regimen sc route daily dose	First dose initiated (hours)	Duration therapy (days)	Detection method	DVT prox/total (%)	PE T/F (n)
Dosage comparison								
Dechavanne, 1989	RD, MC	122	D 2500 IU x 2 D 5000 IU x 1 UFH 5000 IU x 2 then APTT-adjusted	2	10-13	FUT, V	2.4/4.9 2.4/7.3 7.5/10.0	NR
Placebo comparisons								
Torholm, 1991	RD, DB	112	D 5000 IU x 1 placebo	2	6	FUT, V	0/16 26/35	0 1/0
Jorgensen, 1992	RD, DB, MC (HF)	68	D 5000 IU x 1 placebo	2	6	FUT, V	NR/30 NR/58	0 1/0
Drug comparisons								
Barre, 1987	OP, RD	80	D 2500 IU x 2 UFH 3750 IU x 3 (APTT-adjusted)	2	10	V	5/17.5 5/10.0	0 0
Eriksson, 1988	RD, OP	98	D 2500 IU x 2 Dextran 500ml iv x 4	2	7 3	FUT, V	0/20 12/45	2/0 2/0
Eriksson, 1991	RD, DB	122	D 5000 IU x 1 sc UFH 5000 IU x 2 sc	12 2	10	V, LS	9.5/30 30.5/42	8/0 19/0

Dalteparin (D) in hip surgery and hip fracture (HF)

First author year	Design (surgery)	n	Treatment regimen sc route daily dose	First dose initiated (h preop)	Duration therapy (days)	Detection method	DVT prox/total (%)	PE T/F (n)
Drug comparisons								
Monreal, 1989	RD, DB (HF)	90	D 5000 IU x 2 UFH 5000 IU x3	2	9	V, LS	37/43.7 16.7/20.0	6/0 0
Prolonged prophylaxis after hip surgery								
Danish Group, 1996 (Lassen)	RD, DB, MC (hip)	188	• D 5000 IU x 1 • D 5000 IU x 1 + Placebo	12	35 7 ⌉ 28 ⌋	V, LS	0/4 4.5/9	NR NR
Dahl, 1997	RD, DB, MC (hip)	227	• D 5000 IU x 1 • D 5000 IU x 1 + Placebo D7	12	28 7 ⌉ 21 ⌋	V, LS	4.3/12 10/26	4/0 6/1

Dalteparine in medicine

First author year	Design	n	Treatment regimen sc route daily dose	Duration therapy (days)	Detection method	DVT total (%)	PE T/F (n)
Drug comparisons							
Poniewierski, 1988	RD, DB	192	D 2500 IU x 1 UFH 5000 IU x 3	7-10	Clinical V	0 0	0 0

Dalteparin (D) in treatment of DVT

First author year	Design	n	Treatment regimen daily dose	Duration therapy (days)	Dosage adjustment	Detection method	Outcomes		
							imp %	wors %	PE (n) T/F
Dosage comparisons									
Holmstrom, 1992	RD,OP	101	D 200 IU/kg/ x 1 sc D 100 IU/kg/12h sc	5-7	AXa AXa	V	55 51	0 4	0 0
Alhenc-Gelas, 1994	RD,OP	107	D 100 IU/kg/ x 2 sc D AXa-adjust. x 2 sc	10	BW AXa	V LS	83 75	4.0 1.7	4/0 3/0
Drug comparisons									
Bratt, 1985	OP, RD	54	D 120 IU/kg iv D 240 IU/kg iv UFH infusion	7	APTT APTT APTT	V	77 50	0 0 48	0 0 11
Holm, 1986	RD, DB	56	D 5000 IU x 2 sc UFH 10, 000 IU x 2 sc	7	AXa AXa	V	40 48	4 8	1/0 0
Lockner, 1986	RD, OP	54	D 240 IU/kg q12h iv D 120 IU/kg q12h iv UFH 240 IU/kg q12h iv	5	AXa AXa APTT	V	50 77 48	0 0 11	
Albada, 1989	RD, DB	194	D 15 000 IU/24h iv UFH iv infusion	5-10	AXa AXa	LS x 2 V, IPG	56 51	2 0	3/0 6/1
French Study 1989	MC, OP, RD	66	D 100 IU/kg x 2 sc UFH iv infusion	10 10	AXa APTT	V	NR	NR	0 0
Bratt, 1990	RD, OP	94	D 120 IU/kg x 2 sc UFH iv infusion	5-7	AXa APTT	V	75 61	4.4 6	0 0

Dalteparin (D) in treatment of venous thromboembolism (DVT/PE)

First author year	Design	n	Treatment regimen sc route daily dose	Duration therapy (days or months)	Dosage adjustment	Detection method	Outcomes imp %	wors %	PE (n) T/F
Drug comparisons									
Monreal, 1994	RD, OP	80	D 5000 IU x 2 sc UFH 10,000 IU x 2 sc	at hospital discharge up to 3-6M		Clinical, V		2 DVT 3 DVT	2/0 3/0
Lindmarker, 1994	RD, MC, OP (DVT)	204	D 200 IU/kg x 1 sc UFH iv infusion + OAC	5-9 3M	BW APTT	V	59 61	5 10	NR NR
Luomanmaki, 1996	RD, DB, MC (DVT)	330	D 200 IU/kg x 1 sc UFH iv infusion + OAC	5-10 D1 to 3M	BW APTT	V, LS	51 62	12 7	1/0 0
Meyer, 1995	OP, RD, MC (PE)	55	D120 IU/kg x 2 sc UFH iv infusion	10	BW APTT	LS, PA	93 93	0 0	1 1
Fiessinger, 1996	RD, MC (DVT)	268	D 200 IU/kg x 1 sc UFH iv infusion + OAC	5-10 D1 to 3M	BW APTT	V	68 60	8 11	NR
Holmstrom, 1997	OP, RD (DVT)	164	D 200 IU/kg x 1 sc UFH iv infusion + OAC	5-10 D1 to 3M	BW APTT	V	92 93	2 3	NR
Dosage comparison									
Partsch, 1996	OP, RD (PE)	140	D 200 IU/kg x 1 sc D 100 IU/kg x 2 sc	8-15	BW BW	LS	5.5 27.6	NR NR	1 0

Enoxaparin (E) in major abdominal, neurosurgery (N) or cancer (C) surgery

First author year	Design	n	Treatment regimen sc route daily dose	First dose preop– postop + (hours)	Duration therapy (days)	Detection method	DVT total (%)	PE T/F (n)
Dosage comparison								
Samama M.M.*, **1988**	OP, RD, MC	803	E 60mg x 1 E 40mg x 1 E 20mg x 1	–2	7	FUT	2.9 2.8 3.8	NR — —
No comparison								
Haas, 1994	OP, RD, MC	9919	E 20mg x 1	NR	7	Clinical	0.1	24/3
Drug comparisons								
Samama M.M.*, **1988**	OP, RD, MC	803	E 60mg x 1 UFH 5000 IU x 3 E 40mg x 1 UFH 5000 IU x 3 E 20mg x 1 UFH 5000 IU x 3	–2	7	FUT	2.9 3.8 2.8 2.7 3.8 7.6	NR NR NR NR NR NR
Gazzaniga, 1993	OP, RD, MC	1122	E 20mg x 1 UFH 5000 IU x 2	–2 –2	7/10 7/10	Doppler, IPG	0.5 1.0	3/1 4/3
Nurmohamed, 1995	DB, RD, MC	1427	E 20mg x 1 UFH 5000 IU x 3	–2 –2	10 10	FUT, V	7.5 5.2	2/1 5/0
Bergqvist, 1997	DB, RD, MC (C)	631	E 40mg x 1 UFH 5000 IU x 3	–2 –2	8/12	V	14.4 17.6	0 0
Agnelli, 1998	DB, RD, MC (N)	260	E 40 mg x 1 Elastic stockings	+24	≥ 7	V	17 32	0 1/1

*same study.

Enoxaparin (E) in orthopedic surgery (hip replacement)

First author year	Design	n	Treatment regimen sc route daily dose	First dose preop– postop + (hours)	Duration therapy (days)	Detection method	DVT prox/total (%)	PE T/F (n)
Dosage comparisons								
Planes, 1986	OP	228	E 60mg x 1 E 30mg x 2 E 40mg x 1 E 20mg x 2	–12	≥ 12	V	6/6 0/8 4/8 6/8	0 0 1/1 0
Planes, 1991	DB, RD	118	E 40mg x 1 E 20mg x 2	–12 –12	12	V	5.2/10.5 1.7/1.7	0 0
Spiro, 1994	MC, DB, RD	568	E 10mg x 1 E 40mg x 1 E 30mg x 2	≤ 24	7	V	14/31 6/14 6/11	1/0 1/0 0
Placebo comparisons								
Turpie, 1986	MC, DB, RD	100	E 30mg x 2 Placebo	+12/+24 —	14	FUT, V	4/12 20/42	0
Samama C.M., 1997	MC, RD, DB	153	E 40mg x 1 Placebo	+6	10±2	V	2.6/14.1 16/37.3	0 0
Drug comparisons								
Planes, 1988	MC, DB, RD	228	E 40mg x 1 UFH 5000IU x 3	–12	14	V	7.5/12.5 18.5/25	0 1/0
Danish study group, 1991	OP, MC, RD	219	E 40mg x 1 Dextran x 4	–12	7	V	1.8/6.5 5.4/21.6	0 0
Levine, 1991	MC, DB, RD	665	E 30mg x 2 UFH 7500 x 2	+12/+24	≤ 14	V	5.4/19.4 6.5/23.2	0 2/0
Colwell, 1994	OP, MC, RD	604	E 30mg x 2 E 40mg x 1 UFH 5000 IU x 3	≈ +24	≤ 7	V	2/6 4/21 7/15	0 0 1/0
Avikainen, 1995	OP, RD	167	E 40mg x 1 UFH 5000 IU x 3	–12	10	US, V	1.2/ 4.8/	0 1

Enoxaparin (E) after orthopedic surgery (hip replacement)

First author year	Design	n	Treatment regimen sc route daily dose	First dose preop– postop + (hours)	Duration therapy (days)	Detection method	DVT prox/total (%)	PE T/F (n)
Anesthesia comparisons								
Planes, 1991 (4th trial)	MC, RD	188	spinal E 40mg x 1	≥ +12	12	V	6/17	NR
			spinal E 20mg/E 40mg x 1	+1/D1	12	V	6.7/11.7	NR
			general E 40mg x 1	–2	12	V	6.5/6.5	NR
Samama C.M., 1997	MC, RD, DB (Spinal anest.)	153	E 40mg x 1 Placebo	+6	10	V	14.1 37.3	0 0
Prolonged prophylaxis after hip surgery								
Planes, 1996	DB, RD	179	E 40mg x 1 Placebo	–12	≈ 35 ≈ 20	V V	5.9/7.1 7.9/19.3	0 0
Bergqvist, 1996	DB, RD	233	E 40mg x 1 Placebo	–12	31 21	V V	7/18 24/39	0 2

Enoxaparin (E) in orthopedic surgery (knee arthroplasty)

First author year	Design	n	Treatment regimen sc route daily dose	First dose preop– postop + (hours)	Duration therapy (days)	Detection method	DVT prox/total (%)	PE T/F (n)
Placebo comparison								
Leclerc, 1992	MC, DB, RD	129	E 30mg x 2 Placebo	+24	14	V, IPG	0/19 20/65	0 1/0
Drug comparisons								
Faunø, 1994	MC, DB, RD	185	E 40mg x 1 UFH 5000 IU x 3	–12	6-9	V	3/23 5/27	0 0
Leclerc, 1996	MC, DB, RD	417	E 30mg x 2 Warfarin	+12 +12	14	V	12/37 10/52	1/0 3/0

Enoxaparin (E) in orthopedic surgery (major trauma)

First author year	Design	n	Treatment regimen sc route daily dose	First dose preop– postop + (hours)	Duration therapy (days)	Detection method	DVT prox/total (%)	PE T/F (n)
Drug comparison								
Geerts, 1996	MC, DB, RD	265	E 30mg x 2 UFH 5000 IU x 2	≤ +36 ≤ +36	14 14	V V	6.2/31 14.7/44.1	1/0 0

Enoxaparin (E) in the treatment of DVT

First author year	Design (surgery)	n	Treatment regimen daily dose	Duration therapy (days)	Venogram		3 month-follow-up	
					Improv +no change (%)	Wors (%)	Recurrences DVT + PE (%)	Death (%)
Drug comparisons								
Simonneau, 1993	OP, RD, MC	117	E 1mg/kg x 2 sc UFH iv infusion + warfarin	10 from D10	100 91	0 4.0	0 3.0	0.5 3.5
Pini, 1994	OP, RD,	187	E 40mg x 1 sc Warfarin	D11 to D90 D11 to D90	— —	— —	6.0 4.0	4.3 3.2
Levine, 1996	OP, RD, MC hospital vs home treat.	500	E 1mg/kg x 2 sc UFH iv infusion + Warfarin	at least 5D at least 5D D2 to D90	— —	— —	5.3 6.7	4.4 6.7
Spiro, 1997	OP, RD, MC	900	E 1mg/kg x 2 sc E 1.5mg/kg x 1 sc UFH iv infusion + Warfarin	5-8 D1 to D90	— — —	— — —	2.9 4.4 4.3	2.2 3.7 3.1
Leroyer, 1997	OP, MC, RD	216	E 1mg/kg x 2 sc + OAC E 1mg/kg x 2 sc + OAC	≈ 8 D1-D90 14 D10-D90	— —	— —	0 0.9	4.0 2.0

Enoxaparin (E) in medicine

First author year	Design	n	Treatment regimen sc route daily dose	Duration therapy (days)	Detection method	DVT total (%)	PE T/F (n)
Placebo comparison							
Dahan, 1986	RD, DB	253	E 60mg x 1 Placebo	10 10	FUT	3 9.1	1/1 3/3
Drug comparisons							
Bergmann, 1996	RD, DB, MC	423	E 20mg x 1 UFH 5000 IU x 2	10 10	FUT	4.2 4.5	1/0 0
Lechler, 1996	RD, DB, MC	959	E 40mg x 1 UFH 5000 IU x 3	7 7	B-mode, V	0.3 1.3	0 2/0

Nadroparin (N) in major abdominal surgery (MA), neurosurgery (N) or cancer (C)

First author year	Design (surgery)	n	Treatment regimen sc route	First dose preop– postop + (hours)	Duration therapy (days)	Detection method	DVT prox/total (%)	PE T/F (n)
Placebo comparisons								
Pezzuoli, 1989	MC, RD, DB, (MA)	4498	N 7500 AXa ICU (0.3ml) Placebo 0.3ml	–2	7	autopsy	—	2/2 4/4
Nurmohamed, 1996	MC, RD, DB, (N)	385	N 7500 AXa ICU (0.3ml)	+18/24	≥ 10	V	6.9/18.7	0
Drug comparisons								
Kakkar, 1985 1st part	MC, RD, DB, (MA)	400	N 0.3ml x 1 UFH 5000 IU x 2	–2 –2	7	FUT, V	/2.5 /7.5	0 1/1
2nd part	OP, MC	1007	N 0.3ml x 1	–2	9	FUT, V	/2.9	0
E.F.S., 1988	MC, RD (MA)	1909	N 0.3ml x 1 UFH 5000 IU x 3	–2 –2	7	FUT, V	/2.8 /4.5	2/0 5/1
Bounameaux, 1993	RD, SB (MA)	194	N 0.3ml x 1 D 2500 IU x 1	–2	9	V	/16.3 /32.3	
Eurin, 1994	OP, MC, RD, (MA)	480	N 0.3ml x 1 UFH 5000 IU x 3	+2 +2	7	Doppler, IPG	0.4 0	0 0
No comparison								
Paoletti, 1989	OP (N)	97	N 7500 AXa IU (0.3ml)	≈ 3D	8	Clinical ± Doppler, V	0	?
Marassi, 1993	OP, RD (C)	61	N 7500 AXa IU (0.3ml) no treatment	pre an +12h	≥ 7	FUT ± V	7 35	0 0

N 0.3ml corresponds to ≈ 3000 AXa IU or 7500 AXa ICU   D= dalteparin

Nadroparin (N) in orthopedic surgery (hip/knee replacement)

First author year	Design (surgery)	n	Treatment regimen sc route	First dose preop– postop + (hours)	Duration therapy (days)	Detection method	DVT prox/total %	PE T/F (n)
Drug comparisons								
Leyvraz, 1991	OP, MC, RD, (hip)	409	N 40/ 60IU/kg x 1 (time surgery and BW-adjusted)	−12	10	V	2.9/12.6	1/0
			UFH APTT-adjust.	−12			13.1/16.0	4/1
Ghat, 1992	MC, RD, DB, (hip)	341	N 0.4ml x 1	−12	16	V	10.3/33.1	2/0
			UFH 5000 IU x 3	−12			19.7/34.3	6/2
Hamulyak, 1994	MC, RD, SB, (hip)	672	N 60AXa IU/kg x 1	−12	10	V	6.2/13.8	0
			Acenocoumarol (INR 2-3)	preop			4.6/13.8	0
	(knee)		N 60 AXa IU/kg x 1	−12	10		7.7/24.6	0
			Acenocoumarol (INR 2-3)	preop			9.8/37.7	0
Timing injection comparison								
Palareti, 1996	MC, RD, DB (hip)	131	N 0.3/0.4ml x 1	−12	14	V	10.8/41.5	0
			N 0.3/0.4ml x 1	+12			6.1/36.4	0

Nadroparin (N) in traumatology

First author year	Design (surgery)	n	Treatment regimen sc route	First dose preop– postop + (hours)	Duration therapy (days)	Detection method	DVT prox/total %	PE T/F (n)
Regimen comparison								
Haentjens, 1996	OP, MC, RD, (hip fracture)	215	N 0.3ml x 1	preop	42	Doppler, IPG, V	0	**1/0**
			N 60 AXa IU/kg	preop			2.8	2/1
Placebo comparison								
Kujath, 1993	OP, RD (plaster cast)	253	N 0.3ml x 1	after	16±10	IPG, US	4.8	0
			no prophylaxis	injury			16.5	0
N 0.3ml corresponds to ≈ 3000 AXa IU								

Nadroparin (N) in the treatment of DVT

First author year	Design	n	Initial Treatment	Duration therapy sc route	Detection method (days)	Outcomes (% pts) improv. %	worse %	Follow-ups (months) TE (n) recurrences/ fatal PE
Drug comparisons								
Collaborative European Study, 1991	OP, MC, RD	154	N 85 IU/kg x 2* UFH infusion iv + OAC or sc UFH	10 D10 to ?	V	73 60	27** 40**	3 months 0
Prandoni, 1992	OP, RD	170	N 85 IU/kg x 2* UFH infusion iv + OAC	10 D7-6M	V	94 83	6 16	6 months 12/3
Lopaciuk, 1992	OP, MC, RD	134	N 85 IU/kg x 2* UFH x 2 sc. APTT-adjust + OAC	10 D7-D90	V	85 82	12 18	3 months 0 2/1
Koopman, 1996	OP, MC RD	400	N 85 IU/kg x 2 UFH infusion iv + OAC	6-8 D1-D90	Doppler, V			3 months 14/2 17/1
Regimen comparison								
Charbonnier, 1998	MC, RD, DB	651	N 85 IU/kg x 2 sc N 170 IU/kg x 1 sc	4-10	V			3 months 17/6 11/2

* In these studies, nadroparin units were expressed in AXa IC units. For a better comprehension these units have been expressed here in IU.
** The authors have mixed "unchanged or worsened."

Nadroparin (N) in medicine

First author year	Design	n	Treatment regimen sc route daily dose	Duration therapy (days)	Detection method	Thromboembolism	
						Total dvt (n)	PE (n)
Drug comparisons							
Forette, 1995	OP, MC, RD,	295	N 0.3ml x 1 UFH 5000/ 7000 IU x 2	28	Doppler, V	3 4	0 1
Harenberg, 1996	MC, RD, DB	1436	N 0.3ml x 1 UFH 5000 IU x 3	10 10	US, V	2 1	4 (1 fatal) 3
Placebo comparison							
Bergmann, 1996	MC, RD, DB	2474	N 0.3ml x 1 placebo	21	PE, autopsy	—	10 (0.8%) 17 (1.3%)

Parnaparin (P) in major abdominal surgery

First author year	Design (surgery)	n	Treatment regimen sc route daily dose	First dose initiated (h preop)	Duration therapy (days)	Detection method	DVT total (%)	PE T/F (n)
Placebo comparison								
Valle, 1988	RD, DB	100	P 3200 AXa IU Placebo 0.3ml	2	7	D±V	0 6	0 0
No comparison								
Tartaglia, 1989	OP	92	P 3200 AXa IU P 6400 AXa IU	2	7	Clinical ± V	2 4.5	0 0
Drug comparisons								
Salcuni, 1988	OP, RD	73	P 6400 AXa IU UFH 5000 IU x 3	2	7	D	5.7 14.7	1/0 2/0
Verardi, 1988	OP, MC		P 3200 AXa IU P 6400 AXa IU UFH 5000 IU x 2 UFH 5000 IU x 3	2	7	FUT, D ± V, US	3.6 1.7 5.2 7.1	1/0 0 0 3/0
Garcea, 1992	OP, RD	85	P 3200 AXa IU UFH 5000 IU x 3	2	7	FUT, D ± US, V	0 2.2	0 0
Chiapuzzo, 1988	OP	140	P 3200 AXa IU UFH 5000 IU x 3	2	7	D	7.1 10.0	0 0
Limmer, 1994	RD	203	P 2500 AXa U UFH 5000 IU x 3	24 and 2	8	FUT	3.9 5	NR
Dosage comparison								
Becchi, 1993	OP, RD, MC	195	P 1600 AXa IU P 3200 AXa IU P 6400 AXa IU	2	7	IPG	13 5 3	NR

Parnaparin (P) in traumatology (hip fracture)

First author year	Design	n	Treatment regimen sc route daily dose	First dose preop – postop + (h)	Duration therapy (days)	Detection method	DVT prox/total (%)	PE T/F (n)
Drug comparison								
Pini, 1989	OP, RD	49	P 3200 AXa IU UFH 5000 IU x 3	before surgery	14	FUT, IPG ± V	8/20 4/29	0 1/0

Reviparin (R) in major abdominal surgery

First author year	Design	n	Treatment regimen sc route daily dose	First dose initiated (h preop)	Duration therapy (days)	Detection method	DVT total (%)	PE T/F (n)
Drug comparison Kakkar, 1997	MC, RD, DB	1342	R 1750 IU x 1 UFH 5000 IU x 2	−2	≥ 5	FUT ± V	4.6 4.2	1/1 3/2

Reviparin (R) in orthopedic (hip) surgery

First author year	Design surgery	n	Treatment regimen sc route daily dose	First dose initiated (h preop)	Duration therapy (days)	Detection method	DVT prox/total (%)	PE T/F (n)
Drug comparison Planes, 1993	RD, DB	416	R 4200 IU x 1 Enox* 40mg x 1	−10	≥ 10	V	6/10 6/9	2/0 0

*Enox: enoxaparin

Reviparin (R) in the treatment of DVT and/or PE

First author year	Design	n	Initial treatment route	Duration therapy (days)	Dosage adjustment	Detection method	Outcomes (% pts) 3 month-follow-up		
							TE	MB	Deaths
Drug comparison Columbus, 1997	OP, MC, RD	1021	R 90 IU/kg x 2 sc UFH iv infusion	6 6	BW APTT	V, US PA, LS	5.3 4.9	3.1 2.3	7.1 7.6

Tinzaparin (T) in prophylaxis of DVT in major abdominal surgery

First author year	Design (surgery)	n	Treatment regimen sc route daily dose	First dose initiated (h preop)	Duration therapy (days)	Detection method	DVT total (%)	PE T/F (n)
Placebo comparison **Bergqvist, 1996**	MC, RD, DB	80	T 3500 IU x 1 placebo	≤ +24	≥ 5	FUT ± V	8.3 21.1	0 1/
Drug comparison **Leizorovicz, 1991**	MC, RD, DB	1290	T 2500 IU x 1 T 3500 IU x 1 UFH 5000 IU x 2	−2	7-10	FUT ± V	3.7 1.6 1.6	4/0 1/0 2/0

Tinzaparin (T) in orthopedic surgery (hip and knee)

First author year	Design (surgery)	n	Treatment regimen sc route daily dose	First dose initiated (h preop/postop)	Duration therapy (days)	Detection method	DVT prox/total (%)	PE T/F (n)
Placebo comparison **Lassen, 1991**	MC, RD, DB (hip)	190	T 50 IU/kg x 1 placebo	−2	7	V	26/31 36/45	1/1 1/0
Drug comparisons **Matzsch, 1991**	OP; MC, RD (hip)	219	T 50 IU/kg x 1 dextran x 5	−2	7	V	3.6/17 2.8/28.7	2/0 0
Hull, 1993	MC, RD, DB (hip) (knee)	1207 796 641	T 75 IU/kg x 1 warfarin T 75 IU/kg x 1 warfarin	+18/24 D0 +18/24 D0	14 14	V V	4.8/20.8 3.8/23.2 7.8/45 12.3/55	0 0 0 0

Tinzaparin (T) in traumatology

First author year	Design	n	Treatment regimen sc route daily dose	First dose initiated (h preop/postop)	Duration therapy	Detection method	DVT prox/total (%)	PE T/F (n)
Drug comparison (historical) **Green, 1994**	OP	40	T 3500 IU x 1 UFH	+72	8 weeks	V, LS	10/15 /20	2/1 2/2

Tinzaparin (T) in the treatment of DVT and PE

First author year	Design	n	Treatment regimen daily dose	Duration therapy (days)	Detection method	3 months follow-up TE recurrences (%)
Drug comparisons **Hull, 1992**	MC, RD, DB (DVT)	432	T 175 IU/kg x 1 UFH iv infusion + Warfarin	5-6 D2-D90	V LS	2.8% (1 fatal PE) 6.9% (4 fatal PE)
Simonneau, 1997	OP, MC, RD (PE)	612	T 175 IU/kg x 1 UFH iv infusion + OAC	≥ 5 ≥ 5 D2-D90	LS, PA US, V	5.9% (3 fatal PE) 7.1% (3 fatal PE)

8

Low molecular weight heparins

in prophylaxis
and treatment
of arterial thrombosis

8.1

Reconstructive vascular surgery and peripheral arterial disease

Low-molecular weight heparin versus aspirin and dipyridamole after femoropopliteal bypass grafting

AUTHORS	EDMONDSON R.A., COHEN A.T., DAS S.K. et al.
REF	Lancet 1994; 344: 914-918

STUDY	Open-label, multicenter, randomized
CENTERS (n)	8
COUNTRY	United Kingdom
PATIENTS (n)	*included* 200
	evaluated 200

PATIENTS AND TYPE OF SURGERY

Patients with proven arterial occlusive disease stratified before randomization for disabling claudication or salvage surgery. Femoropopliteal bypass surgery (vein, dacron or polytetrafluoroethylene-PTFE-grafts)

ACUTE PHASE TREATMENT **Dalteparin** sc daily dose: 2500 AXa IU o.d.
first injection: 2h preop
treatment duration: 7 days, then,

randomization for:

LONG-TERM TREATMENT **Dalteparin** same regimen for the next 3 months

or

ASA (300mg) + Dipyridamole (100mg)
three times daily for the next 3 months

ASSESSMENTS

❑ Graft occlusion on D7 assessed by Doppler and confirmed by angiography or duplex ultrasonography.
❑ Thrombectomy.
❑ Bleeding complications.
❑ Death.
❑ Follow-up 1-3-6-12 months.

EDMONDSON R.A. et al. 1994

	Dalteparin 2500 AXa IU x 1	ASA + Dipyridamole	p
Patients (total)	94	106	
Operated for:			
disabling claudication	53	54	
limb salvage	41	52	
Total graft patency in all patients			
6-month	87.3% ⌐	72.0% ⌐	log rank test
12-month	79.5% ⌐	64.1% ⌐	0.02
Graft patency in patients with:			
• Surgery for claudication			
6-month	90.1% ⌐	82.7% ⌐	log rank test
12-month	84.7% ⌐	78.2% ⌐	NS
• Salvage surgery			
6-month	84.4% ⌐	59.0% ⌐	log rank test
12-month	81.5% ⌐	45.3% ⌐	< 0.001
Major bleeding	0	0	
Death (within 10 months)	9 (4 vascular disease)	2 (2 vascular disease)	

COMMENTS

❑ Long-term prophylaxis (3-month) with LMWH appeared to be better than association ASA/dipyridamole in maintaining graft patency in patients undergoing salvage surgery.

❑ The risk of graft occlusion with ASA/Dipyridamole was over three times that with LMWH.

❑ No major bleeding events in either group.

❑ This study did not take into account the thrombogenic impact of the graft material.

A randomized controlled trial
of a low molecular-weight-heparin (enoxaparin) to prevent deep-vein thrombosis
in patients undergoing vascular surgery

AUTHORS	FARKAS J.C., CHAPUIS C., COMBE S. et al.
REF	Eur. J. Vasc. Surg. 1993; 7: 554-560

STUDY	Open-label, randomized, controlled
CENTERS (n)	1
COUNTRY	France
PATIENTS (n)	included 269
	evaluated 233

TYPE OF SURGERY
Aorto-iliac aneurysm repair/aorto-femoral bypass/femoro-popliteal or distal bypass

ANESTHESIA
General ≈ 85%, regional ≈ 15%
Surgery duration: 4-8h

STUDY DRUG	**Enoxaparin**	sc daily dose: 40mg o.d. (4200 AXa IU)
		• first injection: 20mg preop (at least 6h preop)
		• second injection: 40mg D0
		treatment duration: 10 days

REFERENCE DRUG	**UFH**	sc daily doses: 7500 IU b.i.d.
		• first injection: 5000 IU preop (at least 6h)
		• second injection: 7500 IU D0
		treatment duration: 10 days

Almost all patients received heparinization (50 IU/kg IU) prior to clamping
Authorized intraoperative use of protamine

ASSESSMENTS
❑ DVT: Duplex scanning at any time if clinical suspicion; if positive, venography within 48h. Duplex scanning between D7 and D10
❑ PE: clinical symptoms confirmed by angiography.
❑ Postoperative hemorrhage, wound hematomas.
❑ Arterial graft potency: duplex-scanning or angiography D7-D10.
❑ One-month follow-up.

FARKAS J.C. et al. 1993

	Enoxaparin 40mg x 1		UFH 7500 IU x 2		p
Total DVT (Duplex-scan) D7-D10	10	8.2%	4	3.6%	NS
Aorto-iliac aneurysm	39		36		
DVT	4	10.2%	2	5.5%	NS
Aorto-femoral bypass	36		35		
DVT	4	11.1%	1	2.8%	NS
Femoro-popliteal or distal bypass	47		40		
DVT	2	4.2%	1	2.5%	NS
Arterial thrombosis	7		6		
Postoperative hemorrhage	3		3		
Minor bleeding	9		5		
One-month follow-up (DVT/PE)	0		0		

COMMENTS

❑ In major vascular surgery this enoxaparin regimen appeared to be safe and effective even though UFH 7500 IU b.i.d. seemed to be more effective than enoxaparin 40mg o.d.

❑ This study was the first which reported the incidence of DVT after major and peripheral vascular surgery in patients receiving a prophylactic regimen with LMWH or UFH.

Prevention of deep venous thrombosis in vascular surgical procedures by LMW-Heparin

AUTHORS	GOSSETTI B., IRACE L., GATTUSO R. et al.
REF	Int. Angio. 1988; 7 (Supp 3): 325-27

STUDY	Open-label
CENTERS (n)	1
COUNTRY	Italy
PATIENTS (n)	included 40

INCLUSION CRITERIA

Patients with atherosclerotic lesions of lower limb arteries necessitating aorto-femoral bypass or femoro-popliteal bypass with dacron or autologous saphenous vein

ANESTHESIA

Not stated

STUDY DRUG	**Parnaparin**	sc daily dose: 8000 AXa IU o.d. first injection: day before surgery treatment duration: 8 days
REFERENCE DRUG	**None**	

ASSESSMENTS
- ❏ DVT: clinical examination, Doppler, echotomography, FUT.
- ❏ Patency of prosthetic graft.

GOSSETTI B. et al. 1988

	Parnaparin 8000 AXa IU x 1	
Patients	40	
Occluded prosthetic grafts	0	
DVT (FUT)	1 (at D2 with dacron graft)	2.5%

COMMENTS

❏ Despite the limited number of patients and the lack of control group, this study suggested that a "strong" prophylactic regimen (8000 IU) prevented formation of thrombi either in the operated leg or in the grafts (dacron in 65% of the cases).

Clinical assessment
of low molecular weight heparin effects
in peripheral vascular disease

AUTHORS	CALABRO A., PIARULLI F., MILAN D. et al.
REF	Angiology J. Vasc. Dis.1993 (March); 188-195

STUDY	Double-blind, placebo-controlled
CENTERS *(n)*	1
COUNTRY	Italy
PATIENTS *(n)*	*included* 36
	evaluated 36

INCLUSION CRITERIA

Atherosclerotic patients with chronic obstructive arteriopathy of the lower limbs

STUDY DRUG	**Parnaparin**	sc daily dose: 15,000 AXa U o.d.
		treatment duration: 6 months

REFERENCE DRUG	**Placebo**	sc daily injection
		treatment duration: 6 months

ASSESSMENTS

❏ Plasma viscosity.

❏ Resting and post-ischemic flow with strain gauge plethysmography of the leg.

❏ Treadmill test for absolute and initial claudication distances.

CALABRO A. et al. 1993

	Parnaparin 15,000 AXa U x 1	Placebo	p
Patients	18	18	

Absolute claudication:
    distance* (in meters ± SD)
    at entry
    at 6-month
	
	300±100
	450±60
		
		290±50
		290±60
			
			NS
			0.04

Initial claudication:
    distance (in meters ± SD)
    at entry
    at 6-month
	
	150±50
	245±60
		
		140±50
		140±50
			
			NS
			0.07

Resting flow (RF) entry/6-month	no significant variation		
Post-ischemic flow (PF) entry/6-month	no significant variation		

* Values extrapolated from figure.

COMMENTS

❏ This study was selected for:

i) the unusual indication (peripheral vascular disease) and

ii) for the administered long-term treatment (6 months).

❏ No local or general intolerance reactions were reported.

❏ The encouraging results obtained in this study confirmed those obtained on 27 patients treated with the same product, same dosage (expressed as 8000 IU) and published by Palmieri G et al in Int. Angio. 1988; 7 (Supp 3): 41-47.

Expert comments

PIER GIORGIO SETTEMBRINI, R. DALLATANA, M CARMO. *DVT and graft patency after vascular surgery*

Vascular surgery is generally considered to carry a low risk of postoperative DVT. But this evaluation may not be entirely accurate. In fact, 25-30% of patients with vascular (arterial) disease have thrombophilia. It has been emphasized that antiphospholipid (aPL) antibodies are detected in the serum of a large percentage (25-30%) of such patients (1).They had undergone previous peripheral vascular surgery nearly twice (1.8) as often and experienced thrombotic complications 5.6 times more often than those without aPL. Finally, arterial graft patency was of shorter duration in patients with aPL (average : 17 months) than in those without aPL (average : 50 months) (p<0.003). Furthermore, even though there is minimal trauma to soft tissue in vascular surgery, temporary ischemia which occurs during vessel clamping necessary to perform vascular anastomosis, acute ischemia prior to vascular reconstruction, and postoperative limb edema all can contribute to alterations of venous flow which can promote the onset of a DVT.

In a prospective study, Olin (2) showed that incidence of DVT without prophylactic heparin was 18% in 50 patients who had undergone surgery for an aneurysm of the abdominal aorta. Evidence of DVT was obtained by venography of the lower limbs in all patients on postoperative day 5, apart from clinical symptoms which sometimes were completely lacking. Previous reports have shown different incidences of DVT ranging from 1.5 to 40%, all of which were obtained by I125 scanning (3-8). However, while this procedure shows a high sensitivity for calf vein thrombosis, it yields 30% false negative results in cases of venous thrombosis of the femoro-iliac axis.

Amputation of a lower limb carries a potentially high rate of DVT, mainly because of extended pre- and postoperative bedrest and surgical trauma. Moreover, concomitant risk factors for DVT, such as diabetes, sepsis, and malignant tumor, are often present in such patients. A prospective study by Yeager (9) showed a 12.5% incidence of DVT, involving 72 patients who had undergone major amputation of a lower extremity above or below the knee. In these patients, a color duplex scan was carried out before the operation and prior to discharge from the hospital. These patients did not receive heparin prophylaxis, except for 9 who received anticoagulant therapy for other diseases. In conclusion, DVT in vascular surgery is a relevant problem. Moreover, the risk of exposure to DVT in vascular patients is not limited solely to hospital stay, but continues up to 30 days after surgery. Even though it has been well-established that a favorable outcome following arterial reconstruction depends primarily on surgical technique and distal vascular resistance, there is no doubt that antithrombotic or anti-platelet therapy can be useful to maintain the patency of a vascular reconstruction itself.

In a recent report by Edmonson (10) two groups of patients were matched by evaluating the vascular graft patency. The first group was given low molecular weight heparin (LMWH), and the second aspirin (ASA) + dipyridamole: in the former group 78% of patients and in the latter only 64% of patients showed one year graft patency (p= 0.02). A possible explanation of this better patency can be related to the antiproliferative effects of heparin on smooth muscle cells of vessel walls (11-13).

Heparin compounds appear to act by reducing intimal hyperplasia, which often causes graft thrombosis. In particular, Wilson (13) reported that LMWH reduces intimal hyperplasia in the aorta of rats by 60% when a balloon catheter was introduced, in comparison with untreated rats. Heparin is widely employed in vascular surgery, both unfractionated and fractionated heparin administered during surgery, by intravenous or intra-arterial injection, in order to prevent graft and arterial thromboses. It is easy to handle and can readily be neutralized by protamine sulfate.

Wilson (14) used LMWHs during 16 operations in major vascular surgery (abdominal aortic aneurysm or aortic obstructions), differentiating three groups of patients based on route of injection of heparin (intravenous, intra-aortic before clamping the aorta, intra-aortic after clamping the aorta) and by evaluating its impact on coagulation by blood samples collected from a femoral vessel. Heparin was found to be highly effective in the lower limb circulation of patients who received heparin by aortic injection before clamping the aorta, in comparison to intravenous injection ($p < 0.05$). Heparin seems to act by reducing intimal hyperplasia.

In the randomized study of Edmonson (10), graft patency was examined in a femoro-popliteal bypass procedure of 200 patients with peripheral arterial disease of the lower extremities. All patients were treated with subcutaneous dalteparin (2500 AXa IU) for seven days and were further subdivided into two groups; the first group continued the same treatment for 3 months, the second received 300 mg ASA + 100 mg dipyridamole for 3 months. All patients were followed for 12 months. Long-term prophylaxis with LMWH appeared to be more effective than the combination of ASA+dipyridamole. The overall 1 year patency rate with LMWH was 78% versus 64% for the other group (log rank test 0.02). A further differentiation in outcome of patients who underwent surgery for claudication or for limb salvage showed a significant difference in the latter group between the two treatments (81% patency rate in the LMWH treated group versus 45% in the ASA+dipyridamole group; log rank test < 0.001). No difference was observed in terms of postoperative bleeding.

The question can then be raised regarding the real advantages of use of LMWH vs UF heparin in vascular surgery. Currently, only one study has compared the two types of prophylactic treatment in reconstructive arterial surgery (aorto-femoral or femoro-popliteal bypass procedures) (15). More than 200 patients received prophylaxis with enoxaparin 40 mg daily or calcium-heparin 7500 units twice daily for 10 days. Results reported did not demonstrate any significant differences between the two groups with regard to postoperative DVT (even though its incidence was slightly lower in patients treated with calcium heparin) as well as postoperative bleeding or graft thromboses.

Conclusion

Heparin therapy is indicated in vascular surgery to protect vascular anastomoses and preserve graft patency from thrombosis. It appears that the use of LMWH for three months after surgery improves long-term patency of vascular reconstructions in comparison to routine treatment with antiplatelet drugs, without gastric adverse events or allergic reactions, even though a daily injection for an extended period may cause discomfort for the patient.

LMWH did not show better efficacy than unfractionated heparin in preventing graft thrombosis or DVT, but appears easier to use because of a single daily injection. Moreover, LMWH does not require laboratory monitoring of coagulation. Additional well-controlled studies are needed to better define the advantages of LMWH vs newer antiplatelet drugs.

REFERENCES

1) Taylor LM Jr, Chitwoood RW, Dalman RL et al. Antiphospholipid antibodies in vascular surgery patients. A cross-sectional study. Ann Surg 1994; 220: 544-51

2) Olin JW, Graor RA, O'Hara P et al. The incidence of deep vein thromboses in patients undergoing abdominal aortic aneurysm resection. J Vasc Surg 1993; 18: 1037-41

3) Angelides NS, Nicolaides N, Femandes J et al. Deep venous thromboses in patients having aortoiliac reconstruction. Br J Surg 1997; 64: 517-8

4) Cass AJ, Jennings SA, Greenhalgh RM. Leg swelling after aortic surgery. Int Angiol 1986; 5: 207-8

5) Jenning S, Cass AJ, Heater BP et al. Coagulation changes during major surgery and relationship to postoperative deep vein thromboses. J Cardiovasc Surg 1981; 22: 327-9

6) Reilly N, McCabe CJ, Abbott WM et al. Deep venous thrombosis following aortoiliac reconstructive surgery. Arch Surg 1982; 1 1 7: 12 1 0-1 1

7) Satiani B, Kuhns M, Evans WE. Deep venous thrombosis following operations on the abdominal aorta. Surg Gynecol Obstet 1980; 151: 241-5

8) Schoon IM, Holm J, Lindberg B, et al. Hemodynamic findings before and after resection of abdominal aortic aneurysm. Acta Chir Scand 1984; 150: 451-6

9) Yeager RA, Moneta GL, Edwards JM et al. Deep vein thrombosis associated with lower extremity amputation. J Vasc Surg 1995; 22: 612-5

10) Edmonson RA, Cohen AT, Das SK et al. Low-molecular weight heparin versus aspirin and dipyridarnole after femoropopliteal bypass grafting. Lancet 1994; 344: 914-18

11) Clowes AW, Karnovsky MJ Suppression by heparin of smooth-muscle cell proliferation in injured arteries. Nature (Lond) 1977; 265: 625-6

12) Guyton JR, Rosenberg RD, Clowes AW et al. Inibition of rat arterial smooth cell proliferation by heparin. In vivo studies with anticoagulant and non anticoagulant heparin. Circ Res 1980; 46: 625-33

13) Wilson NV, Salisbury JR and Kakkar VV. Effect of low molecular weight heparin on intimal hyperplasia. Br J Surg 1991; 78: 1381-83

14) Wilson NV, Melissari E, Standfield NJ et al. Intraoperative antithrombotic therapy with low molecular weight heparin in aortic surgery. How should it be administered? Eur J Vasc Surg 1991; 5: 565-9

15) Farkas JC, Chapuis C, Combe S et al. A randomized controlled trial of a low molecular weight heparin, enoxaparin, to prevent deep vein thrombosis in patients undergoing vascular surgery. Eur J Vasc Surg 1993; 7: 554-560

8.2
Angioplasty/stenting
and
restenosis

Pharmacological therapy after coronary angioplasty. Early experience with low molecular weight heparin for prophylaxis of reocclusion

AUTHORS	SCHMIDT T., TEBBE V., SCHRADER J. et al.
REF	Klin. Wochenschr 1990; 68: 294

STUDY	open pilot
CENTERS *(n)*	1
COUNTRY	Germany
PATIENTS *(n)*	*included* 22
	evaluated 22

INCLUSION CRITERIA

Patients with coronary stenosis dilated by PTCA

OBJECTIVE

To compare the rate of restenosis (defined as reduction of the residual stenosis diameter of more than 50%) in patients treated with either LMWH or

STUDY DRUG	**Dalteparin**	mean sc dose ≈ 80 IU/kg o.d.
		dose adjusted on AXa activity ranging between
		0.3-0.6 IU/ml measured 2h after injection
		first injection: after PTCA (time not stated)
		treatment duration: 3 months

REFERENCE DRUG	**ASA**	100-300 mg/day
		treatment duration: 3 months

ASSESSMENTS

❏ Coronary angiogram before and 3 months after angioplasty.

❏ Symptoms of unstable angina, MI during the 3-month follow-up.

SCHMIDT T. et al. 1990

	Dalteparin ≈ 80 IU/kg x 1	**ASA** 100-300mg
Patients	11	11

Stenosis area (% ± SD)
  initial
  just after PTCA
  3 months after PTCA
	
	85.1±12.7
	39.5±25.9
	48.5±29.3
		
		88.4±10.0
		44.3±17.8
		70.6±28.4

Restenosis (% of patients)	27%	45%

Diameter stenosis (% ± SD)
  initial
  just after PTCA
  3 months after PTCA
	
	64.8±18.7
	26.0±17.7
	35.6±25.8
		
		68.9±15.0
		26.4±13.1
		53.6±27.0

Restenosis (% of patients)	27%	55%

COMMENTS

❑ This pioneering study (in this indication) suggested that a prolonged treatment with a LMWH appeared to be better than ASA in preventing restenosis.

Low molecular weight heparin in prevention of restenosis after angioplasty.
Results of enoxaparin restenosis (ERA) trial

AUTHORS	FAXON D.P., SPIRO T.E., MINOR S. et al.
REF	Circulation. 1994; 90: 908-914

STUDY	Multicenter, double-blind, randomized, placebo-controlled
CENTERS *(n)*	9
COUNTRY	United States
PATIENTS *(n)*	*randomized* 459
	evaluated 357
	(with angiography at 26±12W)

INCLUSION CRITERIA

Patients undergoing successful angioplasty after a first angiogram for angina (90%) (class II-IV) or for previous myocardial infarction (10%)

STUDY DRUG	**Enoxaparin**	sc daily dose: 40mg o.d. (0.4ml)
		first injection: within 24h post procedure
		treatment duration: 28 days

REFERENCE DRUG	**Placebo**	0.4ml sc o.d.
		first dose within 24h procedure

UFH during angioplasty adjusted to ACT ≥ 300 sec. + ASA 325mg for both groups 1 day before procedure and during 28 days of treatment.

ASSESSMENTS
- ❑ Clinical observation at 1, 4 , 24 weeks.
- ❑ Second angiogram 6 months after PTCA (24±4W).
- ❑ Bleeding complications.
- ❑ Adverse events.

FAXON D.P. et al. 1994

	Enoxaparin 40mg x 1	Placebo	p
Six-month follow-up			
Evaluable patients	181	176	
% of patients with restenosis (2nd angiogram)	52%	51%	NS
Patients with asymptomatic restenosis	27%	29%	
Angina (occurrence/worsening)	27%	29%	
Myocardial infarction	2%	2%	
Minor bleeding	48%	34%	<0.001
Thrombocytopenia	9 4%	7 3%	

COMMENTS

❑ Treatment with enoxaparin 40mg sc o.d. for one month did not prevent restenosis after angioplasty.

❑ In EMPAR study [814 patients, enoxaparin associated with Maxepa (omega-3 polyunsaturated fatty acid) for the prevention of angioplasty restenosis] similar results were observed despite a higher enoxaparin dosage (30mg sc b.i.d.) maintained 6 weeks in association with Maxepa (CAIRNS J.A. et al. Circulation. 1996; 94: 1553-1560).

Low-molecular-weight heparin and elective stenting: the ENTICES Trial

AUTHORS	ZIDAR J.P., BERKOWITZ S.D., GREENBERG C.S. et al.
REF	Am. Heart J.1998; 134: S81-S87

STUDY Multicenter, open-label, randomized

CENTERS (n) 7
COUNTRY United States

PATIENTS (n) *included* 123

PATIENTS
with documented ischemia or chest pain scheduled to undergo Palmaz-Schatz stenting

PRIMARY OBJECTIVE
To evaluate the physiological effect and efficacy of enoxaparin and antiplatelet agents versus conventional therapy

STUDY DRUG **Enoxaparin** sc daily doses: 30 mg b.i.d. for BW < 70 kg
40mg b.i.d. for BW 70-100 kg
60mg b.i.d. for BW > 100 kg
first injection: 2h after sheath removal

CONVENTIONAL THERAPY
• Ticlopidine 250 mg b.i.d.
• Dipyridamole 75 mg t.i.d. from D0 up to D30
• Dextran 40 iv infusion
• UFH 2500 IU iv bolus after sheath removal
   then 10 IU/kg/h APTT-adjusted
• Warfarin 10 mg/D after procedure then INR 2-3-adjusted
treatment duration: 30 days

For all patients: ASA 325 mg indefinitely

ASSESSMENTS
❑ Coronary angiograms before and after stenting success defined as ≤ 50% of residual stenosis with TIMI grade 3 flow, thrombosis with TIMI grade 0 or 1 flow, repeat angiogram if AMI suspected.
❑ Hematology samples baseline, before sheath removal at discharge (3 days) and 10 days after stenting.
❑ ECG after stenting and in cases of suspected AMI.
❑ In-hospital complications: major bleeding, stroke, vascular complications.

ZIDAR J.P. 1998

	Enoxaparin BW-adapted x 2		Conventional therapy		p
Patients	79		44		
Procedural data					
final diameter stenosis	7%		7%		
transient closure	3%		5%		
embolization	0%		2%		
dissection	10%		10%		
stent deployment	97%		95%		
angiographic success	99%		93%		
clinical success	95%		81%		
In-hospital complications					
severe bleeding	0%		2%		
retroperitoneal hematoma	0%		5%		
30-day follow-up					
death	0		5		
AMI	3	4%	5	11%	NS
stent thrombosis	0	0%	3	7%	0.04
6-month follow-up					
death	1		2		
AMI	3	4%	7	16%	0.04
bypass surgery	1	1%	4	9%	NS

COMMENTS

❑ The antiplatelet agents association (ticlopidine plus aspirin) with a LMWH (enoxaparin) provided safe and effective antithrombotic therapy following coronary stent placement.

❑ The so called "conventional therapy" seems today very heavy. So, this studied triple association should be compared with the new standard therapy aspirin plus ticlopidine as it will be done in ATLAST study.

❑ Hemobiological markers (not reported here) did not appear to predict clinical oucomes.

Effect of nadroparin, a low molecular weight heparin, on clinical and angiographic restenosis after coronary balloon angioplasty.
The FACT study

AUTHORS	LABLANCHE J.M., McFADDEN E.P., MENEVEAU N. et al.
REF	Circulation 1997; 96: 3396-3402

STUDY	Multicenter, double-blind, randomized, placebo-controlled
CENTERS (n)	12
COUNTRIES	France, Belgium, Spain
PATIENTS (n)	*included* 359
	evaluated 269

INCLUSION CRITERIA

Patients with angina and/or evidence of myocardial ischemia scheduled for angioplasty when stenosis, documented on a recent angiogram, was superior to 50%

STUDY DRUG **Nadroparin** sc daily dose: 0.6ml (5800 AXa IU) o.d.
first injection: 3 days before angioplasty
treatment duration: 3 months
(self-administered, home treatment)

REFERENCE DRUG **Placebo**

For both groups:

• during procedure UFH iv bolus 10,000 IU then
iv bolus 5000 IU 1h later
• ASA 250 mg/day D3 up to 3 months

ASSESSMENTS

❑ Angiographic quantitative analysis performed before, just after, 24h after and 3 months after angioplasty
❑ Angiographic restenosis defined as a residual stenosis of < 50% after angioplasty that became ≥ 50% at follow-up.
❑ MI, CABG surgery, repeat angioplasty, death (6-month follow-up).

LABLANCHE J.M. et al. 1997

	Nadroparin 0.6ml x 1		Placebo x 1	
Patients	131		138	
Minimal luminal diameter (mm ± SD)				
before PTCA	0.78±0.29		0.82±0.28	
after PTCA	1.74±0.45		1.84±0.39	
at follow-up	1.37±0.66		1.48±0.59	
Net gain at 3-month	0.59±0.65		0.66±0.59	
Stenosis (%)				
before PTCA	72±10		71±9	
at follow-up	52±21		79±19	
Clinical endpoints at 6-month:				
death	1	0.6%	3	1.7%
AMI	7	4.0%	4	2.2%
CABG	19	10.9%	8	4.5%
repeat PTCA	26	14.9%	53	29.6%

COMMENTS

❑ Pretreatment with a relatively high nadroparin dose (about 6000 IU/day) continued for 3 months after angioplasty had no beneficial effect on restenosis or on adverse clinical outcomes.

❑ These negative results confirmed those obtained by Amman et al. on a limited number of patients (n=20), where a recurrent stenosis > 50% was observed in 30% of nadroparin-treated patients [Semin. Thromb. & Hemost. 1993; 19 (Supp) 160-163].

Low molecular weight heparin (reviparin) in percutaneous transluminal coronary angioplasty. Results of a randomized, double-blind, unfractionated heparin and placebo-controlled, multicenter trial (Reduce Trial)

AUTHORS	KARSCH K.R., BREISACK M.B., BAILDON R. et al.
REF	JACC. 1996; 28: 1437-1443

STUDY	Multicenter, randomized, double-blind
CENTERS (n)	26
COUNTRIES	Europe, Canada
PATIENTS (n)	randomized 612
	evaluated 500
	for protocol analysis

INCLUSION CRITERIA

Patients with stable or unstable angina and presenting a single lesion. Suitable PTCA for coronary obstruction planned for all patients

STUDY DRUG   **Reviparin**   initial treatment
- 7000 IU iv bolus before PTCA then,
- 10,500/20h infusion after PTCA followed by

prolonged treatment: 3500 IU sc b.i.d.

treatment duration: 28 days

REFERENCE DRUG   **UFH**   initial treatment

UFH doses:
- 10,000 IU iv bolus before PTCA then,
- 24,000 IU/20h infusion after PTCA

prolonged treatment: placebo saline injections b.i.d.

treatment duration: 28 days

ASA 100mg/day from D1 up to D28 for all patients

ASSESSMENTS
- ❏ Primary endpoint: death/MI/urgent reinterventions (repeat PTCA, CABG, stent) in the first 30 days after procedure.
- ❏ Restenosis incidence one month after angioplasty.

KARSCH K.R. et al. 1996

	Reviparin bolus infusion then 3500 AXa IU x 2		**UFH** infusion, then placebo		**p**
Patients	306		306		
Total exclusions	79	25.8%	93	30.4%	
Total primary events (ITT)	102	33%	98	32%	NS
Acute events occurring within 24h					
Death	0		0		
Non-fatal MI	4	1.3%	3	1.0%	
Urgent revascularization (repeat PTCA/stent)	8	2.7%	22	7.2%	0.003
Events occurring after PTCA					
Death	1		1		
Non-fatal MI	8	2.6%	4	1.3%	
Urgent revascularization	81	26.5%	68	22.3%	NS
Major bleeding (within 35 days)	7	2.3%	8	2.6%	NS
Restenosis	89	33.0%	86	34.4%	NS

COMMENTS

❑ The administration of reviparin resulted in an appreciable reduction in acute events mainly in the stent implantation group.

❑ Complete absence of benefit on restenosis despite the long-term treatment (28 days).

Expert comments

GYÖRGY ACSADY. *Clinical remarks on the effect of some LMWHs in prevention of restenosis after PTCA and in peripheral vascular diseases*

Since the introduction of percutaneous transluminal coronary angioplasty (PTCA) in 1979, one of the main problems has been early restenosis. Rates of restenosis after successful PTCA are between 22 and 52% within the first 6 months based on the clinical signs. The majority of restenosis appears to occur within 3 months and necessitates a repeat intervention in 20 to 25% of patients.

The prophylactic effect of 4 various LMWH preparations (enoxaparin, reviparin, nadroparin, dalteparin) was investigated for the prevention of restenosis after balloon dilatation of the stenosed coronary arteries, and negative results have been observed.

Unfractionated heparin was administered either before or during and after the PTCA for the patients in all of the trials. Acetylsalicylic acid was administered in altering doses (100-325 mg/day) with placebo in the control groups.

Angiography was performed just before and immediately after angioplasty and at follow-up. At angiographic follow-up, the mean minimal lumen diameter and the mean residual stenosis in the LMWH groups did not differ from the corresponding values in the control groups. Likewise there was no difference in combined major cardiac-related clinical events (death, myocardial infarction, target lesion revascularisation) either. In conclusion, none of the different types of LMWHs tested could reduce the incidence of angiographic restenosis or the occurrence of a clinical event within 3-6 months after successful PTCA.

Possible explanations for the lack of benefit of the treatment:

1 - Restenosis is a multifactorial process that involves elastic recoil, platelets deposition, thrombus formation, inflammation, smooth muscle cell proliferation, and matrix organization. Heparin is used routinely during angioplasty to prevent a thrombotic abrupt vessel closure.

2 - Heparin has pharmacological actions that are potentially useful in reducing restenosis. In addition to its anticoagulant and antithrombotic effects, heparin has been shown to limit neointimal proliferation in vitro as well as in animal models of balloon injury. The doses of unfractionated heparin that can safely be administered to humans are limited by the potential occurrence of bleeding complications. The pharmacological profiles of LMWHs differ from those of unfractionated heparin, with a longer half-life and greater bioavailability. Cell culture data demonstrated that the dose-dependent antiproliferative properties of LMWHs are more potent and are basically independent of their ability to bind antithrombin III. LMWHs have shown as great or greater antiproliferative activity in vitro and in vivo than unfractionated heparin. Nevertheless it is also possible that the systemically or subcutaneously injected doses of LMWH or the duration of therapy might not have been sufficient to reduce the local arterial proliferative actions.

3 - Finally, it is possible that mechanisms other than intimal hyperplasia are also important in restenosis. Experimental data and results of intravascular ultrasound studies carried out in humans suggest that late remodeling may be more important than intimal hyperplasia in causing restenosis.

The parnaparin's effect in peripheral vascular diseases was also assessed. The small sample sizes, however, does not seem to be enough for valid conclusions. Two establishments are remarkable:

a) parnaparin caused a statistically significant increase in claudication time with parallel increase in the absolute walking distance and in the interval free of pain.

b) the administration of the drug led to a marked reduction in blood viscosity.

In conclusion, further pharmacologic studies are required to clarify this mechanism of action.

We can suppose that LMWHs repair the collateral circulation by the reduction of blood viscosity, by its antithrombotic effect and by the inhibition of the intimal proliferation in the collateral vessels.

8.3
Acute
coronary syndromes

Acute myocardial infarction (AMI)
Left ventricular (LV) mural thrombosis
Atrial fibrillation

Unstable, stable angina

Expert Comments

Safety of high doses of low molecular weight heparin (Fragmin) in acute myocardial infarction. A dose-finding study

AUTHORS	NESVOLD A., KONTNY F., ABILDGAARD U. et al.
REF	Thromb. Res. 1991; 764: 579-587

STUDY	Open-label, dose-finding
CENTERS (n)	1
COUNTRY	Norway
PATIENTS (n)	included 72

INCLUSION CRITERIA
Patients with MI verified by ECG and with twice the upper limit of normal value of ASAT and CK

OBJECTIVE
To verify whether a LMWH at doses producing plasma levels ranging between 0.6-1 AXa IU/ml may reduce the incidence of left mural thrombosis after an AMI treated with or without streptokinase (SK 1.5 MU) and ASA

STUDY DRUG	**Dalteparin**	sc daily ascending doses:	previous thrombolysis
	group I	240 AXa IU/kg in 3 injections	no
	group II	240 AXa IU/kg in 2 injections	no
	group III	300 AXa IU/kg in 3 injections	no
	group IV	300 AXa IU/kg in 3 injections	yes
	group V	300 AXa IU/kg in 2 injections	no
	group VI	300 AXa IU/kg in 2 injections	yes
	group VII	360 AXa IU/kg in 3 injections	no

when previous thrombolytic treatment, the first dalteparin injection was not given until 8h after SK infusion.

treatment duration: 6-10 days

ASSESSMENTS
- ❏ Echocardiography at D3 or D4 post MI for the detection of left ventricular thrombosis.
- ❏ Blood biochemistry   ❏ Bleeding complications.

NESVOLD A. et al. 1991

	Dalteparin IU/kg/24h		
Dosages	240	300	360
Patients	10	57	5

AXa levels (U/ml)*
2-4h after administration
    peak value
    range
	0.7
	(0.3-0.8)
		1
		(0.7-1.8)
			0.8
			(0.6-1.1)

Minor bleeding complications during the study	3/72 (4.2%) (all in patients who received SK+ASA)		
Left ventricular mural thrombosis (47 AMI patients)	3/47 (6%) (all of these 3 patients received 300 IU/kg)		
Death	1 cardiogenic stroke on D2 after 300 IU/kg		

* read from figures.

COMMENTS
- This trial was designed to determine a regimen producing AXa plasma level ranging between 0.6-1 U/ml. The daily dosage of 300 IU/kg subdivided in 2 injections appeared safe but, interestingly, minor hemorrhage occurred in patients receiving ASA.
- Initial SK and subsequent ASA indication did not influence plasma concentrations.
- In this limited number of patients, bleeding complications were not related to AXa level even over 1.5 AXa IU/ml.
- Low incidence of left mural thrombosis in patients treated with dalteparin in comparison to overall admitted incidence of 25-45% reported in AMI patients.

Anticoagulant effects of low-molecular-weight heparin following thrombolytic therapy in acute myocardial infarction: a dose-finding study

AUTHORS	STRANDBERG L.E., KAHAN T., LUNDIN P. et al.
REF	Haemostasis 1996; 26: 247-257

STUDY	Open-label, pilot
CENTERS (n)	1
COUNTRY	Sweden
PATIENTS (n)	included 20
	evaluated 20

OBJECTIVE

To define a sc dose of dalteparin associated with a peak of AXa activity ranging between 0.6-1.0 IU/ml following thrombolytic therapy (streptokinase) in patients with AMI

STUDY DRUG

4 hours after completion of streptokinase infusion:

Dalteparin sc daily doses b.i.d. of:

- 50 IU/kg or
- 75 IU/kg or
- 100 IU/kg

treatment duration: 6 days

REFERENCE DRUG

Control group no anticoagulant treatment after thrombolysis

ASA for all patients

ASSESSMENTS

- ❏ Plasma concentration of AXa activity.
- ❏ APTT values.
- ❏ Adverse events
- ❏ Major/minor bleeding.

STRANDBERG L.E. et al. 1996

	Dalteparin IU/kg x 2			Control
	50 IU	75 IU	100 IU	
Patients	5	5	5	5

AXa activity (IU/ml) at D6:
   mean value 4h after administration
   (range)
   mean value before administration
   (range)
	0.26
	(0.14-0.46)
	0.07
	(0.0-0.15)
		0.49
		(0.30-0.63)
		0.14
		(0.02-0.33)
			0.79
			(0.59-1.00)
			0.51
			(0.34-0.82)	

APTT (sec) at D6:
   mean value 4h after administration
   (range)
   mean value before last administration
   (range)
	28
	(23-30)
	24
	(20-28)
		30
		(21-47)
		25
		(21-33)
			33
			(27-36)
			28
			(22-31)	

Adverse events:
   major hemorrhage
   hematomas at injection site
   urogenital bleeding
	0
	5
	2
		0
		5
		4
			0
			5
			2
				0
				0
				0

COMMENTS

❑ AXa activity is dose-dependent.

❑ No serious adverse events have been observed on this small number of patients.

❑ The authors suggested that a dalteparin dose slightly higher than 100 AXa IU/kg twice daily could be required in order to achieve the presumed therapeutic range of 0.6-1.0 IU/ml.

Randomized trial of low molecular weight heparin (Dalteparin) in prevention of left ventricular thrombus formation and arterial embolism after acute anterior myocardial infarction: The Fragmin in Acute Myocardial Infarction (FRAMI) study

AUTHORS	KONTNY F., DALE J. ABILDGAARD U. et al.
REF	J. Am. Coll Cardiol. 1997; 30: 962-969

STUDY	Multicenter, randomized, double-blind, placebo-controlled
CENTERS (n)	13
COUNTRY	Norway
PATIENTS (n)	*randomized* 776
	evaluated 517 for primary endpoint
	776 for safety and secondary endpoint

INCLUSION CRITERIA

Randomization on a 24h/day basis of patients with ECG changes (Q waves or ST elevation) suggestive of an evolving anterior Q wave MI in patients receiving or not receiving thrombolytic agent (streptokinase for more than 90% of the patients)

STUDY DRUG	**Dalteparin**	sc daily doses: 150 IU/kg b.i.d.
		first injection: • 8h after thrombolytic therapy
		• or immediately after randomization in patients not receiving thrombolytic agent
		treatment duration: 9±2 days
REFERENCE DRUG	**Placebo**	saline, volume BW-adjusted b.i.d.
		treatment duration: 9±2 days
ASA 160mg for both groups		

ASSESSMENTS

❑ LV mural thrombus formation diagnosed by echocardiography on D9±2 and arterial embolism (stroke), (primary endpoint).

❑ Reinfarction, total and cardiac mortality (secondary endpoint).

❑ Minor/major hemorrhage.

KONTNY F. et al. 1997

	Dalteparin 150 IU/kg x 2		Placebo sc saline x 2		p
Patients	388		388		
Evaluable echocardiography	247		270		
LV mural thrombosis + arterial thromboembolism	34+1	14.2%	59+0	21.9%	0.03
Total arterial embolism (ischemic stroke)	4/388	1.0%	5/388	1.3%	NS
Reinfarction	6/388	1.6%	8/388	2.1%	NS
Major hemorrhage	11 (3 cerebral of which 2 fatal)	2.8%	1	0.3%	0.006
Death	21	5.4%	23	5.9%	NS

COMMENTS

❑ Dalteparin 150 IU/kg twice daily significantly reduced LV thrombus formation in acute anterior MI but was associated with increased hemorrhagic risk (all major events occurred in dalteparin group).

❑ Most patients with major hemorrhage in the dalteparin group received SK and ASA.

❑ High plasma dalteparin levels (1.1 to 2.0 IU/ml) in patients with a major hemorrhage. The mean plasma concentration was 0.91±0.40 IU/ml on day 7, 4h after the injection. This plasma level did not differ between patients with and without LV thrombus.

Reduction of reinfarction and angina with use of low molecular weight heparin therapy after streptokinase (and heparin) in acute myocardial infarction

AUTHORS	GLICK A., KORNOWSKI R., MICHOWISCH Y. et al.
REF	Am. J. Cardiol. 1996; 77: 1145-1148

STUDY	Open-label, randomized, two parallel groups
CENTERS (n)	1
COUNTRY	Israel
PATIENTS (n)	*included* 103

INCLUSION CRITERIA

AMI patients treated by streptokinase and UFH iv (PTT 2-2,5), ASA 100mg/day for 5 days

OBJECTIVE

To examine whether continuing anticoagulant therapy by enoxaparin can prevent recurrent myocardial ischemic

STUDY DRUG   **Enoxaparin**   sc dose: 40mg o.d.
treatment duration: from D5 up to D30 after AMI
(ASA continued?)

REFERENCE DRUG   **Control**   no treatment
(ASA continued?)

ASSESSMENTS

❏ 6-month follow-up for recurrent myocardial ischemic events: unstable angina/reinfarction/death.

❏ Bleeding complications.

❏ Adverse events.

GLICK A. et al. 1996

	Enoxaparin 40mg x 1		Control		p
Patients	43		60		
Six-month follow-up					
Reinfarction	2	4.6%	13	21.6%	0.01
"Early" angina (0-30D)	4	9.3%	12	20.0%	NS
"Late" angina (>30D)	0		1	2.3%	NS
Total angina events	4	9.3%	13	21.6%	NS
Total cardiac events	6	14.0%	26	43.0%	< 0.001
Death	0		1	1.6%	NS
Major bleeding	0		0		
Thrombocytopenia	0		0		

COMMENTS

❑ This study suggested that long-term prophylaxis with enoxaparin can prevent recurrent myocardial ischemic events, mainly reinfarction.

❑ These results support the biological hypothesis of coagulation activation for at least 3 weeks after AMI onset.

❑ If these results were confirmed, all AMI patients treated with streptokinase should receive LMWH for at least one month after AMI.

Fraxiparine for the prevention of left ventricular thrombosis after non-thrombolysed myocardial infarction: the FRATIV trial (French)

AUTHORS	CHARBONNIER B. for the FRATIV group
REF	Arch. Mal. Cœur; 1997; 90: 1215-1221

STUDY	Open-label, multicenter, pilot, non comparative
CENTERS (n)	13
COUNTRIES	France, Italy, Spain, the Netherlands
PATIENTS (n)	*included* 148
	evaluated 119

INCLUSION CRITERIA

AMI patients; less than 3 days without thrombolytic treatment and without left mural thrombosis (LMT)

OBJECTIVE

To determine an effective dose for the prevention of LMT

STUDY DRUG **Nadroparin** iv bolus 0.3ml (2850 AXa IU) followed by sc daily dose:
- 60 IU/kg (Goup I)
- 100 IU/kg (Group II)

first injection: after bolus (time not stated)

treatment duration: 10 days

REFERENCE DRUG **None**

+ ASA 100-250mg/day for all patients

ASSESSMENTS
- ❏ Echocardiography at entry and at D10±1 for left mural thrombosis (primary endpoint).
- ❏ Hemorrhage, thromboembolic events, death (secondary endpoint).
- ❏ Daily clinical surveillance.

CHARBONNIER B. et al.1997

	Group I **Nadroparin** 60 IU/kg x 1	Group II **Nadroparin** 100 IU/kg x 1	p
Patients included	79	69	
evaluable	62	57	
Left ventricular mural thrombosis	7/56 12.5%	9/51 17.6%	NS
Recurrent MI	1	0	
Stroke	1	0	
Atrial fibrillation	1	0	
Death	3	6	
Major hemorrhage	0	0	

COMMENTS

❑ The determination of the most effective dose was not conclusive even though the two regimens of nadroparin appeared to reduce the incidence of left mural thrombosis since literature data reported an incidence of 30-40% of left ventricular mural thrombosis in patients with anterior MI not receiving anticoagulant therapy.

❑ The authors suggested that a higher daily dosage (200 IU/kg) could be more suitable.

Low molecular weight heparin
as an adjuvant to thrombolysis for acute myocardial infarction
the FATIMA study

AUTHORS	CHAMULEAU S.A.J. , DE WINTER R.J., LEVI M. et al. on behalf of FATIMA STUDY GROUP
REF	Heart 1998; 80: 35-39

STUDY	Open-label, pilot
CENTERS (n)	1
COUNTRY	The Netherlands
PATIENTS (n)	included 30
	evaluated 30

OBJECTIVE

To study the pharmacokinetics (based on AXa activity) and safety of nadroparin as adjuvant therapy with a thrombolytic agent (t-PA) in patients with AMI
Nadroparin target therapeutic range: 0.35-0.70 IU/ml

STUDY DRUG   **Nadroparin**

- iv bolus 100 IU/kg just before thrombolytic treatment (Actilyse® 100 mg, accelerated regimen), then
- sc daily doses: BW-adjusted (in two injections):

    9500 IU for BW < 50 kg

    14,000 IU for BW 50-70 kg

    19,000 IU for BW > 70 kg

first injection: 6h after thrombolysis

treatment duration: ≥ 3 days

Carbasalate calcium 300mg on admission then 100mg daily

ASSESSMENTS

❏ AXa activity measured 12 hourly between 6 and 72h.

❏ Bleeding complications.

❏ Coronary angiography at D5 for evaluation of patency.

CHAMULEAU S.A.J. et al. 1998

	Nadroparin BW-adjusted dose x 2				
Patients	30				
Time (hours) after treatment	6*	12	24	48	72
AXa mean value (IU/ml)	0.28	0.50	0.52	0.53	0.54
± SD	0.20	0.10	0.14	0.21	0.21
Bleeding complications					
major	0				
minor	2				
Patients with 80% patency rate	24 (5 with TIMI flow 0; 1 with TIMI flow 1)				

* After the first injection of nadroparin.

COMMENTS

❑ The plasma AXa target range 0.35-0.70 IU/ml was reached with a total daily dosage corresponding to about 250 AXa IU/kg (125 IU/kg twice daily).

❑ The safety of this treatment after a thrombolytic regimen was good (no major hemorrhage).

❑ Efficacy, in terms of patency rates, appeared to be satisfactory (even in absence of comparison group).

Prophylaxis of embolic events in patients with atrial fibrillation using low molecular weight heparin

AUTHORS	HARENBERG J., WEUSTER B., PFITZER M. et al.
REF	Semin. Throm. Hemost. 1993; 19 (Supp 1): 116-121

STUDY	Open-label, randomized, two parallel groups
CENTERS (n)	2
COUNTRY	Germany
PATIENTS (n)	*included* 75
	evaluated 75

INCLUSION CRITERIA

Patients with chronic non rheumatic atrial fibrillation with or without previous cerebral or peripheral embolism in whom oral anticoagulants were contraindicated

STUDY DRUG	**Nadroparin**	sc daily dose: 7500 AXa ICU o.d. = 0.3ml
		treatment duration: 4 to 6 months
REFERENCE DRUG	**None**	

ASSESSMENTS

❑ Clinical signs of thromboembolic events during a 6-month follow-up.
❑ Laboratory analyses.
❑ Death.

HARENBERG J. et al. 1993

	Nadroparin 0.3ml x 1		Control		p
Patients	35		40		
With previous thromboembolic events (TE)	15	42.8%	7	17.5%	0.03
Total TE (during 6 months)	3	8.6%	8	20.0%	chi²*
Fatal PE	1	2.8%	5	12.5%	p =
New TE in patients with previous TE	1	6.6%	3	43.0%	0.0001
Total death	6	17.1%	11	27.5%	

* Global test performed by the reviewer; on the contrary, considering each item, no significant difference was observed.

COMMENTS

❑ Interesting study for the use of a LMWH in long-term treatment in patients with chronic non rheumatic atrial fibrillation with contraindications to oral anticoagulants. Despite the small number of patients, a prophylaxis with a LMWH may be regarded as an effective and safe alternative therapeutic regimen (drug-related side effect did not occur during the 6-month treatment period).

Low-molecular-weight heparin during instability in coronary artery disease

AUTHORS	FRISC Study
REF	Lancet. 1996; 347: 561-568

STUDY	Multicenter, double-blind, randomized, placebo-controlled parallel-groups
CENTERS *(n)*	23
COUNTRY	Sweden
PATIENTS *(n)*	*randomized* 1506
	evaluated 1493 (intention-to-treat)

INCLUSION CRITERIA
Chest pain within 72h with increased angina pectoris or angina at rest with a suspicion of MI and at least one of ECG change: ST segment depression and/or T-wave inversion without Q-waves

STUDY DRUG	Dalteparin	• acute phase: 120 AXa IU/kg b.i.d. (maximum 10000 IU b.i.d.) treatment duration: 5-8 days
		• prolonged treatment: 7500 AXa IU o.d. (0.3ml) treatment duration: 35-45 days

REFERENCE DRUG	Placebo (saline)	• acute phase: BW-adjusted volume not exceeding 1ml b.i.d. prolonged treatment: 0.3ml o.d.

ASA 300mg as starting dose, then 75mg/day
ß-blockers-calcium antagonists, organic nitrates at libidum for all patients

ASSESSMENTS
- ❏ Primary endpoint: death and MI at D6.
- ❏ Secondary endpoint: death, MI, revascularization procedures, need for heparin infusion, separate or composite endpoints at D6, D40 and D150.
- ❏ Major bleeding.

FRISC study. 1996

	Dalteparin 120 AXa IU/kg x 2 7500 AXa IU x 1		Placebo		p
Patients	738		755		
Death, MI					
D6 (primary endpoint)	13	1.8%	36	4.8%	0.001
D40	59	8.0%	81	10.7%	NS
D150	102	14.0%	116	15.5%	NS
Death, MI, revascularization					
D6	16	2.2%	43	5.7%	0.001
D40	133	18.0%	179	23.7%	0.005
D150	296	40.6%	326	43.6%	NS
Death, MI, revascularization or intravenous heparin					
D6	40	5.4%	78	10.3%	0.01
D40	151	20.5%	194	25.7%	0.01
D150	312	42.7%	337	45.1%	NS
Major bleeding during:					
acute treatment	6	0.8%	4	0.5%	NS
prolonged treatment	2	0.3%	2	0.3%	NS

COMMENTS

❑ Treatment with dalteparin 120 AXa IU/kg sc b.i.d. in addition to aspirin significantly reduced the rate of new cardiac events (death and MI) during the acute phase of treatment.

❑ This protection was maintained for at least 40 days i.e. during all the treatment period for the secondary endpoint (death, MI, need for revascularization procedure)

❑ The incidence of major bleeding was not significantly different from placebo during both the acute phase of treatment and extended treatment.

Comparison of low-molecular-weight heparin with unfractionated heparin acutely and with placebo for 6 weeks in the management of unstable coronary artery disease - Fragmin in unstable coronary artery disease study (FRIC)

AUTHORS	KLEIN W., BUCHWALD A. HILLIS S.E. et al.
REF	Circulation. 1997; 96: 61-68

STUDY	Multicenter, randomized, parallel groups
Two phases:	• open; acute phase
	• double-blind: prolonged treatment
CENTERS (n)	81
COUNTRIES	Austria, Canada, Germany, Italy, The Netherlands, Norway, Spain, United Kingdom, United States
PATIENTS (n)	*randomized* 1499
	evaluated 1482 (intention-to-treat)

INCLUSION CRITERIA

Clinical criteria for unstable coronary disease: chest pain within 72h
At least one of ECG abnormality:
ST depression and/or T-wave inversion without corresponding Q-wave

STUDY DRUG	**Dalteparin**	• acute phase D1 to D6: 120 AXa IU/kg b.i.d. • prolonged treatment D6 to D45: 7500 AXa IU o.d.
REFERENCE DRUG	**UFH**	• acute phase D1 to D6: iv bolus 5000 IU then, infusion 1000 IU/h adjusted to APTT values (x 1.5 control); the infusion could be stopped after 48h and replaced with sc 12,500 IU b.i.d. • prolonged treatment D6 to D45: saline 0.3ml

ASA 75 to 165mg/D started as soon as possible and continued throughout the study
antianginal medications according to standard practice for all patients

ASSESSMENTS

❑ Primary endpoint: death/MI/recurrent angina between D6 and D45.
❑ Secondary endpoint: death/MI/recurrent angina during the acute phase (D1 to D6) or revascularization procedures and ischemia during exercise testing during all periods
❑ Major/minor bleeding.

FRIC study. 1997

Acute phase D1 to D6	Dalteparin sc 120 AXa IU/kg x 2		UFH iv infusion or sc injections x 2		p
Patients	751		731		
Death/MI/recurrent angina	69	9.3%	55	7.6%	NS
Death/MI	29	3.9%	26	3.6%	NS
Revascularization	36	4.8%	39	5.3%	NS
Major bleeding	8	1.1%	7	1.0%	NS
Prolonged treatment D6 to D45	Dalteparin 7500 AXa IU x 1		Placebo 0.3ml x 1		p
Patients	562		561		
Death/MI/recurrent angina *	69	12.3%	69	12.3%	NS
Death/MI	24	4.3%	26	4.7%	NS
MI	17	3.1%	20	3.6%	NS
Recurrent angina	60	10.8%	57	10.3%	NS
Revascularization	76	14.3%	76	14.2%	NS
Major bleeding	3	0.5%	2	0.4%	NS
Minor bleeding	28	5.1%	15	2.8%	NS

* Primary endpoint.

COMMENTS
- ❑ No difference between dalteparin subcutaneous BW-adjusted dose and UFH (infusion) during the acute phase.
- ❑ Prolonged treatment with dalteparin at a lower once daily dose did not confer any additional benefit over aspirin alone.
- ❑ Considering the results of FRISC and FRIC studies for patients treated with dalteparin, relevant variations were observed in the incidence of events (death/MI/recurrent angina or death/MI) higher at D6 and lower at D45 in FRIC compared with FRISC.

A comparison of low-molecular-weight heparin with unfractionated heparin for unstable coronary artery disease

AUTHORS	COHEN M., DEMERS C., GURFINKEL E.P. et al. for the ESSENCE Group
REF	N. Engl. J. Med. 1997; 337: 447-452

STUDY	Multicenter, prospective, randomized, double-blind
CENTERS (n)	176
COUNTRIES	10 (North and South America, Europe)
PATIENTS (n)	*randomized* 3171

INCLUSION CRITERIA

Patients with rest angina or non-Q-wave myocardial infarction within 24h of the last episode of angina (without ST elevation) 70% within 12h.
One-third female patients, 46% of patients had prior MI

STUDY DRUG	**Enoxaparin**	sc daily doses: 1mg/kg b.i.d. treatment duration: 48h up to 8 days median duration: 2.6 days
REFERENCE DRUG	**UFH**	iv bolus 5000 IU then continuous iv infusion APTT-adjusted (x 2 control values) treatment duration: 48h up to 8 days median duration: 2.6 days

ASA and standard therapy for all patients

ASSESSMENTS

- ❏ Primary outcome: composite triple endpoint of death, heart attack (MI), recurrent angina at D14.
- ❏ Secondary endpoint: triple endpoint at D2 and D30 and double endpoint (death or MI) at D2, D14 and D30.
- ❏ Major/minor hemorrhage.

Essence group. 1997

	Enoxaparin 1mg/kg x 2		UFH iv infusion		Risk reduction	p
Patients	1607		1564			
Death+MI+recurrent angina (triple composite endpoint)						
D2 (48h)	99	6.2%	115	7.4%	16.2%	NS
D14*	266	16.6%	309	19.8%	16.2%	0.02
D30	318	19.8%	364	23.3%	15.0%	0.02
Death D2	8	0.5%	7	0.4%		NS
D14	36	2.2%	36	2.3%		NS
D30	47	2.9%	57	3.6%		NS
MI D2	11	0.7%	14	0.9%		NS
D14	51	3.2%	70	4.5%		NS
D30	62	3.9%	81	5.2%		NS
Recurrent angina D2	83	5.2%	99	6.3%		NS
D14	207	12.9%	243	15.5%		0.03
D30	252	15.7%	281	18.0%		NS
Need for revascularization (D30)		27.0%		32.2%		0.001
Major bleeding (D30)	102	6.5%	107	7.0%		NS

* Primary endpoint.

COMMENTS

❏ The primary combined triple endpoint (death, MI, recurrent angina) was significantly reduced at D14 with enoxaparin 1mg/kg b.i.d. administered for a short period (2.6 days). This protection was maintained up to D30.

❏ Half of the UFH patients were inadequately treated since the first day of treatment.

Dose-ranging trial of enoxaparin for unstable angina: results of TIMI 11 A

AUTHORS	TIMI 11 A. Trial investigators
REF	J.A.C.C. 1997; 29 : 1474-1482

STUDY	Open-label, dose-ranging
CENTERS (n)	45
COUNTRY	United States
PATIENTS (n)	included 630
	evaluated 630

INCLUSION CRITERIA

Patients with evidence of ischemic heart disease and unstable angina/non-Q-wave myocardial infarction

OBJECTIVE

To evaluate the safety of two dosages of enoxaparin administered in-hospital and to outpatients during 14 days

STUDY DRUG   **Enoxaparin**

- In-hospital phase: sc daily doses: iv bolus 30 mg followed by: 1.25 mg/kg b.i.d. or 1.0 mg/kg b.i.d. for at least 48h then,
- Outpatient phase: sc fixed b.i.d. doses 60 mg for BW $\geq$ 65 kg 40 mg for BW < 65 kg

total duration treatment: 14 days

ASA 325 mg at enrollment and 100 to 300 mg thereafter

ASSESSMENTS

- ❏ Major hemorrhage occurring within two weeks.
- ❏ Total death/myocardial infarction/recurrent ischemia requiring revascularization at D14.
- ❏ AXa activity.

TIMI 11 A. 1997

In-hospital dose	Enoxaparin				p
	1.25 mg/kg x 2		1.0 mg/kg x 2		
Patients	321		309		
Total major hemorrhage	21	6.5%	6	1.9%	0.004
in hospital	18		4		
at instrumented site	17	5.3%	5	1.6%	0.01
in outpatients	3		2		
Fourteen-day clinical outcomes					
death	7	2.2%	2	0.6%	NS
MI	7	2.2%	9	2.9%	NS
revascularization	4	1.2%	5	1.6%	NS
total events	18	5.6%	16	5.2%	NS
AXa activity IU/ml at peak (range)					
for BW-adjusted dose	1.6 (1.1-1.8)		1.1 (1.0-1.2)		< 0.05
in patients with major hemorrhage	1.8 (1.6-2.1)		1.2 (1.2-1.9)		

COMMENTS

❏ This pilot study suggested that the lower initial BW-adjusted dose (1mg/kg) is safer than the higher dose.

❏ In both dose regimens, patients undergoing a procedure had a significantly higher rate of major hemorrhage.

❏ Patients with major hemorrhage had a higher AXa plasma activity than patients without hemorrhage mainly in the higher dose regimen.

❏ The clinical outcome events at 14 days were similar in the two dosage regimens.

❏ A large trial TIMI 11 B including 200 centers with 4000 patients has been carried out. After an initial iv bolus, the dosage of enoxaparin is 1mg/kg b.i.d. during the in-hospital acute phase of treatment, followed by a fixed dose of 40mg b.i.d. for BW < 65kg and 60mg b.i.d. for BW ≥ 65kg during 35 days (see first results on the following pages).

The TIMI 11B trial:
low-molecular-weight heparin as a new antithrombotic
strategy for unstable angina

AUTHORS	ANTMAN E.M. for the TIMI 11B trial
REF	XXth European Congress of Cardiology, Vienna 1998 (oral presentation)

STUDY	Multicenter, randomized, double-blind
CENTERS (n)	200
COUNTRIES	United States, Canada, South America, Europe
PATIENTS (n)	randomized 4021
	analysed 3910

INCLUSION CRITERIA
Patients with unstable angina or non-Q-wave (NQW) MI within 24 hours with documented history or with ECG modifications.
58% of patients with unstable angina (UA)
35% with NQW MI
4% with QW AMI

OBJECTIVE
To test the hypothesis that treatment with enoxaparin during both the acute and chronic phases of UA is superior to UFH during the acute phase only

STUDY DRUG	Enoxaparin	*acute phase:*	initial iv bolus 30mg then,
			sc dose 1mg/kg o.d. D1 up to D8
		mean treatment duration: 4.6 days	
		chronic phase: up to D43	60mg b.i.d. for BW ≥ 65kg
			40mg b.i.d. for BW < 65kg

REFERENCE DRUG	UFH	*acute phase:*	iv regimen : bolus 70 U/kg
		infusion 15 U/kg/h APTT-adjusted	
		(x 1.5-2.5) during ≥ 72h	
	Placebo	*chronic phase:* saline sc route b.i.d. up to D43	
ASA for all patients			

ASSESSMENTS
- ❏ Primary endpoint: combined death, MI, severe recurrent ischemia requiring urgent revascularization at D43.
- ❏ Safety: major bleeding or serious adverse events.

TIMI 11B. 1998 (oral presentation)

	Enoxaparin	UFH	Relative risk reduction	p
Acute phase (D1 up to D8)	iv bolus 30mg 1mg/kg x 2	iv infusion		
Patients	1953	1957		
D14　Death	2.2%	2.8%		
MI	4.2%	5.3%		
Revasc.	9.6%	11.1%		
Triple combined endpoint	14.2%	16.6%	15%	0.03
Death + MI	5.7%	6.8%		
Chronic phase (D43)	**Enoxaparin** 40-60mg x 2	**Placebo** sc saline x 2		
Patients	1179	1185		
D43: triple combined endpoint (primary endpoint)	17.3%	19.6%	12%	0.049
Major hemorrhage				
up to 72h	0.8%	0.7%		
at hospital	1.1%	1.0%		NS
in outpatients	1.5%	2.9%		0.02

COMMENTS
- ❑ In acute phase, the efficacy of enoxaparin - based on a triple endpoint, death, MI, urgent revascularization - was superior to UFH.
- ❑ Only 60% of the patients were included in the chronic phase.
- ❑ The prolonged treatment did not add clinical benefit but increased bleeding risk.
  (Please note that these results may be slightly different in the final publication).

Low molecular weight heparin versus regular heparin or aspirin in the treatment of unstable angina and silent ischemia

AUTHORS	GURFINKEL E., EUSTAQUIO J., MEJAIL R. et al.
REF	J. Am. Coll. Cardiol. 1995; 26: 313-318

STUDY	Randomized, single-blind comparing 3 treatments
CENTERS (n)	1
COUNTRY	Argentina
PATIENTS (n)	randomized 219 evaluated 211

INCLUSION CRITERIA

Resting chest pain within 24h, confirmed underlying ischemic heart disease

EXCLUSION CRITERIA

Acute Q or non-Q-wave myocardial infarction angioplasty within 3 months

STUDY DRUG	• **Nadroparin** + **Aspirin**	≈ 80 IU/kg twice daily by sc route 200mg/day orally treatment duration 5-7 days (hospital stay)
REFERENCE DRUGS	• **UFH** + **Aspirin**	iv bolus 5000 IU then continuous infusion 400 IU/kg/day (APTT-adapted x 2 fold control values) 200mg/day orally
	• **Aspirin** + **Saline iv, infusion**	200mg/day orally treatment duration 5-7 days (hospital stay)

+ *Standard antianginal therapy*

ASSESSMENTS

❑ Recurrent angina, AMI, urgent intervention, major bleeding, death during hospital stay.
❑ Silent ischemia, minor bleeding.

GURFINKEL E. et al. 1995

	Group I **Nadro** 80 IU/kg x 2 + **ASA**		Group II **UFH** iv infusion + **ASA**		Group III **Saline** infusion + **ASA**	
Patients	68		70		73	
In-hospital events						
Recurrent angina	14	21.0%●	31	44.0%■	27	37.0%●■
AMI	0		4	6.0%	7	9.5%●
Urgent reinterventions	1	1.5%●	7	10.0%	9	12.0%●■
Major bleeding	0	—	2	3.0%	0	—
Death	0		0		0	
Total events	15	22.0%●	44	63.0%■	43	59.0%●■

● p < 0.05 between groups I and III.
■ p < 0.05 between groups I and II.

COMMENTS
- ❏ First published study which compared the efficacy of a LMWH to UFH in the acute phase of unstable angina.
- ❏ Despite the small number of patients, the incidence of in-hospital total events clearly indicated that treatment with a high subcutaneous dose of nadroparin plus aspirin resulted in a significantly better outcome than either iv heparin plus ASA or ASA alone.

Unstable angina and heparin therapy:
comparative study between a low molecular weight heparin (Fraxiparine®)
and unfractionated heparin

AUTHORS	LEIZOROVICZ A. for the FRAXIS investigators
REF	XXth European Congress of Cardiology, Vienna, 1998, (oral presentation)

STUDY	Multicenter, double-blind, 3 parallel groups		
CENTERS (n)	179		
COUNTRIES	17 (Europe, Argentina)		
PATIENTS (n)	*randomized*	3468	
	analyzed	3449	

INCLUSION CRITERIA
Patients with unstable angina or non-Q-wave MI with chest pain at rest (5-30min duration) within 48h or aggraved effort angina ECG modifications: ST depression, T W inversion, ST elevation not requiring thrombolysis.
UA: 76% of patients, NQW MI: 16%, MI: 2.7%

OBJECTIVE
To compare the efficacy of standard heparin

STUDY DRUG	**Nadroparin**	D1: initial iv bolus ≈ 85 AXa IU/kg then 85 AXa IU/kg b.i.d. sc injection for Gr 1: from D2 up to D6 (5.2±2) for Gr 2: from D2 up to D14 (12±4)
REFERENCE DRUG	**UFH**	initial iv bolus 5000 IU followed by iv infusion 1250 IU/h APTT-adjusted (x 1.5-2)

Antiplatelet agents: ASA or ticlopidine for all patients

ASSESSMENTS
- ❑ Primary endpoint: combined death, MI, refractory or recurrent angina at D14 for all groups.
- ❑ Secondary endpoint: above combined endpoint for both nadroparin treated groups at D6 and 3-month vs UFH group and comparison of nadroparin treated-6 days vs nadroparin treated-14 days at D14 and 3-month.
- ❑ Incidence of serious events: major hemorrhage.

FRAXIS, 1998 (oral presentation)

	Nadroparin iv bolus, 85 AXa IU/kg x 2		UFH iv bolus + infusion	p
	6 days	14 days		
Patients	1158	1141	1140	
Death, MI, refractory/recurrent angina at:				
• D6 (secondary endpoint)	13.8%	15.8%	14.9%	NS
• D14 (primary endpoint)	17.8%	20.0%	18.1%	NS
• 3 months (secondary endpoint)	22.3%	26.2%	22.2%	NS
death + MI	8.6%	8.9%	7.9%	NS
death	4.2%	4.4%	3.6%	NS
CABG, PTCA	28.6%	30.0%	29.4%	NS
Major hemorrhage				
6 days	0.7%	1.3%	1.1%	
14 days	1.5%	3.5%	1.6%	
3 months	1.9%	4.0%	2.4%	

COMMENTS

❑ Similar effect on the combined endpoint death MI, refractory/recurrent angina at D6 for nadroparin treated-6D and UFH.

❑ Prolonging LMWH treatment up to 2 weeks did not add clinical benefit and increased the risk of bleeding.

(Please note that these data may slightly differ in the final publication).

Benefit of adding low molecular weight heparin to conventional treatment of stable angina pectoris
A double-blind, randomized, placebo-controlled trial

AUTHORS	MELANDRI G., SEMPRINI F., CERVI V. et al.
REF	Circulation. 1993; 88: 2517-2523

STUDY	Double-blind, randomized, placebo-controlled
CENTERS (n)	1
COUNTRY	Italy
PATIENTS (n)	*included* 29
	evaluated 29

INCLUSION CRITERIA

Patients with stable exercise induced angina and angiographically proven coronary artery disease

STUDY DRUG	**Parnaparin**	sc daily dose: 15,000 AXa U o.d. (corresponding to 6400 AXa IU) treatment duration: 3 months
REFERENCE DRUG	**Placebo**	saline sc injection

+ Beta and calcium blockers associated with nitrates and ASA (325mg) for all patients

---

ASSESSMENTS

❏ Treadmill exercise tests at entry and after 3 months.

❏ ECG before and during exercise performed 4h after last treatment; evaluation of ST depression by blind evaluation.

❏ Biochemistry analyses.

MELANDRI G. et al. 1993

		Parnaparin 15,000 AXa U x 1	Placebo saline injection
Patients		15	14
Mean values ± SD of :			
AXa levels U/ml (4h after inj.)	1st month	0.37±0.24	—
	3 months	0.42±0.23*	—
APTT(s) 4h after injection	baseline	24±4	22±2
	at 3 months	36±9*	24±4
Fibrinogen (mg/DL)	at entry	387±90	346±60
	at 3 months	333±6	345±56
Fibrinopeptide A (ngml)	at entry	5±6	7±8
	at 3 months	3±4	3±2
Bleeding time (s)	at entry	400±164	425±151
	at 3 months	484±172	413±139
Time to 1 mm ST depression (s)	at entry	285±126	271±133
	at 3 months	346±168*	304±117
Time to peak exercise (s)	at entry	409±130	356±144
	at 3 months	441±142*	396±139
Peak ST depression (mm)	at entry	2.3±0.5	2.1±0.9
	at 3 months	1.9±0.6*	2.1±0.8

* $p < 0.01$ between baseline and the following data.

COMMENTS

❏ Interesting study for the hemostatic variables monthly followed during 3 months.

❏ Prolonged parnaparin treatment significantly reduced fibrinogen levels but did not increase bleeding time.

❏ Patients assigned to parnaparin showed an improvement in both the time to 1-mm ST depression and the peak ST segment depression.

❏ A LMWH sc administered during a 3-month period may be useful in addition to ASA and conventional antianginal therapy to treat stable angina.

Expert comments

ROBERT GABOR KISS, GYÖRGY BLASKO. *Low molecular weight heparins in acute coronary syndromes*

Acute Coronary Syndromes (ACS) are one of the most significant morbidity factors of the industrialized world. Regarding our current understanding of the development of ACS, a uniform process, the completely/incompletely occlusive coronary thrombus growing on the underlying plaque rupture plays a pivotal role. The degree of occlusion, and therefore the appearance of the actual clinical syndrome depends exclusively on the lability of the thrombus formed, instead on the stenosis of the underlying atherosclerotic plaque (which was mostly non-significant before the plaque rupture). A brief occlusion, similar to the "Folts cyclic flow reduction" results in unstable angina pectoris (UAP), a definite occlusive clot leads to Q-type acute myocardial infarction (AMI) in the clinical scenario. A complete, but transient occlusion (20-120 min) regards the non-Q AMI. Revealing the pathogenesis of ACS, strategies containing antiplatelet/antithrombotic drugs are the ultimate way to treat these sicknesses as an exclusive medical treatment, or in a combination of practices opening and/or dilating the related artery (thrombolysis, angioplasty) reconstructing the original blood flow, which is one of the most important factors to keep the platelet shear force low.

Antiplatelet drugs (aspirin, thienopyridines, GP IIb/IIIa receptor blocking agents) are probably the most effective agents to reduce clinical events in ACS in a combination of different antithrombins (unfractionated heparin (UFH) low molecular weight heparins (LMWH) and hirudin derivatives). Hirudin and its derivatives have been very attractive in a theoretical or experimental setting; clinical studies are less promising and/or are ongoing with these agents.

LMWHs can be more widely used, replacing the conventional UFH therapy in ACS, because of their specific advantages: better bioavailability, with a better dose-response; longer half-life, which allows b.i.d. subcutaneous bolus treatment; less risk of thrombocytopenia; more sustained release of tissue-factor pathway inhibitor.

AMI (Q-type). Indication: infarct-related vessel patency

As an adjunctive treatment of thrombolytics, heparin (UFH) is obligatory during and after t-PA administration, furthermore, heparinization is widely used after streptokinase treatment, however, the usage of IV UFH after streptokinase is debated and controversies of insignificant results coming mainly from the GUSTO I. trial make this indication questionable. IV infusion of a short-acting antithrombotic compound, UFH, with the possibility of prompt and complete neutralization with protamine in such a critical clinical situation, like the first 1-2 days of AMI treated with fibrinolytics or angioplasty is still widely used. At present, clear advantages of LMWHs, like easy, subcutaneous administration, lack of blood sampling for dose-adjustment, less risk for heparin-associated thrombocytopenia (HAT) still do not make LMWHs the drug of choice in the setting of peri and early postprocedural anticoagulation in thrombolysis or in primary balloon angioplasty, when IV lines are used, frequent blood-sampling is not available for other laboratory measurements, and the duration of heparin treatment is less than the usually observed 5-10 days to induce HAT. However, results of the REDUCE and ENTICES trials open a perspective to use LMWH as a periprocedural heparin of coronary angioplasty and stent placement, with a better antithrombotic profile. Small, but promising trials with LMWHs after thrombolysis in AMI are already published. The FATIMA study used nadroparin as an adjunctive drug for thrombolysis with tissue-type plasminogen activator and revealed an 82% infarct-related artery patency (TIMI-flow 2+3). Significantly less total cardiac event was observed in an interesting study with enoxaparin given up to 30 days after thrombolysis with streptokinase. Large-scale study to evaluate the superiority of LMWHs on UFH treatment concerning the infarct vessel patency is not published yet.

AMI. Indication: intracardiac thrombus prevention

Concerns in AMI, like mural thrombus and/or systemic embolization, atrial fibrillation, large anterior AMI with poor left ventricular function are indications of anticoagulant treatment. In the FRAMI study, a high dose (150 IU/kg b.i.d.) of a LMWH, dalteparin was used, resulting slightly less mural thrombosis, but a higher bleeding risk in patients treated with streptokinase. Studies, like FRATIV, showed that LMWHs in their therapeutic dose are equally useful and safe to prevent intracardiac clot formation in these settings, and the ease and safety of LMWHs can provide a better and comfortable way of embolus prevention before switching to warfarin.

Unstable angina and non-Q AMI. Indication: prevention of definite coronary occlusion

In UAP and non-Q AMI the thrombotic coronary occlusion is incomplete and/or transient. In avoiding the development of the definite occlusion of the artery with plaque rupture, aspirin and UFH alone were effective to prevent coronary events. The combination of these traditional drugs showed a synergistic effect regarding the event-free survival (Theroux). Considering the 30 days event-free survival, 8% of the UAP and non-Q AMI patients still developed recidive AMI or died despite combined aspirin and UFH treatment (GUSTO II).

A wide variety of different antiplatelet and antithrombotic compounds are currently under clinical investigation or already declared beneficial. RGD-mimicking small molecules as platelet GP IIb/IIIa receptor antagonists resulted a modest, but significant effect; a monoclonal antibody abciximab against this receptor was strikingly positive, but at present, it was tried mostly under intracoronary interventions only. Hirudin or hirudin derivatives showed a borderline effect in GUSTO IIb compared to UFH, studies as OASIS-2, HERO-2 are still ongoing. Thrombolytics are not the drug of choice in these clinical situations (TIMI 3b).

Low molecular weight heparins are already studied and declared positive in UAP and non-Q AMI. First, Gurfinkel published the results of a small study, where nadroparin was given to patients with UAP. During the first week, nadroparin-treated patients showed significantly less cardiac events than controls. This study has limitations, the case number investigated is seemingly lower than is usually sufficient to study such a clinical problem as UAP, where the event rate is less than 10%. The other possible limitation of this study is that results regarding events in the first week only are certainly not enough to tell anything relevant concerning the late or even intermediate oucome, because as we learned from other LMWH and UFH studies in UAP, events became more frequent after cessation of the study drug, yielding a "thrombotic rebound phenomenon".

Two large-scale and well-conducted studies with dalteparin are already published. Results of the FRISC study repeated the information coming from Theroux in 1988, that parenteral antithrombotic treatment with a heparin in UAP and non-Q AMI is clearly beneficial compared to placebo. Two subcutaneous injections daily of a full, therapeutic dose of a LMWH, dalteparin, could significantly prevent cardiac events. However, switching to a smaller, preventive dose given up to 40 days could not prevent the diminishment of the benefit of the early phase dalteparin administration, which was pertinent at 6 days, borderline at 30 days and completely eroded at 6 months.

Regarding the other dalteparin study, the FRIC study used UFH in the control arm.

The FRIC study clearly proved that a LMWH given in a full dose b.i.d. subcutaneously could provide the same benefit as the IV UFH infusion in patients with UAP or non-Q AMI. Kaplan-Meier curves of the LMWH and UFH treated patients revealed equipotent chances of these treatments in any time-points.

The ESSENCE trial compared the clinical effect of enoxaparin to UFH in UAP and non-Q AMI. Less composite cardiac events were observed in the enoxaparin group at day 14 and 30. The bleeding risk was similar. Quality control problems concerning the poorly achieved therapeutic APTT-levels in the UFH-arm could diminish the positive results.

Other large-scale LMWH studies, such as the TIMI IIb and the FRAXIS, are currently ongoing.

In UAP and non-Q AMI, LMWHs became a useful therapeutic alternative of UFH. LMWHs are at least as effective as UFH in these diseases, and patients treated with LMWH can enjoy the relative comfort of a b.i.d. subcutaneous injection, instead of hanging on an iv line, having less venipunctures for blood samples, and furthermore facing a lower risk of HAT.

ALEXANDER G. TURPIE. *Considerations on LMWHs in acute coronary ischemic syndromes*

The acute coronary ischemic syndromes including unstable angina, non-Q-wave myocardial infarction and transmural myo-cardial infarction are the most common causes of morbidity and mortality in the Western world. Partial or complete coronary artery occlusion is responsible for most clinical manifestations of acute coronary ischemia. Antithrombotic therapy with or without revascularization has been extensively studied in patients with acute coronary ischemic syndromes. The role of aspirin in reducing both fatal and non-fatal myocardial infarction in the early stages of unstable angina is well estab-lished and the long-term risk of death or myocardial infarction in patients with acute coronary syndromes is reduced by ap-proximately 50% with regular aspirin use. In acute transmural myocardial infarction, aspirin alone reduces mortality by 25%.

Anticoagulants such as heparin play a key role in inhibiting the generation of thrombin, the enzyme which is central for the formation of fibrin. In a series of trials in patients with unstable angina and non-Q-wave myocardial infarction, standard heparin has been shown to decrease the frequency of myocardial infarction and to reduce overall mortality particularly when used in combination with aspirin. Heparin is also used to maintain coronary patency in patients who receive tissue plasminogen activator for thrombolysis. However, standard heparin has a number of limitations. In particular, its anticoagulant effect is unpredictable and after subcutaneous injection, it has poor bioavailability. Low molecular weight heparins (LMWH), offer a number of pharmacological and pharmacokinetic advantages over standard heparin with a predictable anticoagulant response, high bioavailability and long plasma half-life. Importantly, with LMWHs, a therapeutic anticoagulant effect can be achieved by once or twice daily subcutaneous injections at fixed, weight-adjusted doses.

The studies of low molecular weight heparin in acute unstable angina, non-Q-wave myocardial infarction and acute transmural myocardial infarction are summarized in this section.

Low molecular weight heparins (nadroparin, dalteparin and enoxaparin) have been evaluated in clinical trials in acute coronary syndromes, the most important of which have been in patients with unstable angina and non-Q-wave myocardial infarction. The results of these studies indicate that low molecular weight heparins are effective in reducing major ischemic outcomes in such patients and have established their role in the treatment of unstable angina.

In a small open trial, nadroparin reduced the risk of ischemic outcomes compared with aspirin alone or a combination of aspirin and standard heparin. Dalteparin has been evaluated in two large clinical trials in the management of unstable angina. The Low-Molecular Weight Heparin (Fragmin) During Instability in Coronary Artery Disease (FRISC) trial showed that dalteparin resulted in a 63% reduction in risk of death or acute MI compared with aspirin alone. The Fragmin in Unstable Coronary Artery Disease (FRIC) trial showed that dalteparin was as effective as intravenous heparin. Enoxaparin resulted in a statistically significant 16% reduction in the combined outcome of death, MI and recurrence of angina in comparison with standard heparin in the Efficacy and Safety of Subcutaneous Enoxaparinin non-Q-wave Coronary Events (ESSENCE) trial. Recent data reported at the American College of Cardiology in March 1998 show that the benefit seen with enoxaparin is maintained at one year.

The results of the FRAXIS trial using nadroparin in unstable angina were presented in the summer of 1998 and showed that nadroparin was as effective as iv UFH with a 6-day treatment. A prolonged treatment of up to 2 weeks did not improve clinical benefit. There is accumulating evidence that LMWHs are safe and effective alternatives to standard heparin in coronary artery disease and that they offer practical and therapeutic advantages.

LARS WALLENTIN. *Low molecular weight heparins in acute coronary syndromes*

Background

The success in exchanging standard heparin for low molecular weight heparin (LMWH) in deep vein thrombosis (DVT) had been ongoing for many years before a corresponding interest was awakened in cardiac diseases. Although standard heparin had been used for many years for the prevention of recurrences of ischemia, reocclusion and reinfarction in acute myocardial infarction and unstable angina, very few seemed to realize the potential benefits of LMWH for these indications. The concept of platelet and thrombin activity as the major underlying mechanisms for thrombotic coronary occlusion might have hampered the interest in FXa inhibition in acute coronary syndromes. Thus, the first studies concerning LMWH in cardiac disease concerned the prevention of thrombi formed during slow flow conditions; e.g. left ventricular mural thrombi after myocardial infarction and thromboembolism in association with atrial fibrillation.

Advantages of LMWH in acute coronary syndromes

The best evidence for a preventive effect of heparin infusions was the reduction of myocardial infarction and ischemic episodes during 5-7 days treatment in unstable coronary syndromes reported in the end of the 1980s (1,2). However, such a long-term regimen has seldom been used in clinical practice and was not even recommended in the current treatment guidelines (3) because of inconvenience and prolongation of bed rest and hospital stay. The disadvantages of standard heparin have been well known for many years; i.e. the limited subcutaneous bioavailability and the short half-life necessitating iv infusions, the avid binding to plasma proteins, the neutralization by platelet factor 4, the variable anticoagulant response for given dose and the narrow safety window (APTT 50-70 seconds) necessitating frequent laboratory monitoring and dose adjustments, the lack of a dose-response effect concerning efficacy, the early rebound after termination of treatment and the risk of thrombocytopenia. In comparison, the following advantages of LMWHs should favor their exchange for standard heparin in most instances; i.e. complete subcutaneous bioavailability, longer half-life allowing sc treatment, less binding to plasma proteins, no neutralization by platelet factor 4, predictible effect when given in fixed dosages, no need for laboratory monitoring and dose adjustments, less rebound after termination of treatment and a very low risk of thrombocytopenia (4). The sc twice daily standard doses can therefore be used in a wider range of patients for longer period of time and even on an outpatient basis.

Dosing of LMWH in acute coronary syndromes

There are only a few dose-finding studies concerning LMWHs in coronary artery diseases. The aim of these has been to reach the highest tolerable dose in order to maintain a 24-hour anti-Xa level comparable to heparin infusion. In 1991, Nesvold et al. found that dalteparin 150 IU/kg body-weight b.i.d. gave peak anti-Xa levels 0.7-1.8 and 120 IU/kg body-weight b.i.d. 0.3-0.8 IU/ml (5). Correspondingly, in 1996 Strandberg et al. reported that dalteparin 100 IU/kg body-weight b.i.d. gave peak level 0.6-1.0 IU/ml and through level 0.3-0.8 IU/ml (6). De Winter (FATIMA 1997) reported that nadroparin around 125 IU/ml b.i.d. gave anti-Xa levels 0.4-0.7 IU/ml. In the largest dose-finding effort the TIMI 11A trialists (1997) reported that enoxaparin 1.25 mg/kg b.i.d. gave peak anti-Xa levels 1.1-1.8 IU/ml and 1.1-1.2 IU/ml with 1.0 mg/kg b.i.d. In this study, patients with the higher dose of enoxaparin 1.25 mg/kg b.i.d. versus the lower 1.0 mg/kg dose in addition to aspirin had an elevated rate of major hemorrhage, 6.5% versus 1.9%. Correspondingly, in the FRAMI (1997) study using dalteparin 150 IU/ml in addition to aspirin starting 8 hours after streptokinase there was a 2.9% of major bleeding versus 0.3% in aspirin only. However, using dalteparin 120 IU/kg b.i.d. in addition to aspirin as in the FRISC (1996) and FRIC (1997) trials, the occurrence of major bleeding was low (0.5-0.8%) and no different than aspirin or aspirin plus heparin respectively.

Based on these studies, it can be suggested that the highest acceptable dose of LMWH in aspirin treated patients with unstable angina or after acute myocardial infarction, is dalteparin 120 IU/kg body-weight b.i.d. or enoxaparin 100mg/kg b.i.d. obtaining peak anti-Xa levels around 0.5-1.1 IU/ml and through levels 0.3-0.8 IU/ml. These anti-Xa levels has also led to substantial reductions in coagulation activity as demonstrated in the FRISC study (7). For long-term outpatient use the doses generally have been kept somewhat lower. There have also been attempts to use once daily dosing in acute coronary syndromes but both the clinical effects (8), the anti-Xa through levels (FRISC 1998, in press) and the reduction of coagulation activity (7) have so far been disappointing. Thus, for treatment and prevention of acute coronary syndromes with LMWHs, a b.i.d. regimen seems preferable.

LMWH in unstable coronary artery syndromes

After a first promising small pilot study of nadroparin in unstable angina (Gurfinkel A. 1995) three larger scale trials have been reported - the FRISC trial in 1996, the FRIC and ESSENCE trials in 1997. The FRISC trial showed a more than 50% reduction in the double end-point of death or myocardial infarction and the triple end-point death, myocardial infarction or revascularization after 5-7 day treatment with dalteparin b.i.d. and aspirin in comparison to aspirin only in patients with unstable angina or non-Q-wave myocardial infarction. Neither the FRIC nor the ESSENCE trials showed any significant difference in any of these end-points during the acute phase comparing respectively enoxaparin or dalteparin to an i.v. infusion of standard heparin for 2-6 days.

Concerning long-term outcome, there was a maintained reduction of the initial benefit in the triple end-point during prolonged treatment with dalteparin 7500 IU/ml o.d. for 5 weeks in the FRISC study while no corresponding benefit of this regimen could be observed in the FRIC study. However, the FRISC study also reported a substantial increase in the initial benefit and a significant reduction in both the double and triple end-points in the high risk sub-group identified by an elevation of troponin-T at inclusion (9). On the other hand, the ESSENCE trial demonstrated a significant reduction in the triple and a positive trend concerning the double end-point after 14 days and remaining until one year without any further treatment than exchanging the i.v. heparin infusion for enoxaparin during the initial 2-3 days in the acute phase.

Because of the differences in long-term outcome between the FRIC and ESSENCE trials, there is an ongoing dicussion whether this discrepancy is related to differences between the compounds or to the design and power of the two trials. At present, it can be concluded that either of these LMWHs used in appropriate dosages twice daily is at least as effective as standard heparin infusions in unstable coronary syndromes.

LMWH in acute myocardial infarction

LMWH has been evaluated in myocardial infarction mainly as a prophylactic against left ventricular mural thrombi. In the FRAMI study (1997), there was a 35% reduction of mural thrombi as shown by echocardiograms. However, there was no difference in the rate of ischemic stroke which was very low in both the dalteparin and the placebo groups, 1.0 and 1.3% respectively. On the other hand, there was an increased risk of major bleeding, including cerebral hemorrhages, 2.9 and 0.3% in the dalteparin and placebo groups respectively. Therefore, the overall clinical outcome does not encourage the use of an aggressive anticoagulant treatment for this indication.

At present, there is a renewed interest for evaluation of LMWHs as adjuvants during and after thrombolysis of acute myocardial infarction in order to augment immediate reperfusion and avoid early reocclusion. There are encouraging results in both areas in a few small pilot studies (10, 11, 12) and larger trials will start during the next year.

Present implications regarding the use of LMWH in acute coronary syndromes

Today, sc LMWH b.i.d. is better documented than i.v. infusions of standard heparin for the prevention of myocardial infarction, recurrence of symptoms and need for urgent revascularization in unstable coronary syndromes i.e. unstable angina or non-ST-elevation myocardial infarction. The use of LMWH instead of i.v. heparin in unstable coronary artery syndromes is considerably more convenient for both the patient and the care providers in hospital. This treatment can also be continued on an outpatient basis. Therefore, this regimen can be recommended for all chest pain patients with a suspicion of an unstable coronary syndrome and signs of ischemia as evidenced by ST-depression or elevation of CKMB or troponin-T provided there are no contraindications. The duration of treatment should probably be related to the estimated risk of future events.

This risk can be evaluated by easily available risk indicators such as increasing age, previous and present manifestations of the coronary artery disease, signs of ischemia at rest (recurring symptoms, dynamic ST-changes during ECG monitoring, elevation of CKMB or troponin-T) or, in stabilized patients, at a pre-discharge stress test; In patients with a low risk, the LMWH treatment can probably be restricted to 3-4 days. However, in higher risk patients, the treatment should be prolonged at least until a coronary angiogram and, if appropriate, revascularization has been performed. Whether the patient will benefit from prolonged treatment with LMWH for several weeks or months will be revealed at the presentation of the results from the FRAXIS, TIMI 11B and FRISC II trials.

REFERENCES

(1) THEROUX P., OUIMET H., McCANS J. et al. Aspirin, heparin, or both to treat acute unstable angina. N. Engl. J. Med. 1988; 319 : 1105-1111

(2) The RISC Group. Risk of myocardial infarction and death during treatment with low dose aspirin and intravenous heparin in men with unstable coronary artery disease. Lancet 1990; 336 : 827-830

(3) Unstable angina: diagnosis and managment. Clinical practice guidelines. U.S. Department of Health and Human Services. AHCPR Publication N°94-0602, 1994

(4) WALLENTIN L. Low molecular weight heparin: a valuable tool in the treatment of acute coronary syndromes. Eur. Heart J. 1996; 17 : 1470-1476

(5) NESVOLD A. KONTNY F. ABILDGAARD U. DALE J. Safety of high doses of low molecular weight heparin (Fragmin) in acute myocardial infarction. A dose-finding study. Thromb. Res. 1991; 64 : 579-587.

(6) STRANDBERG L.E., KAHAN T., LUNDIN P., SVENSSON J., ERHARDT L. Anticoagulant effects of low molecular weight heparin following thrombolytic therapy in acute myocardial infarction; a dose-finding study. Haemostasis 1996; 26 : 247-257

(7) ERNOFSSON M., STREKERUD F., TOSS H., ABILDGAARD U., WALLENTIN L., SIEGBAHN A. Low molecular weight heparin reduces the generation and activity of thrombin in unstable coronary artery disease. Thromb. Haemostais 1998 Mar; 79 (3) : 491-494

(8) CHARBONNIER B. Fraxiparine and prevention of left ventricular thrombosis in non-thrombolyzed myocardial infarction. FRATIV STudy. Arch. Mal. Coeur Vass. 1997 Sep; 90 (9) : 1215-1221

(9) LINDAHL B., VENGE P., WALLENTIN L for the FRISC Study Group. Troponin T identifies patients with unstable coronary artery disease who benefit from long term antithrombotic protection. J. Am. coll. Cariol. 1997; 29 : 43-48

(10) GLICK A., KORNOWSKI R., MICHOWICH Y., KOIFMAN B., ROTH A., LANIADO S., KEREN G. Reduction of reinfarction and angina with use of low molecular weight heparin therapy after streptokinase (and heparin) in acute myocardial infarction. Am. J. Cardiol. 1996; 77 : 1145-1148

(11) FROSTFELT G., AHLBERG G., GUSTAFSSON G., HELMOIUS G., LINDAHL B., NYGREN A., SWAHN E., VENGE P., WALLENTIN L. Low molecular weight heparin maintains flow in successfully reperfused coronary arteries after treatment with streptokinase. Abstract. Eur. Congress Cardiology 1997 and Amer Heart Assoc. 1997

(12) FROSTFELT G., AHLBERG G., HELMIUS G., LINDAHL B., NYGREN A., SIEGBAHN A., SWAHN E., WALLENTIN L. Low molecular weight heparin subcutaneously for 24 hours as an adjuvant to thrombolysis in acute myocardial infarction - a pilot study. Abstract. Eur. Congress Cardiology 1997 and Amer Heart Assoc. 1997

8.4
Management
of acute stroke

Prophylaxis of deep venous thrombosis with a low molecular weight heparin (Kabi 2165/Fragmin ®) in stroke patients

AUTHORS	PRINS M.H., GELSEMA R., SING A.K.
REF	Haemostasis 1989; 19: 245-250

STUDY	Randomized, double-blind, placebo-controlled
CENTERS (n)	1
COUNTRY	The Netherlands
PATIENTS (n)	*included* 60
	evaluated 60

INCLUSION CRITERIA

Patients with severe acute non-hemorrhagic stroke (onset < 72h) controlled by CT scan

STUDY DRUG	**Dalteparin**	sc daily doses: 2500 AXa IU b.i.d.
		treatment duration: 14 days
REFERENCE DRUG	**Saline**	sc daily doses: 0.2ml b.i.d.
		treatment duration: 14 days

ASSESSMENTS

- ❏ CT scan before randomization and at the end of the trial (D14).
- ❏ DVT: FUT daily up to D14; clinical suspicion confirmed by unilateral venography.
- ❏ PE: clinical symptoms.
- ❏ Cerebral bleeding.
- ❏ Death.

PRINS M.H. et al. 1989

	Dalteparin 2500 AXa IU x 2		Placebo 0.2ml x 2		p
Patients	30		30		
Total DVT	6/27	22.2%	15/28	50.0%	0.03
Proximal DVT	2/27	7.4%	3/28	10.0%	NS
PE (clinical)	1	3.3%	2	6.6%	NS
Cerebral bleeding	4/22	18.8%	2/27	7.4%	NS
Cerebral death	5		2		
Total death	9		4		NS

COMMENTS

❑ In non-hemorrhagic stroke patients, dalteparin 2500 AXa IU administered twice daily significantly reduced the frequency of total DVT.

❑ The results of this trial differ from those observed in the Sandset's study.

❑ Because of the small number of patients, safety could not be properly evaluated.

A double-blind and randomized placebo-controlled trial of low molecular weight heparin once daily to prevent deep vein thrombosis in acute ischemic stroke

AUTHORS	SANDSET P. M., DAHL T., STIRIS M. et al.
REF	Semin. Thromb. Hemost. 1990; 16 (suppl): 25-33

STUDY	Randomized, double-blind, placebo-controlled
CENTERS (n)	1
COUNTRY	Norway
PATIENTS (n)	*included* 103
	evaluated 92

INCLUSION CRITERIA

Acute non-hemorrhagic stroke (<72h) confirmed by CT scan before randomization

STUDY DRUG	**Dalteparin**	sc daily dose: BW-adjusted (about 55-65 AXa IU/kg): 3000 to 5500 AXa IU/day o.d.
		first injection: the day of randomization
		treatment duration: 14 days or until discharge
REFERENCE DRUG	**Placebo (saline)**	sc daily dose: BW-adjusted (0.3-0.5ml)

ASSESSMENTS

- ❏ DVT: venography of the paretic limb on D10 to D14 (or at discharge) or ultra sound scanning when venograhy was not possible.
- ❏ Clinical signs of DVT confirmed by IPG on D1, D5 and D14.
- ❏ CT scan before randomization and after venography (D10/D14).
- ❏ Bleeding complications.
- ❏ PE, death.

SANDSET P.M. et al. 1990

	Dalteparin 3000-5000 AXa IU x 1		Placebo x 1		p
Venography performed	42		50		
Total DVT	15	36%	17	34%	NS
Proximal DVT	5	12%	8	16%	NS
Hemorrhagic transformation of brain infarction	4/50	8%	3/52	6%	NS
Major bleeding	0		0		
AXa levels IU/ml (range) 4h after injection at D2	0.42 (0.35-0.49)		—		
PE	0		1 (fatal)		
Death	5/51 (4 thromboembolic events)		1/52		

COMMENTS

❏ This dalteparin regimen (o.d. administration) did not provide effective prophylaxis against DVT in patients with acute ischemic stroke, although plasma AXa activity reached "substantial" prophylactic level. Almost all DVT were asymptomatic.

❏ No increase in hemorrhagic transformation of brain infarction, nor higher incidence of major bleeding in dalteparin treated patients than in placebo group.

Dalteparin
in acute ischemic cerebrovascular disease:
a safety study

AUTHORS	DAHL T., FRIIS P., ABILDGAARD U.
REF	Cerebrovasc. Dis. 1997; 7: 28-33

STUDY	Open-label, non controlled
CENTERS (n)	2
COUNTRY	Norway
PATIENTS (n)	included 60

INCLUSION CRITERIA

Patients with acute ischemic
non hemorrhagic stroke and TIAs:
- stable stroke in 24 patients
- in progression in 23 patients
- serious and frequent TIAs
  in 13 patients

Cerebral CT scan for all patients

STUDY DRUG

Dalteparin
sc daily doses: 100 AXa IU/kg b.i.d.
first injection: mean 39h after onset (2-168h)
reduced by 50% when INR at 2.8
treatment duration: 8-10 days

+

Warfarin
started on D1 or D2 and monitored: INR $\leq$ 3
treatment duration: not stated (<10D ?)

ASSESSMENTS

❑ Hemorrhagic transformation (CT scan performed before treatment and on D7-D10).

❑ Clinical course based on neurological status (Scandinavian Stroke Scale).

❑ Laboratory data.

DAHL T. et al. 1997

	Dalteparin 100 AXa IU/kg x 2 + **Warfarin**	
Evaluable patients	60	
Clinical progression of neurological symptoms for:		
all strokes	6/50	
stroke in progression	6/23	
cardioembolic stroke	0/24	
Clinical worsening (without hemorrhagic transformation)	6	10%
Asymptomatic hemorrhagic transformation at 2nd CT scan	3*	5%
AXa levels IU/ml (range)		
3h after injection	0.58 (0.20-1.20)	
11h after injection	0.25 (0.10-0.80)	

* All these 3 patients have ASA medication prior to dalteparin therapy.

COMMENTS

❑ Despite the surprising association of a LMWH with warfarin in a safety study, this LMWH dosage appeared well tolerated without hemorrhagic transformation in the small number of patients treated.

❑ In patients included because of TIAs, no further cerebro-vascular events were observed; no recurrent stroke or deterioration occurred in patients with stable cardioembolic stroke.

❑ The AXa activity did not differ in patients with or without neurological deterioration.

Low-molecular-weight heparin for the treatment of acute ischemic stroke

AUTHORS	KAY R., WONG K., YU Y. et al. for FISS trial
REF	N. Engl. J. Med. 1995; 333: 1588-1593

STUDY	Multicenter, randomized, double-blind, placebo-controlled
CENTERS (n)	4
COUNTRY	China
PATIENTS (n)	312

INCLUSION CRITERIA
Stroke onset within 48h

EXCLUSION CRITERIA
Evidence of intracranial hemorrhage, major confounding, neurologic illness including previous disabling stroke, imminent death

STUDY DRUG	Nadroparin	• sc daily high doses ≈ 4000 AXa IU x 2 (0.4ml x 2) or • sc daily low dose ≈ 4000 AXa IU o.d. (0.4ml x 1) + 0.4ml saline one sc injection as placebo treatment duration: 10 days
REFERENCE DRUG	Placebo	saline 0.4ml x 2 treatment duration: 10 days

ASA thereafter in both groups

ASSESSMENTS
- ❏ In-hospital initial period: second CT scan (to determine hemorrhagic cerebral events), death.
- ❏ 3 and 6-month outcomes, independence from care/complete recovery/continued dependence on care (Barthel index).
- ❏ Death.

KAY R. et al. 1995

	Nadroparin high dose	Nadroparin low dose	Placebo
Patients	102	101	105
Ten-day outcomes			
Second CT scan	81	81	83
hemorrhagic events	5 (6.2%)	7 (8.6%)	10 (12.0%)
Recurrent ischemic stroke	1	2	5
Total death	7	8	8
Three-month/Six-month outcomes	3M/6M	3M/6M	3M/6M
Independent patients :			
• complete recovery	21/ 29	22/ 26	18/ 20
• incomplete recovery	26/ 26	17/ 22	22/ 17
Dependent patients	41/ 32	46/ 36	52/ 48
Death	12/ 13	15/ 17	15/ 20
*Six-month all poor outcomes**	45 45%	53 52%	68 65%

* $p = 0.005$ by the chi-square for trend.

COMMENTS

❑ In the acute phase of stroke, nadroparin "high dose" did not increase cerebral hemorrhagic events and was superior to placebo in improving the 6-month outcomes (dependency or death) of patients treated within 48h of the onset of symptoms.

❑ There was a significant dose-dependent effect in favor of nadroparin (chi^2 for trend $p=0.005$) for 6-month outcomes.

❑ A larger multicenter, randomized, double-blind trial including 750 patients (FISS bis) did not confirm these promising results (see following pages).

**Fraxiparine®
in ischaemic stroke study**

AUTHORS	HOMMEL M. for the FISS bis Investigators Group
REF	Cerebrovasc. Dis. 1998; 8 (suppl 5) Abst.

STUDY	Randomized, multicenter, double-blind, placebo-controlled
CENTERS *(n)*	≈ 120
COUNTRIES	16 (Canada, Europe, Asia)
PATIENTS *(n)*	*randomized* 767
	analyzed 766

INCLUSION CRITERIA
Patients with non-hemorrhagic ischemic stroke (30% with a previous stroke)
CT scan at entry:
29% with atherosclerosis in large arteries
27% with small vessel occlusion
19% with cardioembolism
25% other

STUDY DRUG	**Nadroparin**	sc daily injections:

- 85 IU/kg o.d. plus one sc injection of saline o.d. or
- 85 IU/kg b.i.d.

first injection: within 24h within stroke onset
treatment duration: 10 days

REFERENCE DRUG	**Placebo**	saline: two daily injections

treatment duration: 10 days

Adjunctive therapy: antiplatelet or oral anticoagulant after acute treatment from D10 up to six months

ASSESSMENTS
- ❑ CT scan at entry, before randomization and at D10±2.
- ❑ Primary end point: combined bad-outcome at 6-month defined as overall mortality and poor functional status: Barthel Index < 85.
- ❑ Neurological impairment, Rankin scale.
- ❑ Clinical observation: cerebral and other hemorrhage, DVT, PE (confirmed by lung scan or angiography).

HOMMEL M. (FISS bis) 1998

| | **Nadroparin** 85 AXa IU/kg | | | | **Placebo** | |
	x 1		x 2			
Patients	271		245		250	
Bad outcome at 6-month	155	57.2%	145	59.2%	142	56.2%
Death	73	26.9%	73	28.6%	68	27.2%
Barthel < 85	82	30.3%	75	30.6%	74	29.6%
Cerebral hemorrhage	10	3.7%	15	6.1%	7	2.8%
Fatal hemorrhage	3	1.1%	7	2.9%	1	0.4%
Total PE	4	1.5%*	5	2.0%	14	5.6%
Fatal PE	2	0.7%	3	1.2%	9	3.6%
Symptomatic DVT	9	3.3%	9	3.7%	5	2.0%

* p= 0.01 vs placebo value

COMMENTS

- These FISS bis results do not confirm the previous one observed in FISS (Kay R. et al) despite the reduction of the mean window-time between onset and first administration (15h vs 27h).
- In FISS, 64% of strokes were in large arteries vs 29% in FISS bis. The mortality was lower in the first study (19% vs 27.2%).
- With the lower (once daily) dosage, the safety regarding cerebral hemorrhage was similar to placebo.
- Interestingly, a significant difference in the incidence of PE was observed in favor of nadroparin once daily regimen.

Expert comments

MARIE-GERMAINE BOUSSER. *LMWHs in the treatment of acute non-hemorrhagic stroke*

The most striking fact in this section devoted to LWMHs in stroke patients is that stroke has been a rather neglected area with insufficient studies in both quantity and quality. Only 4 studies were performed with a total of 535 patients, to which should be added a recent study reported so far as an abstract: "Fraxiparin in ischaemic stroke study (FISS bis)".

The four studies analyzed by the editors widely differ from each other: 2 included 60 patients each, one 103, the most recent one, the Hong Kong study 312. Three studies were randomized, double blind, placebo-controlled, but one was an uncontrolled open study.

Dalteparin was used in 3 studies at different dosages and for different durations: 2500 AXa IU b.i.d. for 14 days in one, 3000 to 5500 AXa IU o.d. in another one. Dalteparin was associated with warfarin in the open study. Nadroparin was used in 2 different doses: 4000 AXa IU o.d. or b.i.d. for 10 days in the Hong Kong study.

Inclusion criteria were also different: all studies excluded hemorrhagic stroke, but 3 studies included only completed ischemic stroke whereas one (the open one) also recruited patients with transient ischemic attacks and stroke in evolution. The delay from stroke onset was < 48 hours in the Hong Kong study and < 72 hours in the 2 other randomized studies.

Assessment was centered on deep venous thrombosis (DVT) and pulmonary embolism (PE) in 2 studies, on tolerance in the dalteparin/warfarin combination study and on stroke outcome in the Hong Kong study.

The efficacy objectives of any antithrombotic treatment in acute stroke are threefold:

1 - Prevention of DVT and PE
2 - Improvement of stroke outcome
3 - Prevention of early recurrence of brain ischemia.

As regards safety there is only one major concern: the risk of intra-cranial bleeding, within the infarcted brain area (hemorrhagic infarct), or in other parts of the brain (intra-cerebral hemorrhage). The least that can be said is that the 4 studies analyzed here do not allow any firm conclusions regarding these 4 points. The risk of DVT and PE was significantly decreased by LMWH in one study, but not in the other; stroke outcome at 6 months was improved with a good dose effect relationship in the Hong Kong study, but there was no significant efficacy at 3 months so that it has been suggested that the results obtained at 6 months might have been due to chance (1); none of the studies assessed the risk of early recurrence of cerebral ischemia. As regards the risk of intra-cranial bleeding, although it can not statistically significantly increased in any of the 4 studies, in all of them the number of intra-cranial hemorrhage was higher in patients treated with LMWH than in those receiving the placebo and this effect was dose-dependent.

What does the recent FISS 2 study (which exactly replicated the Hong Kong study) add to these 4 trials? Unfortunately, it does not confirm the benefit on stroke outcome observed in the Hong Kong study. Nevertheless, it shows a significant decrease in the rate of PE with the 2 doses of nadroparin. It also confirms a dose related (though non significant) risk of symptomatic intra-cranial hemorrhage.

In conclusion, when the results of these studies are put into perspective with trials of other heparin or heparinoid modalities (1,2), two clear conclusions emerge:

1 - Low dose of LMWH and of heparin have statistically significant preventive effect on DVT and PE, without a significant increase in the risk of symptomatic intra-cranial hemorrhage.

2 - High doses significantly increase the risk of intra-cranial hemorrhage.

As regards the effect of stroke outcome, there seems to be no benefit of high doses, but the question is still open, particularly with the results of the IST trial, of a small benefit (equal to that of aspirin) of low doses. There is also a suggestion that the association of low dose heparin and aspirin might be better that each treatment alone. Thus, based on the evidence presently available, low doses of LMWH are indicated in ischemic stroke patients prone to DVT and PE, in hemiplegic or bedridden patients. Aspirin is indicated in addition, given its beneficial (though very moderate) effect on stroke outcome and on prevention of early recurrence of cerebral ischemia (3).

REFERENCES

(1) International stroke trial collaborative group: the International Stroke Trial (IST): a randomized trial of aspirin, subcutaneous heparin, both or neither among 19 435 patients in acute ischemic stroke. Lancet 1997; 349 : 1569-1581

(2) BOUSSER M.G. Aspirin or heparin immediately after a stroke? Lancet 1997; 349 : 1564-1565

(3) CAST (Chinese Acute Stroke Trial) collaborative group: CAST : randomized placebo controlled trial of early aspirin use in 20,000 patients with acute ischemic stroke. Lancet 1997; 349 : 1641-1649

9

Low molecular weight heparins
in pregnancy

Expert Comments

Low molecular weight heparins in pregnancy

ANDRÉ KHER

Anticoagulant therapy during pregnancy

Pulmonary embolism is a major cause of maternal mortality. Moreover, in view of the young age of the women who develop deep vein thrombosis in pregnancy and subsequent deep vein insufficiency, this is likely to raise a significant chronic health problem. The use of anticoagulants during pregnancy is problematic because of the potential adverse effects on mother and fetus.

Warfarin crosses the placenta and is teratogenic when used during the first trimester of pregnancy. The warfarin fetal syndrome consists of nasal and mid-face hypoplasia, with a typical facial appearance, stippled epiphysis, digital hypoplasia and other bone malformations. When used in the second and third trimesters, warfarin produces a risk of both maternal and fetal bleeding.

Unfractionated heparin is thought not to cross the placenta and is therefore most commonly used in pregnancy for the prevention of venous thromboembolism in high risk patients, treatment of venous thromboembolism, prevention of systemic embolism in patients with artificial heart valves, or prevention of venous thromboembolism or miscarriage in patients with the antiphospholipid antibody syndrome. However, with long-term treatment, potential risks of heparin treatment in pregnancy include osteoporosis in the mother and bleeding in both the mother and the fetus.

Unfractionated heparin compared to oral anticoagulants

The results of a pooled evaluation of patients treated during pregancy either with UFH or with oral anticoagulants have been published by Ginsberg (1989). The risk for the fetus of either treatment was calculated as the incidence of adverse events, which was 21.7% for UFH and 27.9% for oral anticoagulants, evaluated in all pregnancies. When healthy premature babies and maternal comorbid conditions were eliminated from the analysis, the incidence of adverse events dropped to 3.6% for UFH, but remained roughly the same for anticoagulants: 26.1%.

With UFH, osteoporosis-related fractures were observed in 2-3%, a reduction in bone density of 5-10% was observed in two series of patients, while in matched controls it was 7%.

LMWHs during pregnancy

Since their introduction, LMWHs have become the anticoagulant treatment of choice during pregnancy. When compared to UFH, LMWHs are at least as effective and safe. They present additional advantages such as adjustment of dosage to body weight only and once daily administration increasing patient acceptability. There is no need for laboratory monitoring, they do not appear to cross the placenta (Forestier et al. 1987,1992, Schneider et al. 1995) and they probably produce fewer adverse events such as osteoporosis and thrombocytopenia than unfractionated heparin.

LMWHs are not yet licensed for use in pregnancy in any country, but a number of reports cases have been published.

LMWHs have been used successfully during pregnancy in patients with antiphospholipid antibodies, protein C deficiency, protein S deficiency and in patients at increased risk of thromboembolism (see tables on following pages).

The influence of LMWHs on bone density during pregnancy, using dual photon absorptiometry of the lumbar spine, has been evaluated in three studies. In the first one (Melissari et al. 1992), 11 cases were compared to controls, and in the second study (Laskin and Ginsberg 1997), 43 patients served as their own controls and were scanned before and after pregnancy. In both studies, no difference was found between cases and controls, and although osteoporosis is assumed as a possible adverse outcome of heparins, no clear-cut evidence was obtained.

In the third study (Nelson-Piercy et al. 1997), the bone density in the spine or hip was more than 1 standard deviation below the mean for age- and sex-matched controls. Nevertheless, no fracture was reported.

It is now well established that using LMWHs during pregnancy, the rate of adverse fetal outcomes is essentially related to comorbid maternal conditions rather than the treatment itself. The frequency of adverse outcomes is similar to the general population. Moreover, there are no demonstrable differences between LMWH preparations. The risk of osteoporosis is low, does not appear to be much different than the risk in controls, and seems to be lower than that of UFH.

The main published papers or reports regarding LMWHs in pregnancy are presented in the following tables.

FIRST AUTHOR YEAR	LMWH	n*	DAILY DOSAGE	DURATION THERAPY (WEEKS)	INDICATIONS	RESULTS COMMENTS
Priollet, 1986	Enoxaparin	1	60/80mg	13 to 34W before	Thrombosis of all saphenous system	No thromboembolism or hemorrhage Normal baby
Harenberg, 1987	Dalteparin	2	5000 IU 10,000 IU	27W before 20W before	DVT Valvular prosthesis	No thromboembolism or bleeding
Baudot, 1988	Enoxaparin	1	80mg	1W before and 4W after delivery	PS deficiency	Normal baby No complication
De Boer, 1989	Dalteparin	1	10,000 IU	36W before	DVT	Healthy baby
Borg, 1991	Dalteparin	8	5000 IU	16W before and 3W after delivery	PC/PS deficiencies	Normal babies No thrombosis No hemorrhage
Melissari, 1992	Dalteparin	11	2500 IU then 5000 IU (20,000 and 22,500 IU in 2 patients)	before and 12W after delivery	Recurrent miscarriages	1 miscarriage 1 early delivery No osteoporosis
Gillis, 1992	Enoxaparin	6	40mg (80mg) 1 patient	12W before and 4W after delivery	Previous DVT/PE	1 fetal death (emergency cesarean)
Sturridge, 1994	Enoxaparin	16	20mg or 40mg	10W before and 4W after delivery	Past history of thromboembolism, thrombophilia, systemic lupus	2 abortions (both involving anticardiolipin syndrome)

* n = number of cases

FIRST AUTHOR YEAR	LMWH	n	DAILY DOSAGE	DURATION THERAPY (WEEKS)	INDICATIONS	RESULTS COMMENTS
Rasmussen, 1994	Dalteparin	24	2500 IU - 10,000 IU	14 to 29W before	Previous and present history of thromboembolism, anticardiolipin syndrome	3 spontaneous abortions Healthy babies
Manoharan, 1994	Dalteparin	5	2500 IU - 5000 IU	15W before and after delivery	Previous DVT	One patient with induced skin reaction Normal babies
Wahlberg, 1994	Dalteparin	184	2500 IU - 16,000 IU	mean: 42.5 days	Previous thrombo-embolism, thrombogenic disposition, miscellaneous	Minor bleeding= 2.2% Clinical DVT: 2.2%
Dulitzki, 1996	Enoxaparin	34	20-80mg 87%: 40mg	median 12W (+ labor and puerperium)	Thromboembolism, antiphospholipid syndrome, active lupus	One thromboembolic event- No significant bleeding. 3 terminations of pregnancy (worsening lupus)
Boda, 1996	Nadroparin	7	2050 to 4100 IU	3W before and 1W after delivery	ATIII-PC-PS deficiencies	No thromboembolic or hemorrhagic complication Healthy babies
Lee, 1996	Nadroparin	2	100 IU/kg x 2	throughout pregnancy	Prosthetic mitral valve	Normal babies No hemorrhagic complication
Hunt, 1997	Dalteparin	32	5000 IU x 1 5000 IU x 2	3W before and 6W after delivery	Previous thrombo-embolism, thrombosis in current pregnancy, antiphospholipid syndrome	No thromboembolic event or excessive hemorrhage 1 case of osteoporosis 4 first trimester pregnancy losses 1 intrauterine death
Horellou, 1997	Enoxaparin Dalteparin Nadroparin	6 3 5	100 IU/kg x 2	3W to 33W (mean 20W) before	ATIII-PC-PS deficiency, APC resistance, previous thrombo-embolism	No thromboembolic events - No fetal adverse effects No bleeding complications

FIRST AUTHOR YEAR	LMWH	n	DAILY DOSAGE	DURATION THERAPY (WEEKS)	INDICATIONS	RESULTS COMMENTS
Schneider, 1997	Certoparin	108	3000 IU	median 12 days	High risk pregnancy	No thromboembolic event - No bleeding complication related to treatment
Nelson-Piercy, 1997	Enoxaparin	50 11	40mg 20mg	3W before and 6W after delivery	Past history of DVT, PE, antiphospholipid syndrome	No thromboembolic event - No bleeding complication - Mild decrease in bone density of 30% in pregnant women
Daskalakis, 1997	Nadroparin	18	6000 IU x 1	from 7W before to 4w after	protein C, protein S, ATIII deficiency recent history of DVT	No thromboembolic event - No adverse maternal effect

REFERENCES

BAUDOT N. et al. Grossesse chez une malade ayant un déficit congénital en protéine S. Intérêt d'une héparine de bas poids moléculaire. La presse médicale 1988; 17 : 1761

BODA Z. et al. Low molecular weight heparin as thromboprophylaxis in familial thrombophilia during the whole period of pregnancy. Thromb. Haemostasis 1996; 76 : 124-128

DE BOER K. et al. Low molecular weight heparin treatment in a pregnant woman with allergy to standard heparins and heparinoid. Thromb. Haemostasis 1989; 61 : 148

BORG J.Y. et al. Thrombosis prophylaxis in protein C or S deficient pregnant women; low molecular weight heparin management using prethrombotic markers as compared to normal pregnancies. Thromb. Haemostasis 1991; 6 : Abst. 1939

DASKALAKIS G. et al. Thrombosis prophylaxis after treatment during pregnancy. Eur. J. Obs. Gynecol. 1997; 74 : 165-167

DULITZKI M. et al. Low molecular weight heparin in pregnancy and delivery: preliminary experience with 41 pregnancies. Obstet. Gynecol. 1996; 87 : 380

FORESTIER F. et al. Absence de passage transplacentaire de la Fraxiparine (héparine de bas poids moléculaire) au cours du troisième trimestre de la grossesse. J. Gynecol. Obstet. Biol. Reprod. 1987; 16 : 981-986

FORESTIER F. et al. Absence of transplacental passage of Fragmin (Kabi) during the second and the third trimesters of pregnancy. Thromb. Haemostasis 1992; 67: 180-181

GILLIS S. et al. Use of low molecular weight heparin for prophylaxis and treatment of thromboembolism in pregnancy. Int. J. Gynecol. Obstet. 1992; 39 : 297-301

GINSBERG J.S., HIRSH J. Anticoagulants during pregnancy. Ann Rev. Med. 1989; 40 : 79-86

HARENBERG. J. et al. Thromboemboliprophylaxe mit niedermolekularem heparin in der schwangerschaft. Geburtsh. Frauenheilkd. 1987; 47 : 15-18

HORELLOU M.H. Treatment of thrombosis with low molecular weight heparins during 15 pregnancies in 14 women. Pregnancy: clinical and therapy. Thromb. Haemostasis 1997; Supp. June, Abst. 2992

HUNT B.J. et al. Thromboprophylaxis with low molecular weight heparin (Fragmin) in high risk pregnancies. Thromb. Haemostasis 1997; 77 : 1-6

LASKIN C., GINSBERG J. Low molecular weight heparin and ASA therapy in women with autoantibodies and unexplained recurrent fetal loss. Society of perinatal obstetricians, Anaheim, 1997 (Abst.)

LEE L.H., LIAUW A.S. Low molecular weight heparin for thromboprophylaxis during pregnancy in 2 patients with mechanical mitral valve replacement. Thromb. Haemostasis 1996; 76 : 627-631

MACKLON N.S. et al. Thrombocytopenia, antithrombin deficiency and extensive thromboembolism in pregnancy: treatment with low molecular weight heparin. Blood Coag. Fibrinolysis 1995; 6 : 672-675

MANOHARAN A. Use of low molecular weight heparin during pregnancy. J. Clin. Pathol. 1994; 47 : 94

MELISSARI E. et al. Use of low molecular weight heparin in pregnancy. Thromb. Haemostasis 1992; 68 : 652-656

NELSON-PIERCY C. et al. Low molecular weight heparin for obstetric thromboprophylaxis: experience of sixty nine pregnancies in sixty one women at high risk. Am. J. Obst. Gynecol. 1997: 176: 1062-1068

PRIOLLET P. et al. Low molecular weight heparin in venous thrombosis during pregnancy. Br. J. Haematol. 1986; 63 : 605-606

RASMUSSEN C. et al. Thromboembolic prophylaxis with low molecular weight heparin during pregnancy. Int. J. Gyn. and Obst. 1994; 47 : 121-125

SCHNEIDER D. et al. Placental passage of low molecular weight heparin (Germ.), Geburtshilfe Frauenheilkd. 1995; 55 : 93-98

SCHNEIDER D. et al. Safety and efficacy of low molecular weight heparin (certoparin) in pregnancy. Thromb. Haemostasis 1997; Supp. June, Abst. 2994

STURRIDGE F. et al. The use of low molecular weight heparin for thromboprophylaxis in pregnancy. British J. Obst. and Gyn. 1994; 101 : 69-71

WAHLBERG B. and KHER A. Low molecular weight heparin as thromboprophylaxis in pregnancy. Haemostasis 1994; 24 : 55-56

Low molecular weight heparins in pregnancy

ZOLTÁN BODA, GYÖRGY BLASKO

Thromboembolic complications during pregnancy are the most common cause of maternal death. Throughout pre-gnancy, anticoagulant administration is indicated for the treatment and prophylaxis of thromboembolic diseases in women with inherited thrombophilia, antiphospholipid-antibody syndrome, prosthetic heart valve. Normal pregnancy is characterized by variable changes in blood coagulation factor levels, suppression of antithrombin (ATIII) and protein S acti-vity although levels of protein C remain normal, with a decrease of fibrinolytic activity. A hypercoagulable state may lead to thromboembolic events in 0.7-2.6% of pregnancies (Bokareva 1996). Administration of heparin in familial thrombophilia during pregnancy provides effective thromboprophylaxis of pregnant women and prevents uteroplacental thrombosis.

Recently, the EPCOT (European Prospective Cohort on Thrombophilia) study has reported an increased number of fetal losses in women with inherited thrombophilia. The risks were greatest for women with ATIII deficiency and for those with combined defects. In women with factor V Leiden mutation, the results suggested the possibility of increased risk of stillbirth (1.2% vs 0.6% of controls) but without excess of miscarriages (Preston 1996). Another study reports second trimester pregnancy loss associated with activated protein C resistance (Rai 1996). Inherited deficiencies of the vitamin K-dependent physiological anticoagulants protein C and protein S have recently been associated with an increa-sed risk for gestational abnormalities. The increased risk was significant in particular for intra-uterine fetal death (Brenner 1997). Patients with a deficiency of ATIII, protein C or Protein S have 70, 33 and 17% incidence of thrombosis during pregnancy, respectively (Toglia 1996).

Low-dose unfractionated heparin (UFH) has a prophylactic effect, but the long-term UFH administration may be complicated by osteoporosis and/or thrombocytopenia. Controlled clinical trials with LMWHs for thromboprophylaxis in pregnancy are missing, however, according to some recent studies, LMWHs do not cross the placental barrier (Melissari 1992, Forestier 1992, Harenberg 1993, Wahlberg 1994). The advantages of LMWHs over UFH are multiple: body weight fixed-dose, no laboratory control, once daily dosage.

LMWHs may offer four other advantages over UFH during pregnancy:

1 - Since LMWHs bind less to PF4, the incidence of LMWH-induced thrombocytopenia is extremely low. Heparin-induced thrombocytopenia (HIT) occurred in 9 of 332 patients who received UFH and in none of 333 patients who

received LMWH (2.7% vs 0%). Eight of the 9 patients with HIT also had one or more thrombotic events (Warkentin 1995). This suggests that thrombotic events associated with HIT and heparin-dependent IgG antibodies are reduced in patients treated with LMWHs.

2 - In spite of long-term use, the risk of heparin-induced osteoporosis may be reduced by the use of LMWHs. Spinal fractures occur less frequently with long-term treatment with LMWHs compared with UFH (Samama 1996). According to our own data (32 pregancies of 27 women with familiar thrombophilia treated with a LMWH throughout pregnancy) there was no case with clinical signs of symptoms of osteoporosis. One of our patients had 3 pregnancies with successful outcomes, and was treated with a LMWH for more than 30 months, but the result of bone-densitometry remained negative after the third delivery (Boda, in press).

3 - The longer plasma half-life of LMWHs has a practical consequency: once daily use is enough for prophylaxis.

4 - Laboratory control is not necessary (but platelet counts are recommended during the first weeks).

Combined use of LMWH (7500 IU once daily) and low dose aspirin (100 mg daily) were effective as a therapeutical approach in pregnancy with antiphospholipid-antibody syndrome. The fetal wastage was 23.5% (4/17) in comparison with 90.2% (37/41) in pregnancies without specific treatment (Serrano 1997).

There are very few reports of the use of LMWHs in pregnant patients with mechanical heart valves. Two cases in which use of nadroparin 100 IU/kg twice daily was successful with no adverse side effects or complications have been published (Lee 1996).

The dose of LMWH as thromboprophylaxis for pregnant women during all pregnancy has great importance. According to theoretical and clinical data (summarized in this review), patients with antithrombin deficiency or combined defects need high doses (1000 IU/kg twice daily). In pregnant patients with protein C or protein S deficiency the recommended dose is 100 IU/kg once daily. For pregnant patients with Factor-V-Leiden, a dose of 50 IU/kg seems to be sufficient. In patients with antiphospholipid-antibody syndrome, high dose of LMWH (100 IU/kg twice daily) together with 100 mg/day ASA (combined antithrombotic treatment) is the best available treatment. For pregnant women with prosthetic heart valves, 100 IU/kg LMWH twice daily are suggested.

Randomized, controlled multicenter studies are needed to assess the general use of LMWHs in pregnant women necessitating thromboprophylaxis.

SCHEMA OF ANTICOAGULANT TREATMENT IN PREGNANT WOMEN WITH THROMBOPHILIA

Before pregnancy :
continuous oral anticoagulation with oral anticoagulant (INR 2.0-3.0)

During all the 40 weeks of pregnancy: LMWH
low risk: 50-100 IU/kg o.d.
high risk: 100 IU/kg b.i.d.
antiphospholipid-antibody: 100 IU/kg b.i.d. and 100 mg ASA daily
prosthetic heart valve: 100 IU/kg b.i.d.

After delivery (one/two weeks)
oral anticoagulants again

REFERENCES

(1) BOKAREVA M.I., BREMME K., BLOMBÄCK M. Arg506-Gln mutation in factor V and risk of thrombosis during pregnancy. Brit. J. Haematol. 1996; 92 : 473-478

(2) BRENNER B., BLUMENFELD Z. Thrombophilia and fetal loss. Blood Reviews 1997; 11 : 72-79

(3) FORESTIER F., SOLE Y., AIACH M. et al. Absence of transplacental passage of Fragmin (Kabi) during the second and the third trimesters of pregnancy. Thromb. Haemostasis 1992; 67 : 180-181

(4) HARENBERG J., SCHNEIDER D., HEILMANN L., WOLF H. Lack of anti-factor Xa activity in umbilical cord vein samples after subcutaneous administration of heparin or low molecular mass heparin in pregnant woman. Haemostasis 1993; 23 : 314-320

(5) LEE L.H., LIAUW P.C.Y. NG A.S.H. Low molecular weight heparin for thromboprophylaxis during pregnancy in 2 patients with mechanical mitral valve replacement. Thromb. Haemostasis 1996; 76 : 628-630

(6) MELISSARI E. PARKER C.J., WILSON N.V. et al. Use of low molecular weight heparin in pregnancy. Thromb. Haemostasis 1992; 68 : 652-656

(7) PRESTON F.E., ROSENDAAL F.R., WALKER I.D. et al. Increased fetal loss in women with heritable thrombophilia. Lancet 1996; 348 : 913-916

(8) RAI R., REGAN L., HADLEY E. et al. Second trimester pregnancy loss is associated with activated protein C resistance. Brit. J. Haematol. 1996; 92 : 489-490

(9) SAMAMA M.M., BARA L., GOUAIN-THIBAULT I. New data on the pharmacology of heparin and low molecular weight heparins. Drugs 1996; 52 : 8-15

(10) TOGLIA M.R., WEG J.G. Venous thromboembolism during pregnancy. N. Engl. J. Med. 1996; 335 : 108-114

(11) SERRANO F., RAMOS P., PINTO G. et al. Pregnancy outcome and primary antiphospholipid antibody syndrome. Thromb. Haemostasis 1997; supp June, 1349 (abstr)

(12) WAHLBERG T.B., KHER A. Low molecular weight heparin as thromboprophylaxis in pregnancy. Haemostasis 1994; 24 : 55-56

(13) WARKENTIN T.E., LEVINE M.N., HIRSH J. et al. Heparin-induced thrombocytopenia in patients treated with low molecular weight heparin or unfractionated heparin. N. Engl. J. Med. 1995; 332 : 1330-1335

10

Low molecular weight heparins
in pediatrics

Low-molecular-weight heparin in pediatric patients with thrombotic disease: a dose-finding study

AUTHORS	MASSICOTTE P., ADAMS M., MARZINOTTO V. et al.
REF	J. Pediatr. 1996; 128: 313-318

STUDY	Open-label
CENTERS (n)	1
COUNTRY	Canada
PATIENTS (n)	included 25
	evaluated 25

INCLUSION CRITERIA

Children, age ranging 0-17 year-old
(9 neonates) requiring anticoagulation for:
- DVT or PE (14 children)
- complications in the central nervous system (9 children)
- congenital heart disease (2 children)

STUDY DRUG **Enoxaparin** starting sc daily dose: 1mg/kg b.i.d.
then AXa-adjusted dose (monitoring at 4h)
AXa level: 0.5-1.0 IU/ml

treatment duration:
- 10 days (5 children)
- 11D-20D (7 children)
- 21D-30D (6 children)
- 30D-60D (4 children)
- over 60D (3 children)

Use of sc catheters

ASSESSMENTS

❑ Recurrent thrombotic events.
❑ Bleeding complications.
❑ Biological monitoring: APTT and AXa activity.

MASSICOTTE P. et al. 1996

	Enoxaparin starting dose ≈ 1mg/kg x 2	
	Neonates	Children
Patients	9	16
Recurrent thromboembolic events during treatment	0	0
Bleeding events	0	2*
Dose requirements in mg/kg (according to AXa level)	1.6 (0.6 U/ml)	1mg (0.5-1 U/ml) 0.5mg (0.35 U/ml) (in 2 children with heart disease)
APTT	minimal effect	

* Requiring transfusion therapy in children with previous gastrointestinal ulcers.

COMMENTS

❑ Interesting study for the use of a LMWH in pediatric patients.

❑ Children seem to need dosage at least equivalent to adult dosage for treating thromboembolic events: 1mg/kg b.i.d.

❑ Neonates seem to need increased dose requirements.

Expert comments

PATRICK MISMETTI. *Use of anticoagulants in pediatric patients*

The indications for using anticoagulants in children have rapidly increased essentially due to the advances in tertiary care pediatrics. These indications include :
- venous thromboembolic diseases where ages of greatest risk for deep vein thrombosis (DVT) and pulmonary embolism were infants less than one year of age and teenagers
  - central venous lines-related thrombosis which represented 40% of DVT in children and over 80% in newborns;
  - inherited prothrombotic complications including deficiencies of AT III, protein C and S, activated protein C resistance etc.;
  - arterial thromboembolic diseases mostly due to cardiac catheterizations and central or peripheral catheters in the intensive care setting
  - umbilical artery catherizations.

Unfractionated heparins (UFH) and oral anticoagulants (OAC) were largely prescribed in pediatrics but they all together presented some limitations:
- first of all, their therapeutic index in infants were directly extrapolated from clinical trials in adults,
- bleeding risk under UFH and OAC is significant in infants since they have frequently serious underlying primary problems,
- the dose of either UFH and OAC to achieve adult therapeutic range is age-dependant with the youngest children having the highest dose requirements. If a higher clearance of UFH in pediatric patients could explain this phenomena, no clear explanation was established for OAC,
- UFH and OAC pharmacodynamic intra- and inter-individual variabilities were great enough to require close supervision and frequent blood samples and dose adjustments despite well-established and specific nomograms for initial dosing,
- finally, limited venous access in pediatric patients hinders safe and effective monitoring with a high incidence of both significant bleeding complications and recurrent thromboembolic diseases especially with OAC treatment (1).

However, some general recommendations in pediatrics have been published (2).
- Arterial and venous thromboembolism in children and newborns have to be treated by iv heparin sufficient to get an antifactor Xa level of 0.3 to 0.7 U/ml. Treatment with oral anticoagulant should be overlapped with heparin for 4 to 5 days and long term anticoagulant therapy should be continued for at least 3 months using oral anticoagulants to prolong the prothrombin time to an INR of 2.0 to 3.0. Indefinite oral anticoagulant therapy should be considered for children with a first recurrence of thromboembolic disease or a continuing risk factors such as antithrombin III, protein C and S deficiencies, central venous line, etc.
- Prophylaxis for cardiac catheterization in children and newborns should be considered with iv heparin doses of 100 to 150 U/kg since aspirin alone cannot be recommended.
- Oral anticoagulant therapy to prolong the INR to 2.5 to 3.5, is strongly recommended for children with mechanical prosthetic heart valves. If systemic embolism occurs despite adequate oral anticoagulant therapy, the addition of aspirin, 6 to 20 mg/kg/d, should be considered. The addition of dipyridamole, 2 to 5 mg/kg/d, to oral anticoagulant therapy is an alternative option.

• Some other less frequent indications for anticoagulant therapy and specific pediatric rules for adaptative control of iv heparin or oral anticoagulants are also well-described in the fourth American College of Chest Physicians' consensus conference on antithrombotic therapy (2).

More recently developed, low molecular weight heparins (LMWHs) could present some advantages in pediatric patients, such as their therapeutic regimen, i.e once daily subcutaneous treatment, a smaller volume per injection and a less intensive monitoring since their pharmacokinetic profile is more reproductible.

Only one dose-finding study has already been published on LMWH in pediatric patients (3). Once again, the recommended therapeutic index was directly extrapolated from data in adults (anti Xa activity between 0.5 and 1 IU/ml). This study has shown some differences between infants and adults with age-dependance of LMWH pharmacokinetic, with the youngest having the highest clearance and so the higher dosage requirements. Moreover, this treatment is only to be supervised twice weekly, suggesting a reproductible pharmacokinetic of LMWH. But the statistical analysis used in this study is powerless to confirm the low pharmacokinetic interindividual variability of LMWH, with regard to the limited venous access and so the small number of blood samples per child. This limited venous access is not yet a problem when using a "population pharmacokinetic approach", well-adapted to sparse sampling time on the condition to evaluate a higher number of patients (4). A precise estimation of the inter- and intra-individual variability is essential to determine the optimal dosing and monitoring of LMWH in children, before carrying out future randomized clinical trials.

In fact, the potential advantages of LMWH for pediatric patients, especially in terms of monitoring, safety and efficacy, require urgent testing in randomized controlled trials in both prophylactic and therapeutic settings.

REFERENCES

(1) ANDREW M., MARZINOTTO V., BLANCHETTE V. et al. Heparin therapy in pediatric patients: a prospective cohort study. Pediatr. Res. 1994; 35 : 78-83

(2) MICHELSON A., BOVILL E., ANDREW M., Antithrombotic therapy in children. Chest 1995; 108 : 506S-522S

(3) MASSICOTE P., ADAMS M., MARZINOTTO V. et al. Low molecular weight heparin in pediatric patients with thrombotic disease: a dose finding study. J. Pediatr. 1996; 128 : 313-318

(4) MISMETTI P., LAPORTE-SIMITSIDIS S., DOUBINE S. et al. Predictive nadroparin calcium (Fraxiparin ®) dosage regimens in neonates and children after cardiovascular surgery. Thromb. Haemost. 1995; 6 : 968

11

Low molecular weight heparins
and osteoporosis

André Kher, Francis Toulemonde p. 448

Heparin-induced osteoporosis

ANDRÉ KHER, FRANCIS TOULEMONDE

Osteoporosis is a rare complication which can ensue after a prolonged heparin treatment.

Reports in the mid-sixties of patients with spontaneous fractures under long-term treatment with heparin, first drew attention to a possible relationship between heparin treatment and osteoporosis (Griffith G.C. et al 1965).

Most of the reported cases of symptomatic osteoporosis with spontaneous fractures occurred in pregnant women treated for recurrent thromboembolism with unfractionated heparin (Hellgren M. et al 1982, De Swiet M. et al 1983, Dahlman T.C. 1993).

The actual incidence of heparin-induced osteoporosis is unknown but according to reported observations, in almost every case, the minimum daily dose of heparin was 15,000 IU administered at least during a 6-month period.

The mechanism of this complication is poorly understood. Heparin-induced osteoporosis is probably multifactorial and various mechanisms have been involved:

- direct heparin activity on bone cells, osteoblastic depression and osteoclastic activation;
- reduction of the calcium ionized fraction causing secondary hyperparathyroidism;
- activation of vitamin D.

It has been postulated that pregnancy predisposes to the development of osteoporosis, while in elderly subjects with age-related osteopenia no such predisposition was found.

Diagnosis

A practical way to evaluate the relationship between heparin and osteoporosis is to use bone density measurements by dual X ray absorptiometry (DXA) of the lumbar spine. Barbour L.A. et al 1994 showed that heparin adversely affected bone density in about one third of exposed pregnant women. These results confirmed those obtained by Ginsberg K.S. et al (1990).

Concerning experimental data on LMWH induced-osteoporosis, the results are contradictory. Murray W (1985) has shown that the loss of bone matrix resulting from a prolonged treatment with heparin on rats was proportional to the molecular weight of the heparin; the LMWH CY216 (nadroparin) did not cause any evidence of osteoporosis either in this study or during the chronic toxicity studies (6 months) carried out on the rat and on the dog with the highest tested doses (twenty-times the clinical dose). The same author (Murray W 1995) compared long-term administration of heparin and LMWH (CY216) on rabbits. Doses of 1500 AXa units/kg for one month did not cause toxic skeletal effects as opposed to UFH which induced clear osteoporotic changes. Similar favorable results were obtained in the rats with dalteparin by Monreal (1990).

On the contrary, Matzch T et al (1990) demonstrated that tinzaparin causes the same osteoporosis-inducing effect as standard heparin when it is administered in AXa equivalent units in rats. In this regard, it must be stressed that the dosages administered were as high as 2000 AXa IU/kg (more than ten-times the clinical dosage).

Data published on osteoporotic risk comparing UFH and LMWH in humans are rare. A double-blind study by Monreal M et al 1994 compared UFH and dalteparin in patients treated for DVT with contraindication to oral anticoagulant. The incidence of fracture was 15% and 2.5% for UFH and LMWH-treated patients respectively.

Melissari et al (1982) performed bone density scans of the lumbar spine and hip in 11 patients treated through the pregnancy with dalteparin (2500+25,000 IU/day) and showed normal mineral bone mass.

Nelson-Piercy and colleagues (1997) observed that after administration of enoxaparin (usually 40mg/day) for 3-9 months, 32% of the pregnant treated women presented bone density values below the mean but all were asymptomatic.

In conclusion, despite the lack of controlled studies, current data suggest that the risk of heparin-induced osteoporosis is reduced with LMWHs.

REFERENCES

BARBOUR L.A. et al. A prospective study of heparin-induced osteoporosis in pregnancy using bone density. Am. J. Obstet. Gynecol. 1994; 170 : 862-869

DAHLMAN T.C. Osteoporotic fractures and the recurrence of thromboembolism during pregnancy and the puerperium in 184 women undergoing thromboprophylaxis with heparin. Am. J. Obstet. Gynecol. 1993; 168 : 1265-1270

DE SWIET M et al. Prolonged heparin therapy in pregnancy causes bone demineralization. Br. J. Obstet. Gynaecol. 1983; 90 : 1129-1134

GINSBERG K.S. et al. Heparin effect on bone density. Thromb. Haemostasis 1990; 64 : 286-289

GRIFFITH G.C. et al. Heparin osteoporosis. Jama. 1965; 193 : 85-88

HELLGREN M. et al. Long-term therapy with subcutaneous heparin during pregnancy. Gynecol. Obstet. Invest. 1982; 13 : 76-89

KHER A., TOULEMONDE F., RABY C., Héparinothérapie au long cours et ostéoporose, Nlle Presse Méd. 1973,2,23,1585-87

MATZCH T. et al. Effects of low molecular weight heparin and unfragmented heparin on induction of osteoporosis. Thromb. Haemostasis 1990; 63 : 505-509

MELISSARI E. et al. Use of low molecular weight heparin in pregnancy. Thromb. Haemostasis 1982; 68 : 652-656

MONREAL M. et al. Comparison of subcutaneous unfractionated heparin with a low molecular weight heparin (Fragmin) in patients with venous thromboembolism and contraindications to coumarin. Thromb. Haemostasis 1994; 71 : 7-11

MONREAL M. et al. Heparin-related osteoporosis in rats. A comparative study between unfractionated heparin and a low molecular weight heparin. Haemostasis 1990; 20 : 204-207

MURRAY W.J.G. Low molecular weight heparin in surgical practice. M. S. Thesis. (London)1985; 4 : 586-591

MURRAY W.J.G. et al. Long-term administration of heparin and heparin fractions and osteoporosis in experimental animals. Blood Coagulation and Fibrinolysis 1995; 6 : 113-118

NELSON-PIERCY C. Review heparin-induced osteoporosis in pregnancy. Lupus 1997; 6 : 500-504

NELSON-PIERCY C. et al. Low molecular weight heparin for obstetric thromboprophylaxis: experience of 69 pregnancies in 61 high risk women. Am. J. Obstet. Gynecol. 1997; 176 : 1062-1068.

12

Low molecular weight heparins
induced thrombocytopenia

André Kher, Francis Toulemonde   p. 452

Heparin/LMWHs-induced thrombocytopenia

ANDRÉ KHER, FRANCIS TOULEMONDE

Among the adverse events related to heparin therapy, thrombocytopenia, in addition to hemorrhage, is the most clinically severe complication. Two types of heparin-induced thrombocytopenia (HIT) with distinct clinical outcomes have been defined: HIT type I and HIT type II.

HIT type I

HIT type I is mainly characterized by a strong decrease in platelet count of the initial value, but generally higher than 100,000/µl, persisting for two or more days without any clinical symptomatology and with no apparent reason other than heparin treatment. HIT type I is relatively common, being observed in about 10% or more of patients treated with heparin (range 0.3-30%). It develops within a few days (less than 5 days) after starting heparin treatment, and is generally of a mild and benign nature. It resolves spontaneously, and in many patients, platelet count returns to normal despite continuing treatment.

HIT type II

HIT type II is characterized not only by severe thrombocytopenia with an absolute reduction of platelet count less than 100,000/ml or a relative decrease of more than 50%, but also with thromboembolism (arterial or venous: white clot syndrome) and adrenal complications in many cases.

Although it is less frequent than HIT type I, this variant is associated with high morbidity (20%) and mortality (30%) (Grenacher et al 1994) and increased hospital stay regardless of the originating clinical situation. With UFH the frequency of HIT type II has been estimated to be about 1-2% and less than 0.1% with LMWHs.

After a first exposure of patients to heparin treatment, this condition is delayed and becomes manifest within 5 to 14 days after starting heparin therapy and it is usually associated with a platelet count between 20,000 and 60,000/µl.

The antibody titers decline over several months; however, early reexposure can result in a catastrophic immediate secondary immune response. Frequently, this strongly reactive immune response is associated with life threatening thromboembolic complications including stroke.

Pathogenesis of HIT type II

Since the observations of Rhodes et al in 1973, it is now widely accepted that HIT is an immunologic reaction caused by an antibody, usually immunoglobulin (IgG class) which activates platelets via their Fc receptors. The antigen recognized by this IgG often consists of a complex of heparin and platelet factor 4 (PF4), a protein of a-granules that binds to, and neutralizes, heparin molecules (mainly those strongly sulfated and with a high molecular weight).

These immune complexes cause not only activation of platelet function but also activation of the coagulation system, expression of tissue factor from endothelial cells. Clinical evidence of this activation in patients with HIT type II included a high risk of venous or arterial thromboembolism.

Low molecular weight heparins and thrombocytopenia

It appears certain that HIT type II occurs much less frequently in patients receiving LMWH (Warkentin T.E. et al 1995). But even though these products interfere less with platelets than UFH due to their lower molecular weight and lower degree of sulfation therefore their decreasing affinity for PF4, they should not be administered to patients with present or previous HIT type II. Furthermore, in vitro studies have demonstrated a high cross reactivity rate (about 80%) between these agents and PF4/ heparin antibody (Chong B.H. et al 1995). Moreover, all LMWHs can induce HIT and cause the same serious and life-threatening complications as unfractionated heparin (Warkentin T.E. et al 1995).

Diagnosis and management of thrombocytopenia

As soon as the clinical diagnosis of HIT is suspected all forms of heparin therapy should be stopped and the adverse clinical event confirmed by laboratory tests. The simplest and most rapid test is the platelet count; in fact, according to Warkentin (1997) "rarely a dramatic clinical event will occur with formation of HIT-IgG without a major fall in the platelet count".

Both functional and immunological assays have been developed to detect HIT-IgG:

• functional tests: their rationale is based on the ability of HIT-IgG to activate normal donor platelets in the presence of heparin. Several test are proposed:

- platelet aggregation test (PAT)
- serotonine release (SRA)
- heparin-induced platelet activation (HIPA)

• immunological tests: their rationale is based on the ability of the HIT - IgG to recognize heparin-PF4 complexes (ELISA technique).

Subsequent management should be guided by the clinical situation.

When immediate acting antithrombotic therapy is mandatory as frequently occurs, three drugs are presently available such as the heparinoid (danaparoid), the r-hirudin (lepirudin) and the synthetic thrombin inhibitor (argatroban) (Walenga J et al 1996).

REFERENCES

BECKER P.S. et al. Heparin-induced thrombocytopenia. Stroke. 1989; 20 : 14-59

CHONG B.H. Heparin-induced thrombocytopenia. Br. J. Haematol. 1995; 89 : 431-439

GREINACHER A. et al. Heparin associated thrombocytopenia: Isolation of the antibody and characterization of a multimolecular PF4-heparin complex as the major antigen. Thromb. Haemostasis 1994; 71 : 247-251

GREINACHER A. Heparin-associated thrombocytopenia. Biomed. Prog. 1994; 7 : 53-56

GRUEL Y. et al. Specific quantification of heparin-dependent antibodies for the diagnosis of heparin associated thrombocytopenia using an ELISA. Thromb. Res. 1991; 62 : 377-387

HARENBERG J. et al. Anticoagulation in patients with heparin-induced thrombocytopenia Type II. Semin. Thromb. Hemost. 1997; 23 : 189-196

RHODES G.R. et al. Heparin-induced thrombocytopenia with thrombotic and hemorrhagic manifestations. Surg. Gynecol. Obstet. 1973; 136 : 409-419

SCHMITT B.P. et al. Heparin-associated thrombocytopenia: a critical review and pooled analysis. Am. J. Med Science 1993; 305 : 208-215

WARKENTIN T.E. et al. Heparin-induced thrombocytopenia in patients treated with low molecular weight heparin or unfractionated heparin. NEJ Med. 1995; 332 : 1330-1335

WARKENTIN T.E. et al. A 14-year study of heparin-induced thrombocytopenia. Am. J. Med. 1996; 101 : 502-507

WARKENTIN T.E. Heparin-induced thrombocytopenia pathogenesis, frequency, avoidance and management. Drug Safety 1997; 17 : 325-341

WALENGA J.M. et al. Relative heparin-induced thrombocytopenia potential of low molecular weight heparins and new antithrombotic agents. Clin. Appl. Thromb. Haemostasis 1996; 2 (Supp) : S21-S27

13

Low molecular weight heparins
and neutralization
by protamine

André Kher, Monique Sarret, Francis Toulemonde   p. 456

Low molecular weight heparins and protamine neutalization

ANDRÉ KHER, MONIQUE SARRET, FRANCIS TOULEMONDE

Since the pioneering studies published by Chargaff and Olson (1937), protamine-sulfate or chloride salt is commonly used to neutralize the effect of excess heparin mainly after cardiopulmonary bypass when full heparin therapy has been administered to avoid clot in extracorporeal circuit.

In fact, this high basic protein is able to chemically combine with the negatively charged heparin molecules forming stable complexes which impede their binding with ATIII, with subsequent loss of their anticoagulant and hemorrhagic properties.

Interestingly, it has been observed that if all the anticoagulant activity of UFH (measured with TT or APTT tests) was totally neutralized in vitro, around 25% of the AXa activity measured after in vivo administration remained present (Michalski et al 1978). This effect has been attributed to the release of components with AXa activity from the vessel wall or to the decrease of binding affinity with decreasing molecular weight of saccharide chains; in fact, below 18 units, they become increasingly resistant to protamine neutralization (Holmer et al 1983).

An important question is whether protamine can reverse the hemorrhage potential as well as the anticoagulant properties of LMWHs since these two effects may not always be synonymous.

It has been observed that a significant proportion of the AXa activity of LMWH (up to 50%) is not neutralized by protamine either in vitro or in vivo although the AIIa activity (expressed as TT or APTT) is totally reversed (Holmer et al 1983, Harenberg et al 1985, Woltz et al 1995).

Several animal studies have shown complete neutralization of the hemorrhagic effect of LMWH by protamine (Doutremepuich et al 1985, Racanelli et al 1985), but these animal models may not accurately reflect the clinical situation. Indeed, Massonet-Castel et al (1986) found protamine of limited effectiveness in controlling bleeding induced by a high dose of a LMWH (enoxaparin) in human extracorporeal circulation.

As stated by Woltz et al, it is unclear whether the residual impairment of hemostasis is still detectable after administration of the theorical "recommended" dose of protamine is associated with a residual bleeding risk.

The relevance of protamine use for stopping excessive bleeding induced by LMWHs is therefore uncertain. Nevertheless, it must be keep in mind that in literature, no mention of severe hemorrhage induced by LMWH has necessitated the use of protamine (with the only exception referred by Farkas et al 1993 in vascular surgery). This fact indirectly underlines the rareness of severe hemorrhage events with LMWH agents.

Since protamine itself can provoke serious adverse reactions, its use cannot be recommended at least in clinical situations not related to extracorporeal circulation. In the rare event of unexpected severe bleeding, LMWH should be stopped and a transfusion of fresh frozen plasma or erythrocyte concentrates can be considered.

REFERENCES

ANDRASSY K. et al. Neutralization of the anticoagulant activity of low molecular weight heparin LU 47311 (clivarin) in man by protamine chloride. Thromb. Res. 1994; 73 : 85-93

BANG C.J. et al. Incomplete reversal of enoxaparin-induced bleeding by protamine sulfate. Haemostasis 1991; 21 : 155-160

CHARGAFF E., OLSON K.B. Studies on the chemistry of blood coagulation. VI. studies on the action of heparin and other anticoagulants: the influence of protamine on the anticoagulant effect in vivo. J. Biol. Chem. 1937; 122 : 153-167

DOUTREMEPUICH C. et al. In vivo neutralization of LMW heparin fraction CY216 by protamine. Thromb. Haemostasis 1985; 11 : 318-322

FARKAS J.C. et al. A randomized controlled trial of a low molecular weight heparin enoxaparin to prevent deep vein thrombosis in patients undergoing vascular surgery. Eur. J. Vasc. Surg. 1993; 7 : 554-560

HARENBERG J. et al. Inhibition of low molecular weight heparin by protamine chloride in vivo. Thromb. Res. 1985; 38 : 11-20

HOLMER E. et al. Neutralization of unfractionated heparin and a low molecular weight heparin fragment by protamine. Thromb Haemostasis 1983; 50 : 103

HOLST J. et la. Protamine neutralization of intravenous and subcutaneous low molecular weight heparins (tinzaparin, logiparin): an experimental investigation in healthy volunteers. Blood Coag. Fibrinlysis 1994; 5 : 795-803

MASSONNET-CASTEL S. et al. Partial reversal of low molecular weight heparin (PK10169) anti-Xa activity by protamine sulfate: in vitro and in vivo study during cardiac surgery with extracorporeal circulation. Haemostasis 1986; 16 : 139-146

MICHALSKI R. et al. Neutralization of heparin in plasma by platelet factor 4 and protamine sulfate. B.J. Haematol. 1978; 38 : 561

RACANELLI A. et al. Biochemical and pharmacologic studies on the protamine interactions with heparin, its fractions, and fragments. Semin. Thromb. Haemostasis. 1985; 11 : 176-190

VAN RYN-Mc KENNA J. et al. Neutralization of enoxaparin-induced bleeding by protamine sulfate. Thromb. Haemostasis. 1990; 63 : 271-274

WOLZT M. et al. Studies of the neutralization effects of protamine on unfractionated and low molecular weight heparin (Fragmin ®) at the site of activation of the coagulation system in man. Thromb. Haemostasis. 1995; 73 : 439-443

14

Low molecular weight heparins

and meta-analyses
(references)

Monique Sarret, Francis Toulemonde   p. 460

Meta-analysis with LMWHs

MONIQUE SARRET, FRANCIS TOULEMONDE

An impressive number of meta-analyses have been published comparing various LMWHs to unfractionated heparin in the prophylaxis and treatment of DVT (see the following references).

According to the more recent meta-analyses, it is shown that LMWHs and UFH do not differ significantly in terms of prevention of thromboembolism but LMWHs have a significantly better safety profile in general surgery (Palmer A.J. et al 1997).

LMWHs are significantly superior to UFH and result in significantly less minor bleeding complications when compared to UFH in orthopedic surgery (Palmer A.J. et al 1997).

Following total knee arthroplasty, LMWHs are more efficacious than either adjusted-UFH dose or warfarin (Howard A.W. et al 1988).

Regarding the treatment of venous thromboembolism, some discrepancies appear between recent meta-analyses: in two reports, the incidence of recurrent thromboembolic events and major bleeding are significantly reduced in LMWH-treated patients (Siragusa S. et al 1996, Lensing A.W. A. et al 1995).

In the report recently published by Dolovich L. and Ginsberg S.S. (1997), these favorable results are somewhat offset by two trials comparing hospital and home treatment. This report indicates that LMWHs are at least as effective as UFH but are unlikely to be superior. This position is shared by another meta-analysis (Mismetti P. 1997). Despite this controversy, all the meta-analyses indicate that LMWHs are associated with a lower mortality rate, particularly in the subgroup of patients with cancer and can be recommended whatever the indications related to venous thromboembolism. The main references concerning the various indications of LMWHs are reported hereafter.

REFERENCES

In prophylaxis of venous thromboembolism

COLLINS R., SCRIMGEOUR A. YUSUF S. et al. Reduction in fatal pulmonary embolism and venous thrombosis by perioperative administration of subcutaneous heparin. N.E.J. Med. 1988; 318 : 1162-1173

DAURES J.P., SCHVED J.F., MOMAS I. et al. Meta-analysis on randomized trials comparing LMWH to standard heparin or to placebo in the prevention of deep vein thrombosis. Rev. Epidem. Santé Publ. 1989; 37 : 363-369

LASSEN M.R., BORRIS L.C., CHRISTIANSEN H.M. et al. Clinical trials with low molecular weight heparins in the prevention of postoperative thromboembolic complications: a meta-analysis. Semin. Thromb. Hemost. 1991; 17 Suppl 3 : 284-290

LEIZOROVICZ A., HAUGH M.C., CHAPUIS F.R. et al. Low molecular weight heparin in prevention of perioperative thrombosis. B.M.J. 1992; 305 : 913-920

BERGQVIST D. Review of clinical trials of LMW Heparins. Eur. J. Surg. 1992; 158 : 67-78

NURMOHAMED M.T., ROSENDAAL F.R., BULLER H.R. et al. Low molecular weight heparin versus standard heparin in general and orthopedic surgery: a meta-analysis. Lancet 1992; 340 : 152-156

SIMONNEAU G., LEIZOROVICZ A. Prophylactic treatment of post-operative thrombosis. A meta-analysis of the results from trials assessing various methods used in patients undergoing major orthopaedic (hip and knee) surgery. Clin. Trial Meta Anal. 1993; 28: 177-191

KAKKAR V.V. Meta-analyse de l'efficacité et de la tolérance de Clivarine et d'autres HBPM en chirurgie générale. Blood Coag. Fibrinolysis 1993; 4 (1) : 523-527

MOHR D.N., SILVERSTEIN M.D., MURTAUGH P.A. Prophylactic agents for venous thrombosis in elective hip surgery. Arch. Inter. Med. 1993; 153 : 2221-2228

JØRGENSEN L.N., WILLE-JØRGENSEN P., HAUCH O. Prophylaxis of postoperative thromboembolism with low molecular weight heparins. Br. J. Surg. 1993; 80 : 689-704

IMPERIALE T.F., SPEROFF T. A meta-analysis of methods to prevent venous thromboembolism following total hip replacement. J. Am. Med. Assoc. 1994; 271 : 1780-1785

KAKKAR V.V. Effectiveness and safety of low molecular weight heparins (LMWH) in the prevention of venous thromboembolism (VTE). Thromb. Haemostasis 1995; 74 : 364-368

PINEO G.F., HULL R.D. Low molecular weight heparin: prophylaxis and treatment of venous thromboembolism. Annu. Rev. Med. 1997; 48 : 79-91

PALMER A.J., SCHRAMM W., KIRCHHOF B. et al. Low molecular weight heparin and unfractionated heparin for prevention of thrombo-embolism in general surgery: a meta-analysis of randomized clinical trial. Haemostasis 1997; 27 : 65-74

PALMER A.J., KOPPENHAGEN K., KIRCHHOF B. et al. Efficacy and safety of low molecular weight heparin, unfractionated heparin and warfarin for thrombo-embolism prophylaxis in orthopaedic surgery: a meta-analysis of randomized clinical trials. Haemostasis 1997; 27 : 75-84

KOCH A., BOUGES S., ZIEGLER S. et al. Low molecular weight heparin and unfractionated heparin in thrombosis prophylaxis after major surgical intervention: update of previous meta-analyses. Br. J. Surg. 1997; 84 : 750-759

HOWARD A.W., AARON S.D. Low molecular weight heparin decreases proximal and distal deep venous thrombosis following total knee arthoplasty. A meta-analysis of randomized trials. Tromb. Haemostasis 1998; 79 : 902-906

In treatment of venous thromboembolism

HOMMES D., BURA A., MAZZOLAI L. et al. Subcutaneous heparin compared with continuous intravenous heparin administered in the initial treatment of deep vein thrombosis. A meta-analysis. Ann. Int. Med. 1992; 116 : 279-284

LEIZOROVICZ A., SIMONNEAU G., DECOUSUS H., BOISSEL J.P. Comparison of efficacy and safety of low molecular weight heparins and unfractionated heparin in initial treatment of deep venous thrombosis: a meta-analysis. B.M.J. 1994; 309 : 299-304

LENSING A.W.A., PRINS M.H., DAVIDSON B.L. et al. Treatment of deep venous thrombosis with low molecular weight heparins. A meta-analysis. Arch. Intern. Med. 1995; 155 : 601-607

HIRSH J., SIRAGUSA S., COSMI B., GINSBERG J.S. Low molecular weight heparins (LMWH) in the treatment of patients with acute venous thromboembolism. Thromb. Haemostasis 1995; 74 : 360-363

HIRSH J. Comparison of the relative efficacy and safety of LMWH and UFH for the treatment of venous thrombosis. Haemostasis 1996; 26 Suppl 4 : 189-198

MISMETTI P., LAPORTE-SIMITSIDIS S., LEIZOROVICZ A., DECOUSUS H. Heparins and curative treatment of venous thromboembolic disease: meta-analyses (Fr). Thérapie 1997; 52 : 47-52

SIRAGUSA S., COSMI B., PIOVELLA F. et al. Low molecular weight heparins and unfractionated heparin in the treatment of patients with acute venous thromboembolism: Results of a meta-analysis. Am. J. Med. 1996; 100 : 269-277

LEIZOROVICZ A. Comparison of the efficacy and safety of low molecular weight heparins and unfractionated heparin in the initial treatment of deep venous thrombosis. An updated meta-analysis. Drugs 1996; 52 Suppl 7 : 30-37

DOLOVICH L., GINSBERG J.S. Low molecular weight heparin in the treatment of venous thromboembolism: an updated meta-analysis. Vessels 1997; 1 : 4-17

Various

ABRAM S.E., HOPWOOD M. Can meta-analysis rescue knowledge from a sea of unintelligible data? Region Anesth. 1996; 21 : 514-516

BAILAR J. The promise and problems of meta-analysis. N.E.J. Med. 1997; 337 : 559-561

CHARLTON B.G. The uses and abuses of meta-analysis. Family Practice 1996; 13 : 397-401

LELORIER J., GREGOIRE G., BENHADDAD A. et al. Discrepancies between meta-analyses and subsequent large randomized, controlled trials. N.E.J. Med. 1997; 337 : 356-342

SPECTOR T.D., THOMPSON S.G., The potential and limitations of metaanalysis. J. Epi. Comm. Health 1991; 45 : 89-92

TOULEMONDE F., KHER A., DOUTREMEPUICH Ch. The difficulties of assessing pulmonary embolism during post surgery prophylaxis. Risks of meta-analysis from clinical trials (F), Presse Méd. 1993, 22, 1, 28-32

15
Conclusions and beyond

GIUSEPPE NENCI. *Concluding this clinical survey on LMWHs*

The history of low molecular weight heparins (LMWHs) began more than 20 years ago, when Anderson observed that heparin chains with a molecular weight of about 5,000 lose their effect on the APTT whereas their anti-Xa activity remains unchanged (1).

The observation prompted many researchers to believe that a more effective inhibition of factor Xa than of thrombin would result in a reduced hemorrhagic effect and/or in a higher antithrombotic ability. Indeed, some of them thought that the antithrombotic activity of heparin was correlated to the inhibition of factor Xa, while its hemorrhagic effect was due to inhibition of thrombin. This hypothesis has been rejected by the dissociation of the anti-Xa activity from the antithrombotic effects in heparin chains with a different molecular weight (2) and by the demonstration that dermatan sulfate, an antithrombin which has no anti-Xa activity, is effective and safe in humans (3).

It is likely that the reduced bleeding induced by LMWHs in comparison with unfractionated heparin (UFH) is due to their pharmacokinetics and to a decreased inhibition of platelet function (4).

An impressive number of studies has accumulated over the past 15 years in the attempt to find a way to overcome several shortcomings of UFH, due to its limited efficacy in orthopedic surgery, induction of thrombocytopenia and/or thrombosis, need for multiple daily injections or continuous infusion, laboratory monitoring for therapeutic dosage and hemorrhagic risk.

Since the therapeutic ratio of LMWHs is higher than the ratio of UFH by a small but clinically significant difference, it was observed that some LMWHs at a given dosage were more effective but not safer than UFH, while others were shown to be safer but not more effective. This is due to the fact that the biochemical and pharmacological characteristics of the various LMWHs are different enough to exert different clinical effects and that their dosage used in the different trials is not strictly comparable, also because of the initial uncertainties in choosing a reference material and common units to measure their biological effects.

This difference in the therapeutic ratio (antithrombotic versus hemorrhagic effect) between the various LMWHs weakens the results of the numerous meta-analyses that followed one another over time, thus highlighting the need to examine the results of the individual studies when they are methodologically correct.

This need has been fulfilled by this book that collects all the studies that have been published as full papers on the use of LMWHs in the prevention and treatment of venous thromboembolism.

The available data have been grouped for each product and each studied indication, and a clear description has also been provided of the pharmacological characteristics, study design, type and number of patients, assessment criteria and results.

In July 1991, Jean Choay presented a survey of the pioneer work made by the Institut Choay, later transformed into the Center Choay of the Sanofi Recherche, in the preparation of the first LMWH (5) and in the isolation, study and synthesis of the heparin pentasaccharide and numerous analogues and derivatives. At that time, it was clear that the superiority of LMWHs over UFH was due to their more predictable anticoagulant effect, fixed therapeutic dosage, fewer effects on platelet function and counts, and longer half-life, thus allowing subcutaneous administration once a day.

In his eyes, the new challenge was represented by the assessment of the efficacy of synthetic heparin oligosaccharides, particularly pentasaccharide, which "represent a new potential in basic and therapeutic science" (6).

Was he right? Time will tell.

REFERENCE

1. Anderson L.O., Barrowcliffe T.W., Holmer E. et al. Anticoagulant properties of heparin fractioned by affinity chromatography in matrix bound antithrombin III and by gel filtration. Thromb. Res. 1976; 9: 575-583.
2. Ockelford P.A., Carter C.J., Mitchell L. et al. Discordance between the anti-Xa avtivity and antithrombonic activities of an ultra-low molecular weight heparin fraction. Thromb. Res. 1982; 28: 401-409.
3. Agnelli C.., Cosmi B., Di Filippo P. et al. A randomized double-blind placebo-controlled trial of dermatan sulphate for prevention of deep vein thrombosis in hip fracture. Tromb. Haemostas. 1992; 67: 203-208.
4. Salzman E., Rosenberg R., Smith M. et al. Effect of heparin and heparin fractions on platelet aggregation. J. Clin. Invest. 1980; 65: 64-73.
5. Choay J., Lormeau J.-C., Sinay P. et al. Anti-Xa active heparin oligosaccharides. Thromb. Res. 1980; 18: 573-578.
6. Choay J. From heparin to pentasaccharide. In: Fraxiparine : current status and future perspectives. Amsterdam Symposium, July 6, 1991.

MICHEL M. SAMAMA. *About LMW Heparins*

More than 10 years after the discovery of LMWHs, their mechanism of action is not fully understood. Their antithrombotic action is said to be related to anti-Xa and/or anti-IIa activity associated with TFPI release. However, other factors are involved, such as anti-IXa activity which may play an important role in their efficacy (1).

It is obvious to medical clinicians and hematologists alike that unfractionated heparin (UFH) is being substantially replaced by low molecular weight heparins (LMWHs) because of the great clinical success of the latter.

The success of these LMWHs resides in several factors :

1. There appears to be less bleeding—though this is not yet well documented.

2. They are at least as effective in efficacy as the UFH, as shown in numerous clinical studies.

3. They are superior to UFH in their pharmacokinetics allowing for fewer injections per day. In prophylaxis situations, they require only one injection daily compared to two or three daily for UFH. However, an important observation is the two- to three-fold faster clearance of anti-IIa activity as compared to anti-Xa activity (2,3). This result obtained by our group and others is puzzling when considering the use of a single subcutaneous injection per day in prophylactic treatment in Europe which is efficacious. If anti-IIa activity is important for the efficacy of LMWHs, then an injection every 12 hours seems in better accordance with the pharmacokinetics of LMWHs. This would invalidate this third point of the need for fewer injections, if true.

For therapeutic situations, however, one or two injections daily are at least as effective as continuous intravenous infusion of UFH and thus more feasible. Despite this greater simplicity, one must always continue to re-evaluate the logic of this usage. The benefit-risk ratio may invalidate its usage. One must not forget to continue to survey the over-all clinical picture, for example, to look for underlying causes of the problem such as neoplasm or congenital or acquired thrombophilia.

4. The therapeutic response is said to be more stable. The LMWHs need little or no monitoring by laboratory tests. They have a long half-life and daily testing is not needed. Measuring the anti-Xa is the test which is used if desired. It does not change with the reagents used and can be expressed in international units in any lab. In contrast, the UFH requires the use of the APTT test which does change its results with different reagents. It really needs a standardization similar to the INR available for prothrombin time testing, but this has not yet been developed. We all know that the APTT changes almost daily (or earlier) even with steady doses of UFH. APTT is not usually modified by the sc administration of LMWHs. However, at high dose when the selected compound has a high anti-IIa activity such as tinzaparin, an important prolongation of APTT is not unfrequent (4).

It has been said that the response to LMWH (as measured by anti-Xa) per kg of weight is very stable, but it has been found to vary actually from patient to patient. In a study during prophylaxis with a standard dose, it was found that only 25% of the observed inter-individual variation could be explained by differences in body weight while other factors accounted for 75% (5). Thus, the results are not really totally predictable.

Despite this, the advantages of LMWH which include seemingly fewer injections and greater simplicity in monitoring do account for their mounting success.

Their use has made prophylactic treatment easier and more frequently prescribed.

For established thrombosis, greater simplicity of treatment and an ever greater feasability of ambulatory treatment are two important advantages of LMWHs. It is important however that simplification of the treatment does not trivialize the disease, venous thromboembolism.

REFERENCES

1. Samama M.M., Bara L., Gerotziafas G.T., Mechanism for the antithrombotic activity in man of low molecular weight heparins (LMWHs), Haemostasis, 1994, 24, 105-117.
2. Bara L., Bloch M.F., Zitoun D. Et al., Comparative effects of enoxaparin and unfractionated heparin in healthy volunteers on prothrombin consumption in whole blood during coagulation, and release of tissue factor pathway inhibitor, Thromb. Res., 1993, 69, 443-452.
3. B. Boneu, C. Navarro, J.P. Cambus, H. Caplain et al., Pharmacodynamics and tolerance of two nadroparin formulation (10250 and 2050 anti-Xa IU.mL-1) delivered for 10 days at therapeutic dose, Thromb. Haemost, 1998, 79, 338-341.
4. Achkar A., Horellou M.H., Conard J., Laaban J.P., Samama M., Allongement du temps de céphaline plus activateur au cours du traitement des accidents thromboemboliques veineux par la tinzaparine, Presse Médicale, 1998, 27, 667-668.
5. Bara L., Leizorovicz A., Picolet H., Samama M., Correlation between anti-Xa and occurrence of thrombosis and haemorrhage in post-surgical patients treated with either logiparin (LMWMH), or unfractionated heparin, Post-surgery logiparin study group, Thromb. Res., 1992, 65, 641-650.

HANS KLAUS BREDDIN. *Present positioning of LMWHs*

This book offers an excellent overview on the large number of clinical trials with low molecular weight heparins (LMWH) in different indications. The single studies are listed in a very concise form and data on study design, endpoints and results are readily available. The explanatory and critical comments to each study are relevant and helpful to the reader. When reading this book some open questions become obvious while others have been clarified by the existing trials.

Prophylaxis of thrombosis in patients at low and medium risk

The effectiveness and safety of LMWH in comparison to unfractionated heparin (UFH) has been established in forty trials. A lower age limit for patients which should receive medical prophylaxis is still not clearly defined. The rare complication of heparin induced thrombocytopenia (HIT) is most likely much less frequent under LMWH than under UFH.

Thrombosis prophylaxis in patients at high risk

Prophylaxis with LMWH in patients with elective hip and knee surgery and also more recently in patients with hip fractures and polytrauma has been very frequently studied in comparison with UFH and has become general practice in many hospitals. An important topic of recent trials has been the duration of prophylaxis in high risk patients. The prolongation of medical prophylaxis in these patients prevents late thrombosis effectively as has been shown in recent trials.

A puzzling question is the large variation in the thrombosis incidence after hip or knee replacement in the different trials. Are these differences caused by divergent interpretations of phlebograms, by different operation techniques or by different regimens of general care in various patient populations? Center effects have been shown in several trials but a full explanation of the apparently large differences in postoperative thrombosis incidence is still lacking.

In the different trials fixed doses usually have been as effective as body weight adjusted doses. Dextran has always been less effective than LMWH. Gradual compression in combination with spinal anesthesia is not sufficient to prevent postoperative deep vein thrombosis.

Several studies have shown that LMWH can be used to prevent thrombosis in medical patients and in elderlies. The value of this form of prophylaxis in the elderly is less convincing than in other indications.

Pediatrics

Here are only limited data available. Adequate dosing of LMWH in different age groups still has to be established by new studies.

Prophylaxis of DVT in vascular surgery

Some small trials have shown that LMWHs prevent DVT as effectively as UFH in patients after vascular surgery.

Treatment of deep venous thrombosis

The treatment of deep venous thrombosis (DVT) with LMWH is as effective as the intravenous use of UFH. Recent studies have been performed in patients which were either hospitalized for a short period of time or primarily treated as outpatients. After a correct diagnosis ambulant treatment of patients with DVT seems feasible. However, clinicians and practitioners frequently ask for more specific advice on which patients still need hospitalization (iliac vein thrombosis, thrombosis with massive oedema, thrombosis ocurring in patients in bed rest?). In recent trials recurrence of DVT and new pulmonary embolism (PE) were primarily assessed clinically and had then to be confirmed by objective methods. It is clear from many previous trials that only a minority of new thrombi or new PE develop clinical symptoms. Whether those recurrences which are symptomatic are more relevant for the patients than those without symptoms remains open. It has become likely that the early change to oral anticoagulants is as effective as a change after prolonged treatment. Treatment with LMWH with a once daily administration is as effective as b.i.d s.c. if the same daily dose is applied. Once daily application seemed even to be better in the recent FRAXODI-trial.

An interesting frequently discussed point is the possible reduction in cancer mortality in patients receiving LMWH. This open question still needs to be answered in the future.

Peripheral arterial occlusive disease (PAOD)

Several trials have made it likely that arterial thrombotic complications in patients with peripheral arterial occlusive disease can be prevented by prolonged prophylaxis with LMWH. The group of patients which will profit from this kind of long-term prophylaxis and its adequate dose and duration still need to be defined. Endpoints can be new arterial occlusions. The walking distance is not a useful parameter in this indication.

Coronary heart disease

In patients with coronary heart disease, as in unstable angina and in patients after percutaneous transluminal coronary angioplasty (PTCA), LMWHs have been studied usually with positive results concerning early thrombotic occlusions but it has become likely that LMWH or any other antithrombotic treatment have to be applied for a longer period of time (30 days? 3 months?) to obtain a long-term benefit by preventing coronary occlusions or reocclusions. Treatment with LMWH does not prevent restenosis.

Intracardial thromboses after MI can be prevented with LMWH, but with a higher risk of hemorrhage.

In unstable angina recent trials have shown divergent results but the ongoing trials may well show that adequate dosage and duration of treatment are effective in this indication. A small trial (Gurfinkel et al) has recently shown, that the combination of a LMWH with aspirin was more effective than either drug alone.

Stroke

It is still fully open whether LMWH are helpful in patients with acute non-hemorrhagic stroke, besides preventing deep venous thromboses.

Pregnancy

There are good reasons to use LMWH in pregnant women with DVT or at a high risk of thrombotic complications. Studies in this area are difficult to perform.

JACK HIRSH. *LMWHs versus newer antithrombotics*

Low molecular weight heparins (LMWHs) are effective for the prevention and treatment of venous thrombosis and pulmonary embolism and for the treatment of patients with unstable angina. The main advantages of LMWHs over unfractionated heparin are their more predictable dose response and their longer plasma half-life. The first advantage allows LMWHs to be administered once daily by subcutaneous injection, while the second makes laboratory monitoring unnecessary. Based on these favorable properties, LMWHs are being used with increasing frequency on an out-patient basis when anticoagulation is required for days to weeks after hospital discharge. For example, it is no longer necessary to delay hospital discharge for patients who require an initial course of heparin for treatment of venous thrombosis or unstable angina.

The future of LMWHs is bright, but it will be influenced by two unrelated issues. These are: 1) the relative efficacy of the different commercial LMWHs; and 2) the relative efficacy and safety of LMWHs versus new antithrombotic agents that are either in the clinic or under development.

Are There Clinically Important Differences in Efficacy or Safety Among Different LMWH Preparations?

There are differences among the LMWHs in their method of preparation, molecular weight distribution, anticoagulant potency (in terms of anti-Xa: anti-IIa ratio) and plasma clearance. It is uncertain, however, whether any of these differences are clinically relevant. To date, clinical trials comparing similar dosages of different LMWHs have been few, and limited to prophylaxis of venous thrombosis. Of these studies, one reported a difference in efficacy while the other reported no difference in efficacy or safety between two different preparations of LMWH. Indirect comparison of studies evaluating LMWH for the treatment of venous thromboembolism fail to show differences between efficacy and safety among five different preparations. In contrast, studies evaluating LMWH for the treatment of unstable angina suggest that there may be differences in efficacy between different preparations. Thus, in one study the efficacy and safety of a LMWH preparation (Dalteparin) was reported to be similar to unfractionated heparin, while in two studies using a different LMWH preparation (Enoxaparin), the LMWH was found to be more effective than unfractionated heparin. Therefore, the question of equivalence of LMWH preparations remains unresolved. It is conceivable that different preparations are equivalent for some indications (e.g, treatment of venous thrombosis), but not for others (e.g, unstable angina).

The Relative Efficacy and Safety of LMWHs and New Antithrombotic Agents

The potential indications for LMWH are: 1) prevention of venous thromboembolism; 2) treatment of venous thromboembolism; 3) treatment of unstable angina; and 4) as a substitute for unfractionated heparin in patients with acute myocardial ischemia who are treated with thrombolytic therapy or with platelet glycoprotein (GPIIb/IIIa) antagonists.

1) Prevention of Venous Thromboembolism

LMWH has a number of potential competitors for this indication. The established rival is hirudin, a direct thrombin inhibitor, that has been shown to be equally safe, but more effective than a LMWH in preventing venous thrombosis after elective hip surgery. In this study hirudin was administered as a twice-daily subcutaneous injection, while LMWH was given once daily subcutaneously. PEG-hirudin has a longer half-life than hirudin and is likely to be effective for venous thrombosis prophylaxis when administered once daily. Other new anticoagulants include a synthetic pentasaccharide, the Nematode Anticoagulant Peptide, NAPc2 and low-molecular-weight oral thrombin inhibitors; all are being evaluated as prophylactic agents in high risk orthopedic surgical patients.

The synthetic pentasaccharide has a longer half-life than LMWHs, is administered subcutaneously once daily and could challenge LMWH for this indication. NAPc2 also has a long half-life; it targets factor Xa and is also administered subcutaneously, once daily, but is less likely to be a competitor for LMWH. Neither of these new anticoagulants have antidotes, which reduces their attractiveness for this indication, particularly since the pentasaccharide has a half-life of about 24 hours and NAPc2 has a half-life of about 48 hours. In addition, the likelihood of their clinical use will be influenced by their cost relative to LMWH. Oral thrombin inhibitors could present the greatest challenge to LMWH if they are at least as effective and safe as LMWH and do not require laboratory monitoring. This expectation is supported by the observation that warfarin, the only established oral anticoagulant, is preferred over LMWH for prophylaxis by some orthopedic surgeons, despite its disadvantages of having a slow onset of action and a requirement for laboratory monitoring. An oral thrombin inhibitor with a rapid onset of action, that can be used without laboratory monitoring, would be attractive for this indication because it would be convenient to use after early hospital discharge in high risk patients.

2) Treatment of Venous Thromboembolism

LMWH is particularly attractive for the treatment of venous thrombosis or pulmonary embolism because : a) it can be used without laboratory monitoring; and b) it can be used out of hospital. Although hirudin has been evaluated for this indication, it is unlikely to replace LMWH. A rapidly acting oral thrombin inhibitor would be a potential rival for LMWH for the early treatment of venous thrombosis or pulmonary embolism, particularly if it could be used without the need for laboratory monitoring.

3) Unstable Angina

Results of contemporary studies indicate that antithrombotic therapy for unstable angina needs to be continued for weeks after the presenting event. LMWH is at least as good as (and possibly better than) heparin for this indication, and is much more convenient to use. The competition comes from hirudin and from GP IIb/IIIa antagonists, both of which are more effective than heparin for the treatment of unstable angina. The improved efficacy of hirudin comes at the price of an increased incidence of bleeding. Since GPIIb/IIIa antagonists are usually given in combination with heparin, LMWH has the potential to be used in unstable angina, either alone or in combination with a GPIIb/IIIa antagonist.

4) Other Indications

LMWH has the potential to replace heparin: a) as an adjunct to GPIIb/IIIa antagonists in patients undergoing percutaneous coronary interventions; and b) as an adjunct to thrombolytic agents in patients with acute myocardial infarction.

Author
and study index

FIRST AUTHOR OR STUDY NAME	YEAR	PRODUCT	INDICATION	PAGE	TABLE
PLANES A.	1996	enoxaparin	prophylaxis orthopedic surgery	164	343
PONIEWIERSKI M.	1988	dalteparin	prophylaxis medicine	226	338
PRANDONI P.	1992	nadroparin	DVT treatment	300	348
PRINS M.H.	1989	dalteparin	stroke, DVT prophylaxis	420	

R

RD Heparin Group	1994	ardeparin	prophylaxis orthopedic surgery	118	333
REDUCE Trial (KARSCH K.R.)	1996	reviparin	cardiology, restenosis	378	

S

SALCUNI P.F.	1988	parnaparin	prophylaxis general surgery	92	350
SAMAMA M. M. (GENOX)	1988	enoxaparin	prophylaxis general surgery	60	341
SAMAMA C.M.	1997	enoxaparin	prophylaxis orthopedic surgery	168	343
SANDSET P.M.	1990	dalteparin	stroke, DVT prophylaxis	422	
SCHMIDT T.	1990	dalteparin	cardiology, restenosis	370	
SIMONNEAU G. (THESEE)	1997	tinzaparin	PE treatment	314	353
SIMONNEAU G. (DVT ENOX)	1993	enoxaparin	DVT treatment	288	344
SPIRO T.E.	1994	enoxaparin	prophylaxis orthopedic surgery	158	342
SPIRO T.E.	1997	enoxaparin	DVT treatment	294	344
STANDBERG L.E.	1996	dalteparin	cardiology, thrombolysis AMI	384	
STEP study (PEZZUOLI G.)	1989	nadroparin	prophylaxis general surgery	78	346

T

TARTAGLIA P.	1989	parnaparin	prophylaxis gynecology	96	350
THERY C.	1992	nadroparin	PE treatment (dose ranging)	304	
THESEE study (SIMONNEAU G.)	1997	tinzaparin	PE treatment	314	353
TIMI 11A	1997	enoxaparin	cardiology, unstable angina	402	
TIMI 11B	1998	enoxaparin	cardiology, unstable angina	404	
TØRHOLM C.	1991	dalteparin	prophylaxis orthopedic surgery	130	337
TURPIE A.	1986	enoxaparin	prophylaxis orthopedic surgery	140	342

V

VALLE I.	1988	parnaparin	prophylaxis general surgery	90	350
VERARDI S	1988	parnaparin	prophylaxis general surgery	94	350

Z

ZIDAR J.P.	1998	enoxaparin	cardiology stenting	374	